Neural Networks in Healthcare:
Potential and Challenges

Rezaul Begg
Victoria University, Australia

Joarder Kamruzzaman
Monash University, Australia

Ruhul Sarker
University of New South Wales, Australia

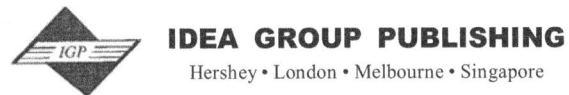
IDEA GROUP PUBLISHING
Hershey • London • Melbourne • Singapore

Acquisitions Editor:	Michelle Potter
Development Editor:	Kristin Roth
Senior Managing Editor:	Amanda Appicello
Managing Editor:	Jennifer Neidig
Copy Editor:	April Schmidt
Typesetter:	Diane Huskinson
Cover Design:	Lisa Tosheff
Printed at:	Integrated Book Technology

Published in the United States of America by
    Idea Group Publishing (an imprint of Idea Group Inc.)
    701 E. Chocolate Avenue
    Hershey PA 17033
    Tel: 717-533-8845
    Fax: 717-533-8661
    E-mail: cust@idea-group.com
    Web site: http://www.idea-group.com

and in the United Kingdom by
    Idea Group Publishing (an imprint of Idea Group Inc.)
    3 Henrietta Street
    Covent Garden
    London WC2E 8LU
    Tel: 44 20 7240 0856
    Fax: 44 20 7379 0609
    Web site: http://www.eurospanonline.com

Library of Congress Cataloging-in-Publication Data

Neural networks in healthcare : potential and challenges / Rezaul Begg,
    Joarder Kamruzzaman, and Ruhul Sarker, editors.
      p. ; cm.
    Includes bibliographical references.
    Summary: "This book covers state-of-the-art applications in many areas
  of medicine and healthcare"--Provided by publisher.
      ISBN 1-59140-848-2 (hardcover) -- ISBN 1-59140-849-0 (softcover)
      1. Neural networks (Computer science) 2. Medicine--Research--Data
  processing. 3. Medical informatics.   I. Begg, Rezaul. II. Kamruzzaman,
  Joarder. III. Sarker, Ruhul.
    [DNLM: 1. Neural Networks (Computer) 2. Medical Informatics Appli-
  cations.   W 26.55.A7 N494 2006]
  R853.D37N48 2006
  610'.285--dc22

                                     2005027413

British Cataloguing in Publication Data
A Cataloguing in Publication record for this book is available from the British Library.

Neural Networks in Healthcare:
Potential and Challenges

Table of Contents

Preface

Artificial neural networks are learning machines inspired by the operation of the human brain, and they consist of many artificial neurons connected in parallel. These networks work via non-linear mapping techniques between the inputs and outputs of a model indicative of the operation of a real system. Although introduced over 40 years ago, many wonderful new developments in neural networks have taken place as recently as during the last decade or so. This has led to numerous recent applications in many fields, especially when the input-output relations are too complex and difficult to express using formulations.

Healthcare costs around the globe are on the rise, and therefore there is strong need for new ways of assisting the requirements of the healthcare system. Besides applications in many other areas, neural networks have naturally found many promising applications in the health and medicine areas. This book is aimed at presenting some of these interesting and innovative developments from leading experts and scientists working in health, biomedicine, biomedical engineering, and computing areas. The book covers many important and state-of-the-art applications in the areas of medicine and healthcare, including cardiology, electromyography, electroencephalography, gait and human movement, therapeutic drug monitoring for patient care, sleep apnea, and computational fluid dynamics areas.

The book presents thirteen chapters in five sections as follows:

- Section I: Introduction and Applications in Healthcare
- Section II: Electrocardiography
- Section III: Electromyography
- Section IV: Electroencephalography and Evoked Potentials
- Section V: Applications in Selected Areas

The first section consists of two chapters. The first chapter, by Kamruzzaman, Begg, and Sarker, provides an overview of the fundamental concepts of neural network approaches, basic operation of the neural networks, their architectures, and the commonly used algorithms that are available to assist the neural networks during learning from examples. Toward the end of this chapter, an outline of some of the common applications in healthcare (e.g., cardiology, electromyography, electroencephalography, and gait data analysis) is provided. The second chapter, by Schöllhorn and Jäger, continues on from the first chapter with an extensive overview of the artificial neural networks as tools for processing miscellaneous biomedical signals. A variety of applications are illustrated in several areas of healthcare using many examples to demonstrate how neural nets can support the diagnosis and prediction of diseases. This review is particularly aimed at providing a thoughtful insight into the strengths as well as weaknesses of artificial neural networks as tools for processing biomedical signals.

Electrical potentials generated by the heart during its pumping action are transmitted to the skin through the body's tissues, and these signals can be recorded on the body's surface and are represented as an electrocardiogram (ECG). The ECG can be used to detect many cardiac abnormalities. Section II, with three chapters, deals with some of the recent techniques and advances in the ECG application areas.

The third chapter, by Nugent, Finlay, Donnelly, and Black, presents an overview of the application of neural networks in the field of ECG classification. Neural networks have emerged as a strong candidate in this area as the highly non-linear and chaotic nature of the ECG represents a well-suited application for this technique. The authors highlight issues that relate to the acceptance of this technique and, in addition, identify challenges faced for the future.

In the fourth chapter, Camps-Valls and Guerrero-Martínez continue with further applications of neural networks in cardiac pathology discrimination based on ECG signals. They discuss advantages and drawbacks of neural and adaptive systems in cardiovascular medicine and some of the forthcoming developments in machine learning models for use in the real clinical environment. They discuss some of the problems that can arise during the learning tasks of beat detection, feature selection/extraction and classification, and subsequently provide proposals and suggestions to alleviate the problems.

Chapter V, by Li, Luk, Fu, and Krishnan, presents a new concept learning-based approach for abnormal ECG beat detection to facilitate long-term monitoring of heart patients. The uniqueness in this approach is the use of their complementary concept, "normal", for the learning task. The authors trained a ν-Support Vector Classifier (ν-SVC) with only normal ECG beats from a specific patient to relieve the doctors from annotating the training data beat by beat. The trained model was then used to detect abnormal beats in the long-term ECG recording of the same patient. They then compared the concept-learning model with other classifiers, including multilayer feedforward neural networks and binary support vector machines.

Two chapters in Section III focus on applications of neural networks in the area of electromyography (EMG) pattern recognition. Tsuji et al., in Chapter VI, discuss the use of probabilistic neural networks (PNNs) for pattern recognition of EMG signals. In this chapter, a recurrent PNN, called Recurrent Log-Linearized Gaussian Mixture Network (R-LLGMN), is introduced for EMG pattern recognition with the emphasis on utilizing temporal characteristics. The structure of R-LLGMN is based on the algorithm of a hidden Markov model (HMM), and, hence, R-LLGMN inherits advantages from both HMM and neural computation. The authors present experimental results to demonstrate the suitability of R-LLGMN in EMG pattern recognition.

In Chapter VII, Tsuji, Tsujimura, and Tanaka describe an advanced intelligent dual-arm manipulator system teleoperated by EMG signals and hand positions. This myoelectric teleoperation system also employs a probabilistic neural network, LLGMN, to gauge the operator's intended hand motion from EMG patterns measured during tasks. In this chapter, the authors also introduce an event-driven task model using Petri net and a non-contact impedance control method to allow a human operator to maneuver robotic manipulators.

Section IV presents two interesting chapters. Kamath et al., in Chapter VIII, describe applications of neural networks in the analysis of bioelectric potentials representing the brain activity level, often represented using electroencephalography plots (EEG). Neural networks have a major role to play in the EEG signal processing because of their effectiveness as pattern classifiers. In this chapter, the authors study several specific applications, for example: (1) identification of abnormal EEG activity in patients with neurological diseases such as epilepsy, Huntington's disease, and Alzheimer's disease; (2) interpretation of physiological signals, including EEG recorded during sleep and surgery under anaesthesia; (3) controlling external devices using embedded signals within the EEG waveform called BCI or brain-computer interface which has many applications in rehabilitation like helping handicapped individuals to independently operate appliances.

The recording of an evoked response is a standard non-invasive procedure, which is routine in many audiology and neurology clinics. The auditory brainstem response (ABR) provides an objective method of assessing the integrity of the auditory pathway and hence assessing an individual's hearing level. Davey, McCullagh, McAllister, and Houston, in Chapter IX, analyze ABR data using ANN and decision tree classifiers.

The final section presents four chapters with applications drawn from selected healthcare areas. Chapter X, by Begg, Kamruzzaman, and Sarker, provides an overview of artificial neural network applications for detection and classification of various gait types from their characteristics. Gait analysis is routinely used for detecting abnormality in the lower limbs and also for evaluating the progress of various treatments. Neural networks have been shown to perform better compared to statistical techniques in some gait classification tasks. Various studies undertaken in this area are discussed with a particular focus on neural network's potential as gait diagnostics. Examples are presented to demonstrate neural network's suitability for automated recognition of gait changes due to ageing from their respective gait-pattern characteristics and their potentials for recognition of at-risk or faulty gait.

Camps-Valls and Martín-Guerrero, in Chapter XI, discuss important advances in the area of dosage formulations, therapeutic drug monitoring (TDM), and the role of combined therapies in the improvement of the quality of life of patients. In this chapter, the authors review the various applications of neural and kernel models for TDM and present illustrative examples in real clinical problems to demonstrate improved performance by neural and kernel methods in the area.

Chapter XII, by Morsi and Das, describes the utilization of Computational Fluid Dynamics (CFD) with neural networks for analysis of medical equipment. They present the concept of mathematical modeling in solving engineering problems, CFD techniques and the associated numerical techniques. A case study on the design and optimization of scaffold of heart valve for tissue engineering application using CFD and neural network is presented. In the end, they offer interesting discussion on the advantage and disadvantage of neural network techniques for the CFD modeling of medical devices and their future prospective.

The final chapter, by Benyó discusses neural network applications in the analysis of two important physiological parameters: cerebral blood flow (CBF) and respiration. Investigation of the temporal blood flow pattern before, during, and after the development of CBF oscillations has many important applications, for example, in the early identification of cerebrovascular dysfunction such as brain trauma or stroke. The author later introduces the online method to recognize the most common breathing disorder, the sleep apnea syndrome, based on the nasal airflow.

We hope the book will be of enormous help to a broad audience of readership, including researchers, professionals, lecturers, and graduate students from a wide range of disciplines. We also trust that the ideas presented in this book will trigger further research efforts and development works in this very important and highly multidisciplinary area involving many fields (e.g., computing, biomedical engineering, biomedicine, human health, etc.).

Rezaul Begg, Victoria University, Australia

Joarder Kamruzzaman, Monash University, Australia

Ruhul Sarker, University of New South Wales, Australia

Editors

Acknowledgments

The editors would like to thank all the authors for their excellent contributions to this book and also everybody involved in the review process of the book without whose support the project could not have been satisfactorily completed. Each book chapter has undergone a peer-review process by at least two reviewers. Most of the authors of chapters also served as referees for chapters written by other authors. Thanks to all those who provided critical, constructive, and comprehensive reviews that helped to improve the scientific and technical quality of the chapters. In particular, special thanks goes to (in alphabetical order): Mahfuz Aziz of the University of South Australia; Harjeet Bajaj of McMaster University; Balazs Benyo of Budapest University of Technology and Economics; Gustavo Camps-Vall of Universitat de Valencia; Paul McCullough of the University of Ulster at Jordanville; Chris Nugent of the University of Ulster at Jordanville; Toshio Tsuji of Hiroshima University; Markad Kamath of McMaster University; Tony Sparrow of Deakin University; Tharshan Vaithianathan of the University of South Australia; and Wolfgang I. Schöllhorn of Westfälische Wilhelms-Universität Münster for their prompt, detailed, and constructive feedback on the submitted chapters.

We would like to thank our university authorities (Victoria University, Monash University, and the University of New South Wales @ADFA) for providing logistic support throughout this project.

The editors would also like to thank the publishing team at Idea Group Inc., who provided continuous help, encouragement. and professional support from the initial proposal stage to the final publication, with special thanks to Mehdi Khosrow-Pour, Jan Travers, Renée Davies, Amanda Phillips, and Kristin Roth.

Finally, we thank our families, especially our wives and children for their love and support throughout the project.

Rezaul Begg, Victoria University, Australia
Joarder Kamruzzaman, Monash University, Australia
Ruhul Sarker, University of New South Wales, Australia
Editors

Section I

Introduction and Applications in Healthcare

Chapter I

Overview of Artificial Neural Networks and their Applications in Healthcare

Joarder Kamruzzaman, Monash University, Australia

Rezaul Begg, Victoria University, Australia

Ruhul Sarker, University of New South Wales, Australia

Abstract

Artificial neural network (ANN) is one of the main constituents of the artificial intelligence techniques. Like in many other areas, ANN has made a significant mark in the domain of healthcare applications. In this chapter, we provide an overview of the basics of neural networks, their operation, major architectures that are widely employed for modeling the input-to-output relations, and the commonly used learning algorithms for training the neural network models. Subsequently, we briefly outline some of the major application areas of neural networks for the improvement and well being of human health.

Introduction

Following the landmark work undertaken by Rumelhart and his colleagues during the 1980s (Rumelhart et al., 1986), artificial neural networks (ANNs) have drawn tremendous interest due to their demonstrated successful applications in many pattern recognition and modeling works, including image processing (Duranton, 1996), engineering tasks (Rafiq et al., 2001), financial modeling (Coakley & Brown, 2000; Fadlalla & Lin, 2001), manufacturing (Hans et al., 2000; Wu, 1992), biomedicine (Nazeran & Behbehani, 2000), and so forth. In recent years, there has been a wide acceptance by the research community in the use of ANN as a tool for solving many biomedical and healthcare problems. Within the healthcare area, significant applications of neural networks include biomedical signal processing, diagnosis of diseases, and also aiding medical decision support systems.

Though developed as a model for mimicking human intelligence into machines, neural networks have an excellent capability of learning the relationship between the input-output mapping from a given dataset without any prior knowledge or assumptions about the statistical distribution of the data. This capability of learning from data without any *a priori* knowledge makes the neural network quite suitable for classification and regression tasks in practical situations. In many biomedical applications, classification and regression tasks constitute a major and integral part. Furthermore, neural networks are inherently nonlinear which makes them more practicable for accurate modeling of complex data patterns, as opposed to many traditional methods based on linear techniques. ANNs have been shown in many real world problems, including biomedical areas, to outperform statistical classifiers and multiple regression techniques for the analysis of data. Because of their ability to generalize unseen data well, they are also suitable for dealing with outliers in the data as well as tackling missing and/or noisy data. Neural networks have also been used in combination with other techniques to tie together the strengths and advantages of both techniques.

Since the book aims to demonstrate innovative and successful applications of neural networks in healthcare areas, this introductory chapter presents a broad overview of neural networks, various architectures and learning algorithms, and concludes with some of the common applications in healthcare and biomedical areas.

Artificial Neural Networks

Artificial neural networks are highly structured information processing units operating in parallel and attempting to mimic the huge computational ability of the human brain and nervous system. Even though the basic computational elements of the human brain are extremely slow devices compared to serial processors, the human brain can easily perform certain types of tasks that conventional computers might take astronomical amounts of time and, in most cases, may be unable to perform the task. By attempting to emulate the human brain, neural networks learn from experience, generalize from previous examples, abstract essential characteristics from inputs containing irrelevant data, and deal with fuzzy situations. ANNs consist of many neurons and synaptic strengths called weights. These neurons and weights are used to mimic the nervous system in the way weighted signals travel through the network. Although artificial neural networks have some functional similarity to biological neurons, they are much more simplified, and therefore, the resemblance between artificial and biological neurons is only superficial.

Individual Neural Computation

A neuron (also called unit or node) is the basic computational unit of a neural network. This concept was initially developed by McCulloch and Pitt (1943). Figure 1 shows an artificial neuron, which performs the following tasks:

a. Receives signals from other neurons.

b. Multiplies each signal by the corresponding connection strength, that is, weight.

c. Sums up the weighted signals and passes them through an activation function.

d. Feeds output to other neurons.

Denoting the input signal by a vector $\mathbf{x}$ $(x_1, x_2, ..., x_n)$ and the corresponding weights to unit j by $\mathbf{w}_j$ $(w_{j1}, w_{j2}, ..., w_{jn})$, the net input to the unit j is given by

$$net_j = \sum_n w_{jn} x_n + w_{j0} = \mathbf{w}_j \mathbf{x} + b \tag{1}$$

The weight $w_{j0}(=b)$ is a special weight called bias whose input signal is always +1.

There are many types of activation functions used in the literature. Activation functions are mostly nonlinear; however, linear activation functions are also used. When neurons are arranged in multiple layers, a network with the linear activation function can be represented as a network of a single layer. Such a network has limited capability since it can only solve linearly separable problems.

Figure 1. Individual neural computation

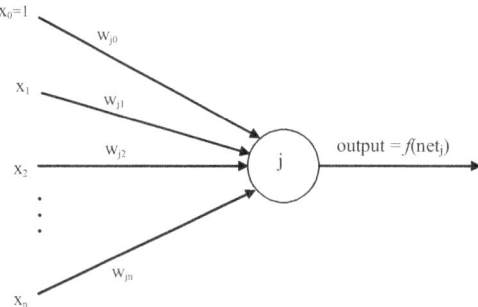

Usually, the final layer neurons can have linear activation functions while intermediate layer neurons implement nonlinear functions. Since most real world problems are nonlinearly separable, nonlinearity in intermediate layers is essential for modeling complex problems. There are many different activation functions proposed in the literature, and they are often chosen to be a monotonically increasing function. The following are the most commonly used activation functions:

Linear $f(x) = x$

Hyperbolic tangent $f(x) = tanh(x)$

Sigmoidal $f(x) = \dfrac{1}{1 + e^{-x}}$

Gaussian $f(x) = \exp(-x^2 / 2\sigma^2)$

Neural Network Models

There have been many neural network models proposed in the literature that vary in terms of topology and operational mode. Each model can be specified by the following seven major concepts (Hush & Horne, 1993; Lippman, 1987):

1. A set of processing units.

2. An activation function of each neuron.

3. Pattern of connectivity among neurons, that is, network topology.

4. Propagation method of activities of neurons through the network.

5. Rules to update the activities of each node.

6. External environment that feeds information to the network.

7. Learning method to modify the pattern of connectivity.

The most common way is to arrange the neurons in a series of layers. The first layer is known as the *input layer*, the final one as the *output layer*, and any intermediate layer(s) are called *hidden layer(s)*. In a multilayer feedforward network, the information signal always propagates along the forward direction. The number of input units at the input layer is dictated by the number of feature values or independent variables, and the number of units at the output corresponds to the number of classes or values to be predicted. There are no widely accepted rules for determining the optimal number of hidden units. A network with fewer than the required number of hidden units will be unable to learn the input-output mapping well, whereas too many hidden units will generalize poorly on any unseen data. Several researchers in the past attempted to determine the appropriate size of the hidden units. Kung and Hwang (1988) suggested that the number of hidden units should be equal to the number of distinct training patterns, while Masahiko (1989) concluded that N input patterns would require N-1 hidden units in a single layer. However, as remarked by Lee (1997), it is rather difficult to determine the optimum network size in advance. Other studies have suggested that ANNs would generalize better when succeeding layers are smaller than the preceding ones (Kruschke, 1989; Looney, 1996). Although a two-layer network (i.e., two layers of weights) is commonly used in most problem solving approaches, the determination of an appropriate network configuration usually involves many trial and error methods. Another way to select network size is to use constructive approaches. In constructive approaches, the network starts with a minimal size and grows gradually during the training (Fahlman & Lebiere, 1990; Lehtokangas, 2000). In feedback network topology, neurons are interconnected with neurons in the same layer or neurons from a proceeding layer.

Learning rules that are used to train a network architecture can be divided into two main types: supervised and unsupervised. In supervised training, the network is presented with a set of input-output pairs; that is, for each input, an associated target output is known. The network adjusts its weights using a known set of input-output pairs, and once training is completed, it is expected to produce a correct output in response to an unknown input. In unsupervised training, the network adjusts its weights in response to input patterns without having any known associated outputs. Through unsupervised training, the network learns to classify input patterns in similarity categories. This can be useful in situations where no known output corresponding to an input exists. We expect an unsupervised neural network to discover any rule that might find a correct response to an input.

Learning Algorithms

During learning, a neural network gradually modifies its weights and settles down to a set of weights capable of realizing the input-output mapping with either no error or a minimum error set by the user. The most common type of supervised learning is backpropagation learning. Some other supervised learning includes: radial basis function (RBF), probabilistic neural network (PNN), generalized regression neural network (GRNN), cascade-correlation, and so forth. Some examples of unsupervised learning, for instance, self-organizing map (SOM), adaptive resonance theory (ART), and so forth, are used when training sets with known outputs are not available. In the following, we describe some of the widely used neural network learning algorithms.

Backpropagation Algorithm

A recent study (Wong et al., 1997) has shown that approximately 95% of the reported neural network applications utilize multilayer feedforward neural networks with the backpropagation learning algorithm. Backpropagation (Rumelhart et al., 1986) is a feedforward network, as shown in Figure 2. In a fully

Figure 2. A three-layer backpropogation network. Not all of the interconnections are shown.

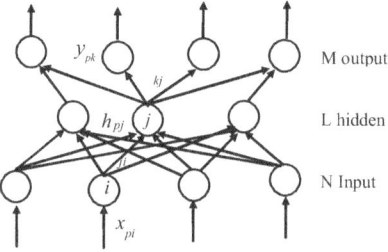

connected network, each hidden unit is connected with every unit at the bottom and upper layers. Units are not connected to the other units at the same layer. A backpropagation network must have at least two layers of weights. Cybenko (1989) showed that any continuous function could be approximated to an arbitrary accuracy by a two-layer feedforward network with a sufficient number of hidden units. Backpropagation applies a gradient descent technique iteratively to change the connection weights. Each iteration consists of two phases: a propagation phase and an error backpropagation phase. During the propagation phase, input signals are multiplied by the corresponding weights, propagate through the hidden layers, and produce output(s) at the output layer. The outputs are then compared with the corresponding desired (target) outputs. If the two match, no changes in weights are made. If the outputs produced by the network are different from the desired outputs, error signals are calculated at the output layer. These error signals are propagated backward to the input layer, and the weights are adjusted accordingly.

Consider a set of input vectors $(\mathbf{x}_1,\mathbf{x}_2,\ldots,\mathbf{x}_p)$ and a set of corresponding output vectors $(\mathbf{y}_1,\mathbf{y}_2,\ldots,\mathbf{y}_p)$ to be trained by the backpropagation learning algorithm. All the weights between layers are initialized to small random values at the beginning. All the weighted inputs to each unit of the upper layer are summed up and produce an output governed by the following equations:

$$y_{pk} = f(\sum_j \omega_{kj} h_{pj} + \theta_k), \tag{2}$$

$$h_{pj} = f(\sum_i \omega_{ji} x_{pi} + \theta_j), \tag{3}$$

where h_{pj} and y_{pk} are the outputs of hidden unit j and output unit k, respectively, for pattern p. ω stands for connecting weights between units, θ stands for the threshold of the units, and $f(.)$ is the sigmoid activation function.

The cost function to be minimized in standard backpropagation is the sum of the squared error measured at the output layer and defined as:

$$E = \frac{1}{2}\sum_p \sum_k (t_{pk} - y_{pk})^2 \tag{4}$$

where t_{kp} is the target output of neuron k for pattern p.

Backpropagation uses the steepest descent technique for changing weights in order to minimize the cost function of Equation (4). The weight update at t-th iteration is governed by the following equation:

$$(t) = \frac{E}{(t)} + \quad (t \quad 1) \tag{5}$$

where   and   are the learning rate and momentum factor, respectively. For the sigmoid activation function, the weight update rule can be further simplified as:

$$\Delta_{\omega kj}(t) = \eta \delta_{pk} h_{pj} + \alpha \Delta_{\omega kj}(t-1) \text{ , for output layer weight} \tag{6}$$

$$\Delta_{\omega ji}(t) = \eta \delta_{pj} x_{pj} + \alpha \Delta_{\omega ji}(t-1) \text{ , for hidden layer weight} \tag{7}$$

$$\delta_{pk} = (t_{pk} - y_{pk}) y_{pk} (1 - y_{pk}) \tag{8}$$

$$\delta_{pj} = y_{pk} (1 - y_{pk}) (\sum_{k} \delta_{pk} \omega_{kj}) \tag{9}$$

δ_{pk} and δ_{pj} are called the error signals measured at the output and hidden layer, respectively.

A neural network with multiple layers of adaptive weights may contain many local minima and maxima in weight space which result in gradients of the error E very close to zero. Since the gradient of E is a factor of weight update in backpropagation techniques, it causes more iterations and becomes trapped in local minima for an extensive period of time. During the training session, the error usually decreases with iterations. Trapping into local minima may lead to a situation where the error does not decrease at all. When a local minima is encountered, the network may be able to get out of the local minima by changing the learning parameters or hidden unit numbers. Several other variations of backpropagation learning that have been reported to have faster convergence and improved generalization on unseen data are scaled conjugate backpropagation (Hagan et al., 1996), Bayesian regularization techniques (Mackay, 1992), and so forth.

Radial Basis Function Network

A radial basis function (RBF) network, as shown in Figure 3, has a hidden layer of radial units and an output layer of linear units. RBFs are local networks, as compared to feedforward networks that perform global mapping. Each radial unit is most receptive to a local region of the input space. Unlike hidden layer units in the preceding algorithm where the activation level of a unit is determined using weighted sum, a radial unit (i.e., local receptor field) is defined by its center point and a radius. Similar input vectors are clustered and put into various radial units. If an input vector lies near the centroid of a particular cluster, that radial unit will be activated. The activation level of the i-th radial unit is expressed as:

$$h_i = exp\left(-\frac{\|\mathbf{x} - \mathbf{u}_i\|^2}{2 s_i^2}\right) \tag{10}$$

where $\mathbf{x}$ is the input vector, $\mathbf{u}_i$ is a vector with the same dimension as $\mathbf{x}$ denoting the center, and s is the width of the function. The activation level of the radial basis function h_i for i-th radial unit is maximum when the $\mathbf{x}$ is at the center $\mathbf{u}_i$ of that unit. The final output of the RBF network can be computed as the weighted sum of the outputs of the radial units as:

$$y_i = \sum_i \omega_i h_i(\mathbf{x})$$

where ω_i is the connection weight between the radial unit i and the output unit, and the solution can be written directly as $\omega = \mathbf{R}^\dagger\mathbf{y}$, where $\mathbf{R}$ is a vector whose components are the output of radial units, and $\mathbf{y}$ is the target vector. The adjustable parameters of the network, that is, the center and shape of radial basis units ($\mathbf{u}_i$, s_i, and ω_i), can be trained by a supervised training algorithm. Centers should be assigned to reflect the natural clustering of the data. Lowe (1995) proposed a method to determine the centers based on standard deviations of training data. Moody and Darken (1989) selected the centers by means of data clustering techniques like k-means clustering, and ss are then estimated by taking the average distance to several nearest neighbors of $\mathbf{u}_i$s. Nowlan and Hinton (1992) proposed soft competition among radial units based on maximum likelihood estimation of the centers.

Probabilistic Neural Network

In the case of a classification problem, neural network learning can be thought of as estimating the probability density function (pdf) from the data. An alternative approach to pdf estimation is the kernel-based approximation, and this motivated the development of probabilistic neural network (PNN) by Specht

Figure 3. A radial basis function network. Not all of the interconnections are shown. Each basis function acts like a hidden unit.

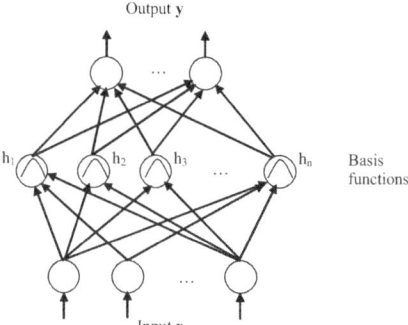

(1990) for classification task. It is a supervised neural network that is widely used in the area of pattern recognition, nonlinear mapping, and estimation of the probability of class membership and likelihood ratios (Specht & Romsdahl, 1994). It is also closely related to Bayes' classification rule and Parzen nonparametric probability density function estimation theory (Parzen, 1962; Specht, 1990). The fact that PNNs offer a way to interpret the network's structure in terms of probability density functions is an important merit of these type of networks. PNN also achieves faster training than backpropagation type feedforward neural networks.

The structure of a PNN is similar to that of feedforward neural networks, although the architecture of a PNN is limited to four layers: the *input layer*, the *pattern layer*, the *summation layer*, and the *output layer*, as illustrated in Figure 4. An input vector **x** is applied to the *n* input neurons and is passed to the pattern layer. The neurons of the pattern layer are divided into K groups, one for each class. The i-th pattern neuron in the k-th group computes its output using a Gaussian kernel of the form:

$$F_{k,i}(\mathbf{x}) = \frac{1}{(2\pi\sigma^2)^{n/2}} \exp\left(\frac{\|\mathbf{x} - \mathbf{x}_{k,i}\|^2}{2\sigma^2} \right) \tag{11}$$

Figure 4. A probabilistic neural network

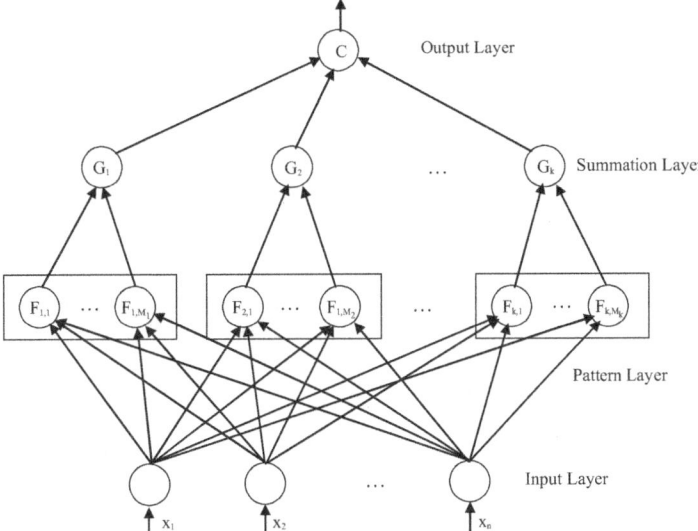

where $\mathbf{x}_{k,i}$ is the center of the kernel, and σ, called the spread (smoothing) parameter, determines the size of the receptive field of the kernel. The summation layer contains one neuron for each class. The summation layer of the network computes the approximation of the conditional class probability functions through a combination of the previously computed densities as follows:

$$G_k(\mathbf{x}) = \sum_{i=1}^{M_k} \omega_{ki} F_{ki}(\mathbf{x}), \quad k \in \{1, \cdots, K\}, \tag{12}$$

where M_k is the number of pattern neurons of class k, and ω_{ki} are positive coefficients satisfying $\sum_{i=1}^{M_k} \omega_{ki} = 1$. Pattern vector $\mathbf{x}$ is classified to belong to the class that corresponds to the summation unit with the maximum output. The parameter that needs to be determined for optimal PNN is the smoothing parameter. One way of doing that is to select an arbitrary set of σ, train the network, and test on the validation set. The procedure is repeated to find the set of σ that produces the least misclassification. An alternative way to search the optimal smoothing parameter was proposed by Masters (1995). The main disadvantages of PNN algorithm is that the network can grow very big and slow to execute with a large training set, making it impractical for large classification problems.

Self-Organizing Feature Map

In contrast to the previous learning algorithms, Kohonen's (1988) self-organizing feature map (SOFM) is an unsupervised learning algorithm that discovers the natural association found in the data. SOFM combines an input layer with a competitive layer where the units compete with one another for the opportunity to respond to the input data. The winner unit represents the category for the input pattern. Similarities among the data are mapped into closeness of relationship on the competitive layer.

Figure 5 shows a basic structure for a SOFM. Each unit in the competitive layer is connected to all the input units. When an input is presented, the competitive layer units sum their weighted inputs and compete. Initially, the weights are assigned to small random values. When an input $\mathbf{x}$ is presented, it calculates the distance d_j between $\mathbf{x}$ and $\mathbf{w}_j$ (weight of unit j) in the competitive layer as:

$$d_j = \| \mathbf{x} - \mathbf{w}_j \|$$

The winner unit c is the one with the lowest distance, such that

$$d_c = \min_j \left(\| \mathbf{x} \quad \mathbf{w}_j \| \right), \text{ for all of unit } j \text{ in the competitive layer.}$$

Figure 5. Architecture of a self-organizing map

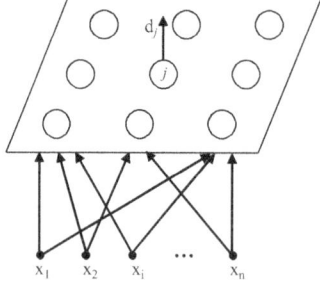

After identifying the winner unit, the neighborhood around it is identified. The neighborhood is usually in the form of a square shape centered on the wining unit c.

Denoting the neighborhood as N_c, the weighs between input i and competitive layer unit j are updated as

$$w_{ji} = \begin{cases} (x_i - w_{ij}) & \text{for unit } j \text{ in the neighbourhood of } N_c \\ 0 & \text{otherwise} \end{cases}$$

where   is the learning rate parameter. After updating the weights to the wining unit and its neighborhood, they become more similar to the input pattern. When the same or similar input is presented subsequently, the winner is most likely to win the competition. Initially, the algorithm starts with large values of learning rate   and the neighborhood size N_c, and then gradually decreases as the learning progresses.

The other notable unsupervised learning algorithm is adaptive resonance theory (ART) by Carpenter and Grossberg (1988), which is not so commonly used in biomedical applications and hence left out of the discussion for the current chapter. Interested readers may consult relevant works.

Overview of Neural Network Applications in Healthcare

One of the major goals of the modern healthcare system is to offer quality healthcare services to individuals in need. To achieve that objective, a key requirement is the early diagnosis of diseases so that appropriate intervention programs can be exercised to achieve better outcomes. There have been many significant advances in recent times in the development of medical technology aimed at helping the healthcare needs of our community. Artificial intelligence techniques and intelligent systems have found many valuable applications to assist in that cause (cf. Ifeachor et al., 1998; Teodorrescu et al., 1998). Specifically, neural networks have been demonstrated to be very useful in many biomedical areas, to help with the diagnosis of diseases and studying the pathological conditions, and also for monitoring the progress of various treatment outcomes. In providing assistance with the task of processing and analysis of biomedical signals, neural network tools have been very effective. Some of such common application areas include analysis of electrocardiography (ECG), electromyography (EMG), electroencephalography (EEG), and gait and movement biomechanics data. Furthermore, neural network's potentials have been demonstrated in many other healthcare areas, for example, medical image analysis, speech/auditory signal recognition and processing, sleep apnea detection, and so on.

The ECG signal is a representation of the bioelectrical activity of the heart's pumping action. This signal is recorded via electrodes placed on the patient's chest. The physician routinely uses ECG time-history plots and the associated characteristic features of P, QRS, and T waveforms to study and diagnose the heart's overall function. Deviations in these waveforms have been linked to many forms of heart diseases, and neural network have played a significant role in helping the ECG diagnosis process. For example, neural networks have been used to detect signs of acute myocardial infarction (AMI), cardiac arrhythmias, and other forms of cardiac abnormalities (Baxt, 1991; Nazeran & Behbehani, 2001). Neural networks have performed exceptionally well when applied to differentiate patients with and without a particular abnormality, for example, in the diagnosis of patients with AMI (97.2% sensitivity and 96.2% specificity; Baxt, 1991).

Electromyography (EMG) is the electrical activity of the contracting muscles. EMG signals can be used to monitor the activity of the muscles during a task or movement and can potentially lead to the diagnosis of muscular disorders. Both amplitude and timing of the EMG data are used to investigate muscle function. Neural networks have been shown to help in the modeling between mechanical muscle force generation and the corresponding recorded EMG signals (Wang & Buchanan, 2002). Neuromuscular diseases can affect the activity of the muscles (e.g., motor neuron disease), and neural networks have been proven useful in identifying individuals with neuromuscular diseases from features extracted from the motor unit action potentials of their muscles (e.g., Pattichis et al., 1995).

The EEG signal represents electrical activity of the neurons of the brain and is recorded using electrodes placed on the human scalp. The EEG signals and their characteristic plots are often used as a guide to diagnose neurological disorders, such as epilepsy, dementia, stroke, and brain injury or damage. The presence of these neurological disorders is reflected in the EEG waveforms. Like many other pattern recognition techniques, neural networks have been used to detect changes in the EEG waveforms as a result of various neurological and other forms of abnormalities that can affect the neuronal activity of the brain. A well-known application of neural networks in EEG signal analysis is the detection of epileptic seizures, which often result in a sudden and transient disturbance of the body movement due to excessive discharge of the brain cells. This seizure event results in spikes in the EEG waveforms, and neural networks and other artificial intelligence tools, such as fuzzy logic and support vector machines, have been employed for automated detection of these spikes in the EEG waveform. Neural networks-aided EEG analysis has also been undertaken for the diagnosis of many other related pathologies, including Huntington's and Alzheimer's diseases (Jervis et al., 1992; Yagneswaran et al., 2002). Another important emerging application of neural networks is in the area of brain computer interface (BCI), in which neural networks use EEG activity to extract embedded features linked to mental status or cognitive tasks to interact with the external environment (Culpepper & Keller, 2003). Such capability has many important applications in the area of rehabilitation by aiding communication for physically disabled people with the external environment (Garrett et al., 2003; Geva & Kerem, 1998). Other related applications of neural networks include analysis of evoked potentials and evoked responses of the brain in response to various external stimuli that are reflected in the EEG waveforms (Hoppe et al., 2001).

Gait is the systematic analysis of human walking. Various instrumentations are available to study different aspects of gait. Among its many applications, gait analysis is increasingly used to diagnose abnormality in the lower limb functions and to assess the progress of improvement as a result of interventions. Neural networks have found widespread applications for gait pattern recognition and clustering of gait types, for example, to classify simulated gait patterns (Barton & Lees, 1997) or to identify normal and pathological gait patterns (Holzreiter & Kohle, 1993; Wu et al., 1998). Gait also changes significantly in aging people with potential risks to loss of balance and falls, and neural networks have been useful in the automated recognition of aging individuals with balance disorders using gait measures (Begg et al., 2005). Further applications in gait and clinical biomechanics areas may be found in Chau (2001) and Schöllhorn (2004).

There are numerous other areas within the biomedical fields where neural networks have contributed significantly. Some of these applications include medical image diagnosis (Egmont-Petersen et al., 2001), low back pain diagnosis (Gioftsos & Grieve, 1996), breast cancer diagnosis (Abbass, 2002), glaucoma diagnosis (Chan et al., 2002), medical decision support systems (Silva & Silva, 1998), and so forth. The reader is referred to Chapter II for a comprehensive overview of neural networks applications for biomedical signal analysis in some of these selected healthcare areas.

References

Abbass, H. A. (2002). An evolutionary artificial neural networks approach for breast cancer diagnosis. *Artificial Intelligence in Medicine, 25*(3), 265-281.

Barton, J. G., & Lees, A. (1997). An application of neural networks for distinguishing gait patterns on the basis of hip-knee joint angle diagrams. *Gait and Posture, 5*, 28-33.

Baxt, W. G. (1991). Use of an artificial neural network for the diagnosis of myocardial infarction. *Annals of Internal Medicine, 115*, 843-848.

Begg, R. K., Hasan, R., Taylor, S., & Palaniswami, M. (2005, January). Artificial neural network models in the diagnosis of balance impairments. *Proceedings of the Second International Conference on Intelligent Sensing and Information Processing*, Chennai, India.

Carpenter, G.A., & Grossberg, S. (1988). The ART of adaptive pattern recognition by a self-organizing neural network. *Computer, 21*(3), 77-88.

Chan, K., Lee, T. W., Sample, P. A., Goldbaum, M. H., Weinreb, R. N., & Sejnowski, T. J. (2002). Comparison of machine learning and traditional classifiers in glaucoma diagnosis. *IEEE Transactions on Biomedical Engineering, 49*(9), 963-974.

Chau, T. (2001). A review of analytical techniques for gait data. Part 2: Neural network and wavelet methods. *Gait Posture, 13*, 102-120.

Coakley, J., & Brown, C. (2000). Artificial neural networks in accounting and finance: Modeling issues. *International Journal of Intelligent Systems in Accounting, Finance & Management, 9*, 119-144.

Culpepper, B. J., & Keller, R. M. (2003). Enabling computer decisions based on EEG input. *IEEE Transactions on Neural Systems and Rehabilitation Engineering, 11*(4), 354-360.

Cybenko, G. (1989). Approximation by superpositions of a sigmoidal function. *Mathematical Control Signal Systems, 2*, 303-314.

Duranton, M. (1996). Image processing by neural networks. *IEEE Micro, 16*(5), 12-19.

Egmont-Petersen, M., de Ridder, D., & Handels, H. (2001). Image processing with neural networks: A review. *Pattern Recognition, 35*, 2279-2301.

Fadlalla, A., & Lin, C. H. (2001). An analysis of the applications of neural networks in finance. *Interfaces, 31*(4), 112-122.

Fahlman, S. E., & Lebiere, C. (1990). The cascade-correlation learning architecture. *Advances in Neural Information Processing Systems, 2*, 524-532.

Garrett, D., Peterson, D. A., Anderson, C. W., & Thaur, M. H. (2003). Comparison of linear, non-linear and feature selection methods for EEG signal classification. *IEEE Transactions on Neural Systems and Rehabilitation Engineering, 11*, 141-147.

Geva, A.B., & Kerem, D. H. (1998). Brain state identification and forecasting of acute pathology using unsupervised fuzzy clustering of EEG temporal patterns. In T. Teodorrescu, A. Kandel, & L. C. Jain (Eds.), *Fuzzy and neuro-fuzzy systems in medicine* (pp. 57-93). Boca Raton, FL: CRC Press.

Gioftsos, G., & Grieve, D.W. (1996). The use of artificial neural networks to identify patients with chronic low-back pain conditions from patterns of sit-to-stand manoeuvres. *Clinical Biomechanics*, *11*(5), 275-280.

Hagan, M. T., Demuth, H. B., & Beale, M. H. (1996). *Neural network design.* Boston: PWS Publishing.

Hans, R. K., Sharma, R. S., Srivastava, S., & Patvardham, C. (2000). Modeling of manufacturing processes with ANNs for intelligent manufacturing. *International Journal of Machine Tools & Manufacture, 40*, 851-868.

Holzreiter, S. H., & Kohle, M. E. (1993). Assessment of gait pattern using neural networks. *Journal of Biomechanics, 26*, 645-651.

Hoppe, U., Weiss, S., Stewart, R. W., & Eysholdt, U. (2001). An automatic sequential recognition method for cortical auditory evoked potentials. *IEEE Transactions on Biomedical Engineering, 48*(2), 154-164.

Hush, P. R., & Horne, B. G. (1993). Progress in supervised neural networks. *IEEE Signal Processing, 1*, 8-39.

Ifeachor, E. C., Sperduti, A., & Starita, A. (1998). *Neural networks and expert systems in medicine and health care.* Singapore: World Scientific Publishing.

Jervis, B. W., Saatchi, M. R., Lacey, A., Papadourakis, G. M., Vourkas, M., Roberts, T., Allen, E. M., Hudson, N. R., & Oke, S. (1992). The application of unsupervised artificial neural networks to the sub-classification of subjects at-risk of Huntington's Disease. *IEEE Colloquium on Intelligent Decision Support Systems and Medicine, 5*, 1-9.

Kohonen, T. (1988). *Self-organisation and associative memory.* New York: Springer-Verlag.

Kruschke, J. K. (1989). Improving generalization in backpropagation networks with distributed bottlenecks. *Proceedings of the IEEE/INNS International Joint Conference on Neural Networks, 1*, 443-447.

Kung, S. Y., & Hwang, J. N. (1988). An algebraic projection analysis for optimal hidden units size and learning rate in backpropagation learning. *Proceedings of the IEEE/INNS International Joint Conference on Neural Networks, 1*, 363-370.

Lee, C. W. (1997). Training feedforward neural networks: An algorithm for improving generalization. *Neural Networks, 10*, 61-68.

Lehtokangas, M. (2000). Modified cascade-correlation learning for classification. *IEEE Transactions on Neural Networks, 11*, 795-798.

Lippman, R. P. (1987). An introduction to computing with neural nets. *IEEE Association Press Journal, 4*(2), 4-22.

Looney, C. G. (1996). Advances in feedforward neural networks: Demystifying knowledge acquiring black boxes. *IEEE Transactions on Knowledge & Data Engineering, 8,* 211-226.

Lowe, D. (1995). Radial basis function networks. In M.A. Arbib (Ed.), *The handbook of brain theory and neural networks.* Cambridge, MA: MIT Press.

Mackay, D. J. C. (1992). Bayesian interpolation. *Neural Computation, 4,* 415-447.

Masahiko, A. (1989). Mapping abilities of three layer neural networks. *Proceedings of the IEEE/INNS International Joint Conference on Neural Networks, 1,* 419-423.

Masters, T. (1995). *Advanced algorithms for neural networks.* New York: John Wiley & Sons.

McCullah, W. S., & Pitts, W. (1943). A logical calculus of ideas immanent in nervous activity. *Bulletin of Mathematical Biophysics, 5,* 115-133.

Moody, J., & Darken, C. J. (1989). Fast learning in networks of locally-tuned processing units. *Neural Computation, 1*(2), 281-294.

Nazeran, H., & Behbehani, K. (2001). Neural networks in processing and analysis of biomedical signals. In M. Akay (Ed.), *Nonlinear biomedical signal processing: Fuzzy logic, neural networks and new algorithms* (pp. 69-97). IEEE Press.

Nowlan, S.J., & Hinton, G.E. (1992). Simplifying neural networks by soft weight-sharing. *Neural Computation, 4*(4), 473-493.

Parzen, E. (1962). On the estimation of a probability density function and mode. *Annals of Mathematical Statistics, 3,* 1065-1076.

Pattichis, C. S., Schizas, C. N., & Middleton, L. T. (1995). Neural network models in EMG diagnosis. *IEEE Transactions on Biomedical Engineering, 42*(5), 486-496.

Rafiq, M. Y., Bugmann, G., & Easterbrook, D.J. (2001). Neural network design for engineering applications. *Computers & Structures, 79,* 1541-1552.

Rumelhart, D. E., McClelland, J. L., & the PDP Research Group (1986). *Parallel Distributed Processing, 1.*

Schöllhorn, W. I. (2004). Applications of artificial neural nets in clinical biomechanics. *Clinical Biomechanics, 19,* 876-98.

Silva, R., & Silva, A. C. R. (1998). Medical diagnosis as a neural networks pattern classification problem. In E. C. Ifeachor, A. Sperduti, & A. Starita (Eds.), *Neural networks and expert systems in medicine and health care* (pp. 25-33). Singapore: World Scientific Publishing.

Specht, D. F. (1990). Probabilistic neural networks. *Neural Networks, 1*(13), 109-118.

Specht, D. F., & Romsdahl, H. (1994). Experience with adaptive probabilistic neural network and adaptive general regression neural network. *Proceedings of the IEEE/INNS International Joint Conference on Neural Networks, 2*, 1203-1208.

Teodorrescu, T., Kandel, A., & Jain, L. C. (1998). *Fuzzy and neuro-fuzzy systems in medicine.* Boca Raton, FL: CRC Press.

Wang., L., & Buchanan, T.S. (2002). Prediction of joint moments using a neural network model of muscle activation from EMG signals. *IEEE Transactions on Neural Systems and Rehabilitation Engineering, 10*, 30-37.

Wong, B.K., Bodnovich, T.A., & Selvi, Y. (1997). Neural network applications in business: A review and analysis of the literature (1988-1995). *Decision Support Systems, 19,* 301-320.

Wu, B. (1992). An introduction to neural networks and their applications in manufacturing. *Journal of Intelligent Manufacturing, 3*, 391-403.

Wu, W. L., Su, F. C., & Chou, C. K. (1998). Potential of the back propagation neural networks in the assessment of gait patterns in ankle arthrodesis. In E.C. Ifeachor, A. Sperduti, & A. Starita (Eds.), *Neural networks and expert systems in medicine and health care* (pp. 92-100). Singapore: World Scientific Publishing.

Yagneswaran, S., Baker, M., & Petrosian, A. (2002). Power frequency and wavelet characteristics in differentiating between normal and Alzheimer EEG. *Proceedings of the Second Joint 24th Annual Conference and the Annual Fall Meeting of the Biomedical Engineering Society (EMBS/BMES), 1*, 46-47.

Chapter II

A Survey on Various Applications of Artificial Neural Networks in Selected Fields of Healthcare

Wolfgang I. Schöllhorn,
Westfälische Wilhelms-Universität Münster, Germany

Jörg M. Jäger,
Westfälische Wilhelms-Universität Münster, Germany

Abstract

This chapter gives an overview of artificial neural networks as instruments for processing miscellaneous biomedical signals. A variety of applications are illustrated in several areas of healthcare. The structure of this chapter is rather oriented on medical fields like cardiology, gynecology, or neuromuscular control than on types of neural nets. Many examples demonstrate how neural nets can support the diagnosis and prediction of diseases. However, their content does not claim completeness due to the enormous amount and exponentially increasing number of publications in this field. Besides the potential benefits for healthcare, some remarks on underlying assumptions are also included as well as problems which may occur while applying artificial neural nets. It is hoped that this review gives profound insight into strengths as well as weaknesses of artificial neural networks as tools for processing biomedical signals.

Introduction

Until now, there has been a tremendous amount of interest in and excitement about artificial neural networks (ANNs), also known as parallel distributed processing models, connectionist models, and neuromorphic systems. During the last two decades, ANNs have matured considerably from the early "first generation" methods (Akay, 2000) to the "second generation" of classification and regression tools (Lisboa et al., 1999) to the continuing development of "new generation" automatic feature detection and rule extraction instruments. Although it is obvious that ANNs have already been widely exploited in the area of biomedical signal analysis, a couple of interesting, and for healthcare reasons, valuable applications of all generations of ANNs are introduced in the following chapter. The selection of applications is arbitrary and does not claim completeness. The chapter is structured rather by medical domains than by type of neural nets or type of signals because very often different types of neural nets were compared on the basis of the same set of data, and different types of signals were chosen for input variables. According to the interdisciplinary character of modern medicine, this structure cannot be totally disjoint and will display some overlappings. However, due to the enormous amount and exponentially increasing number of publications, only a coarse stroboscopic insight into a still growing field of research will be provided.

Cardiology

The versatility of applications of ANNs with respect to their input variables is displayed in the field of applications related to heart diseases. Instead of using electrocardiographic (ECG) data (for a more comprehensive overview of ANN and ECG, see Chapters III-V), laboratory parameters like blood (Baxt, 1991; Baxt & Skora, 1996; Kennedy et al., 1997), angiography (Mobley et al., 2000), stress redistribution scintigrams, and myocardial scintigraphy (Kukar et al., 1999) as well as personal variables including past history (Baxt, 1991; Baxt &

Table 1. Applications of ANNs in cardiology

Authors	Objective	Input	Output	Type of ANN	Results/Remarks
Azuaje et al. (1999)	Coronary disease risk	Poincare plots Binary coded Analog coded	Two, three, and five levels of risk	MLP (144,576,1024/ 70,200,500/30,100, 200/2,3,5)	Even binary coded Poincare plots produce useful results
Baxt (1991); Baxt et al. (1996)	Acute Myocardial infarction (AMI)	20 Items including symptoms, past history, and physical and laboratory findings, e.g., palpitations, Angina, Rales or T-wave inversion	AMI yes/no	MLP (20/10/10/1)	MLP had higher sensitivity and specificity in diagnosing a myocardial infarction than physicians
Dorffner and Porenta (1994)	Coronary artery disease	45 Parameters of the Stress redistribution scintigram (5 segments times 3 views times 3 phases – stress, rest, washout)	Normal/ pathological	1) MLP 2) RBFN 3) Conic section function networks	MLP can be among the poorest methods Importance of initialization in MLP and CSFN
Kennedy et al. (1997)	AMI	39 items, e.g., Blood and ECG parameters derived to 53 binary inputs	AMI yes/no	MLP (53/18/1)	Trained ANN at least as accurate as medical doctors
Kukar et al. (1997)	Ischaemic heart disease (IHD)	77 parameters; IHD data for different diagnostic levels (e.g. signs, symptoms, exercise ECG, and myocardial scintigraphy, angiography)	Classification	1) (semi-)naive Bayesian classifier 2) Backpropagation learning of neural networks 3) Two algorithms for induction of decision trees (Assistant-I and -R) 4) k-nearest neighbors	Improvements in the predictive power of the diagnostic process. Analyzing and improving the diagnosis of ischaemic heart disease with machine learning
Mobley et al. (2004)	Coronary stenosis	11 personal parameters	Stenosis yes/no	MLP (11/36/1)	Specificity 26% Sensitivity 100%
Mobley et al. (2000)	Coronary artery stenosis	14 angiographic variables	Stenosis yes/no	MLP (14/26/1)	ANN could identify patients who did not need coronary antiography

Skora, 1996; Mobley et al., 2004), signs and symptoms (Kukar et al., 1999) or binary and analog coded Poincare plots (Azuaje et al., 1999) were chosen for input. With one exception, all of the selected papers present multilayer perceptrons (MLPs) for diagnosing acute myocardial infarction or coronary stenosis (Table 1). Most intriguingly, the model of coronary disease risk (Azuaje et al., 1999) on the basis of binary-coded Poincare data reveals useful results. The comparison of the performance of MLP with radialbasis function networks (RBFN) and conic section function networks (CSFN) provides evidence for the importance of the initialization of MLPs and CSFNs. With non-optimal initialization, MLPs can be among the poorest methods. Kukar et al. (1999) compares four classification approaches (Bayesian, MLP, decision tree, k-nearest neighbor) for classes of ischaemic heart diseases. The experiments with various learning algorithms achieved a performance level comparable to that of clinicians. A further interesting result in this study was that only ten attributes were sufficient to reach a maximum accuracy. A closer look at the structure of this subset of attributes suggests that most of the original 77 attributes were redundant in the diagnostic process.

Gynecology

Breast Cancer

Breast cancer ranks first in the causes of cancer death among women in developed and developing countries (Parkin et al., 2001; Pisani et al., 1999). The best way to reduce death due to breast cancer suggests treating the disease at an earlier stage (Chen et al., 1999). Earlier treatment requires early diagnosis, and early diagnosis requires an accurate and reliable diagnostic procedure that allows physicians to differentiate benign breast tumors from malignant ones. Current procedures for detecting and diagnosing breast cancer illustrate the difficulty in maximizing sensitivity and specificity (Chen et al., 1999). For data acquisition, versatile diagnostic tools are applied. Correspondingly, most publications about breast cancer diagnosis apply different forms of supervised neural nets (Table 2), in most cases, a three layered MLP with one output node modeling benign or malignant diagnosis.

Abbass (2002) trained a special kind of evolutionary artificial neural network, memetic pareto ANNs on the basis of nine laboratory attributes. Setiono (1996, 2000) took Wisconsin Breast Cancer Diagnosis data as input parameters for a three layered pruned MLP. Buller et al. (1996) and Chen et al. (1999) rely on ultrasonic images for the training of three and four layered MLPs. Input data from radiographic image features are the basis for Fogel et al. (1998), Markey et al. (2003), Ronco (1999), Papadopulos et al., (2004), and Papadopulos et al. (2002) whereby, in all cases, the main amount of image data were reduced either by principal component analysis (PCA) or by selecting characteristic features. Markey et al. (2003) applied a self-organizing map (SOM) for classifying the image data, and Papadopulos et al. (2002) combined a four layered MLP with an expert system.

Lisboa et al. (2003) present a partial logistic artificial neural network (PLANN) for prognosis after surgery on the basis of 18 categorical input data, which include, among others, number of nodes, pathological size, and oestrogen level.

The results of contrasting the PLANN model with the clinically accepted proportional hazards model were that the two are consistent, but the neural network may be more specific in the allocation of patients into prognostic groups using a default procedure.

The probability of relapse after surgery is objective to the MLP model of Gomez-Ruiz et al. (2004). The model is based only on six attributes including tumor size, patient age, or menarchy age and is able to make an appropriate prediction about the relapse probability at different times of follow up. A similar model is provided by Jerez-Aragones et al. (2003). A comparison of a three layered MLP with decision trees and logistic regression for breast cancer survivability is presented by Delen et al. (2004). Cross et al. (1999) describe the development and testing of several decision support strategies for the cytodiagnosis of breast cancer that are based on image features selected by specialist clinicians.

However, the reliability study of Kovalerchuk et al. (2000) shows that the development of reliable computer-aided diagnostic (CAD) methods for breast cancer diagnosis requires more attention regarding the problems of selection of training, testing data, and processing methods. Strictly speaking, all CAD methods are still very unreliable in spite of the apparent and possibly fortuitous high accuracy of cancer diagnosis reported in literature and therefore require further research. Several criteria for reliability studies are discussed next.

Knowledge-based neurocomputation for the classification of cancer tissues using micro-array data were applied by Futschik et al. (2003). Knowledge-based neural nets (KBNN) address the problem of knowledge representation and extraction. As a particular version of a KBNN, Futschik et al. (2003) applied evolving fuzzy neural networks (EFuNNs), which are implementations of evolving connectionist systems (ECOS). ECOS are multilevel, multimodular structures where many modules have inter- and intra-connections. ECOS are not restricted to a clear multilayered structure and do have a modular open structure. In contrast to MLPs, the learned knowledge in EFuNNs is locally embedded and not distributed over the whole neural network. Rule extraction was used to identify groups of genes that form profiles and are highly indicative of particular cancer types.

A whole group of publications in medical literature, including Setiono, (1996, 2000); Downs et al. (1996); Delen et al. (2004); Papadopulos et al. (2002), copes with long assumed disadvantages of MLPs, based on the fundamental theoretical works of Benitez et al. (1997); Castro and Miranda (2002). Mainly, ANNs have been shown to be universal approximators. However, many researchers refuse to use them due to their shortcomings which have given them the title "black boxes". Determining why an ANN makes a particular decision is a difficult task (Benitez et al., 1997). The lack of capacity to infer a direct "human comprehensible" explanation from the network is seen as a clear impediment to a more

Table 2. Applications of ANNs in breast cancer research (? = not specified in reference)

Authors	Objective	Input	Output	Type of ANN	Results/remarks
Abbass (2002)	Breast cancer	9 Attributes: Clump thickness, uniformity of cell size, uniformity of cell shape, marginal adhesion, single epithelial cell size, bare nuclei, bland chromatin, normal nucleoli, mitoses	benign/malignant	1 memetic pareto artificial neural networks (MPANN), (i.e., special kind of Evolutionary ANN)	MPANN have better generalization and lower computational cost than other evolutionary ANNs or back propagation networks
Buller et al. (1996)	Breast cancer	Ultrasonic Image parameters	benign/malignant	2 MLPs: one for malignant, one for benign (27/4/1) (27/14/2/1) compared with experts	Weak when evidence on the image is considered weak by the expert
Chen et al. (1999)	Breast nodules	Ultrasonic images 24-dimensional image feature vector	benign/malignant	MLP (25/10/1)	Accuracy for detecting malignant tumors 95%, sensitivity 98%, specificity 93%
Delen et al. (2004)	Comparison methods Breast cancer survivability	17 predictor variables (race, marital status, histology, tumor size, etc.)	Survived Not survived	1) Decision tree 2) MLP(17/15/2) 3) Log reg	DT: 93.2% ANN: 91.2% Log reg: 89.2% Recommended k-fold cross validation
Downs et al. (1996)	1) Coronary care 2) Breast cancer 3) Myocardial infarction	1) 43 items of clinical or electrocardiographic data 2) 10 binary valued features., e.g., presence/absence of negrotic epithelial cells 3) 35 Items of clinical or ECG data coded as 37 binary inputs	?	Fuzzy ARTMAP	Symbolic rule extraction
Fogel et al. (1998)	Screening features for mammogram	12 radiographic features	Malignant/ non-malignant	MLP (12/1,2/1)	ANNs with only two hidden nodes performed as well as more complex ANNs and better than ANNs with only one hidden node

widespread acceptance of ANNs (Tickle et al., 1998). Knowledge in conventional ANNs like MLPs is stored locally in the connection weights and is distributed over the whole network, complicating its interpretation (Futschik et al., 2003). Setiono (1996, 2000) found that a more concise set of rules can be thus expected from a network with fewer connections and fewer clusters of hidden unit activations. Under some minor restrictions, the functional behavior of radial basis function networks is equivalent to fuzzy interference systems (Jang & Sun, 1993). Analogously, the results of Paetz (2003) are a major extension of

Table 2. Applications of ANNs in breast cancer research (? = not specified in reference) (cont.)

Gomez-Ruiz et al. (2004)	Prognosis of early breast cancer	6 Attributes after cancer surgery (tumor size, patient age, menarchy age, etc.)	Breast cancer relapse	MLP (6/18,16,15,13,12/1)	Predictions about the relapse probability at different times of follow-up
Jerez-Aragones et al. (2003)	Breast cancer relapse	15 personal and laboratory attributes	Breast cancer relapse	1) MLP 2) Decision tree	Control of induction by sample division method
Lisboa et al. (2003)	Prognostic risk groups and management of breast cancer patients (censored data)	18 categorical variables n=1616 cases with variable numbers of missing values	Assignment of a prognostic group index or risk score to each individual record	Partial Logistic Artificial Neural Network (PLANN)	Pathological size and histology are key factors to differentiate the highest surviving-group from the rest and clinical stage Nodes specify lowest-surviving group
Markey et al. (2003)	Breast cancer	Mammographic findings Patient age	1) Classification 2) malignancy	1) 4x4 SOM CSNN profile of each cluster 2) MLP (7/14/1)	25 % specificity 98% sensitivity
Papadopulos et al. (2002)	Detection of micro calcification (mammogram)	Image data PCA data reduction	Micro calcification or not	Hybrid network classifier Expert system + MLP (9/20/10/1)	
Papadopulos et al. (2004)	Micro calcification in mammogram	2048x2048 pixel data reduction PCA	Malignant or benign	1) Rule based classifier 2) MLP (7/15/1) 3) SVM	Performance 0.79-0.83
Ronco (1999)	Breast cancer screening	42 variables: data from familial history of cancer and sociodemographic, gynecoobstetric, and dietary variables	Cancer yes/no	MLP (42/16-256/1)	94.04%positive predictive value and 97.6% negative predictive value Improvement of cost/benefit ratio
Setiono (1996)	Breast cancer diagnosis	Wisconsin Breast Cancer diagnosis (WBCD)	benign/malignant	MLP (Pruned NN)	95% accuracy rate rule extraction
Setiono (2000)	Breast cancer diagnosis	WBCD	benign/malignant	MLP (/3,5/)	Do. improved by preprocessing, e.g., relevant parameters, extracting missing attributes

preliminary work now providing understandable knowledge for classification and generating more performant rules for preventing septic shocks. Rule extraction from neural networks has been in a state of stagnation for the last few years (Tickle et al., 1998); however, the very recent works from Duch et al. (2001), Markowska-Kaczmar and Trelak (2003), and Hammer et al. (2002, 2003) brought new issues back into discussion.

Pregnancy

The applications of ANNs with respect to the subject of pregnancy cover nearly all states of life development from predicting ovulation time (Gürgen et al., 1995) to the prediction of fertilization success (Cunningham et al., 2000) and intrauterine growth retardation (Gurgen, 1999; Gurgen et al., 1997) up to cardiotocography (CTG) (Ulbricht et al., 1998). All investigations listed in Table 3 are based on MLPs with input variables of different numeric scales. The input variables cover the spectrum from symbolic variables (Cunningham et al., 2000) to numeric ultrasound (Gurgen, 1999; Gurgen et al., 1997, 2001), heart rate (Ulbricht et al., 1998) and hormone (Cunningham et al., 2000; Gürgen et al., 1995) parameters. Gurgen et al. (2001), Alonso-Betanzos et al. (1999), and Ulbricht et al. (1998) compare the MLPs with Bayes discriminant analysis (Gurgen, 1999), neurofuzzy-MLPs with neurofuzzy-radial basis functions (Gurgen et al., 2001), and MLPs with Bayes-model, discriminant analysis, Shortliffe/Buchannan-Algorithm (Shortliffe & Buchanan, 1975), as well as with experts (Alonso-Betanzos et al., 1999). Gurgen (1999) achieves the better success rate for predicting intrauterine growth retardation by means of MLPs in comparison to Bayesian based statistical approaches. On the basis of incomplete input data, the results of Alonso-Betanzos et al. (1999) show small advantages for the Shortliffe/Buchanan (SB) algorithm with respect to the false positives. As far as validation against the problem is concerned, it can be seen that presenting a higher level of true positives are three experts, the SB-algorithm, and the ANN.

Image Analysis

General

Automated image analysis is an increasing and important area for the application of ANN pattern recognition techniques. Particularly in healthcare, pattern recognition is used to identify and extract important features in ECTs, MRIs, radiographies, smears, and so forth. Especially with the introduction of film and decreasing radio and photography departments, the role of image analysis is likely to grow. An important step in the analysis of biomedical images is the precise segmentation of the objects of an image. Thereby, the construction of a 3D-model is generally carried out by overlaying contours obtained after a 2D segmentation of each image-slice.

Table 3. Applications of ANNs in research related to pregnancy (? = not specified in reference)

Authors	Objective	Input	Output	Type of ANN	Results/remarks
Alonso-Betanzos et al. (1999)	Pregnancy monitoring with incomplete data	NST parameters, risk factors	Indicators for good or bad/slightly bad moderately bad/quite fetal outcome	1) MLP (8/16/4) 2) Bayes Discriminant 3) ANN 4) Shortliffe/Buchanan (SB) 5) Experts	Best results SB ANN better than experts
Cunningham et al. (2000)	Fertilization	28 parameters: 18 numeric, 10 symbolic	Successful or not	MLP (28/?/1)	Stability problems Results are highly sensitive on training data
Gürgen et al. (1995)	Predicting ovulation time	Luteinizing hormone (LH)	Ovulation time	5 MLPs (1/4-6/1)	Peak error: 0.07-0.12
Gurgen et al. (1997)	Intrauterine growth retardation	Weekly ultrasonic examination parameters (WI, HC, AC, HC/AC, + Gaussian noise in training data)	Normal Symmetric IUGR Assymmetric IUGR	MLP (4,8,12,16/2,3,4,5/3)	Success rate increased from 1st gestational week until the 4th from 61% to 95%
Gurgen (1999)	1) Predicting intrauterine growth retardation (IUGR) and 2) ovulation time on the basis of luteinizing hormone (LH)	1) Week index (WI) Head circumference (HC), Abdominal circumference (AC), HC/AC Between 16th and 36th week 1) LH	1) Symmetric IUGR, normal, asymmetric IUGR 2) Ovulation time	1) MLPs (=1582) 2) Bayes	1) Success rate of 95% 2) Peak error 0.07-0.12 The NN approach is particularly more appropriate than Bayesian-based statistical approaches
Gurgen et al. (2001)	Antenatal fetal risk assessment	4 Doppler Ultrasound Blood flow velocity waveforms	Grade values 0.7-0.95: alarming risk 0.4-0.7: suspicious situation 0-0.4: good fetal conditions	1) MLP 2) Neurofuzzy MLP 3) NF-RBF decision	Sensitivity: 88-100% Specificity: 95-100% PPT: 90-100% PNT: 93-100%
Ulbricht et al. (1998)	Cardiotocogram (CTG)	The baseline of the fetal heart rate and values indicating the microfluctuation	Deceleration No deceleration	MLP (15/3/2)	Correct positive: 72-90% False negative: 20-40%

A comprehensive up-to-date review on image processing and neural networks is provided by Egmont-Petersen et al. (2001), Miller et al. (1992), and Nattkemper (2004). Examples of filtering, segmentation, and edge detection techniques using cellular neural networks (CNN) to improve resolution in brain tomographies and to improve global frequency correction for the detection of microcalcifications in mammograms can be seen in the work of Aizenberg et al. (2001). An ANN was successfully applied to enhance low-level segmentation of eye images for diagnosis of Grave's ophthalmopathy (Ossen et al., 1994). The ANN segmentation system was integrated into an existing medical imaging system. The system provides a user interface to allow interactive selection of images, ANN architectures, training algorithms, and data.

Dellepiane (1999) concentrates on the importance of feature selection in image analysis. The proposed approach, based on the definition of a training set, represents a possible solution to the problem of selecting the best feature set that is characterized by robustness and reproducibility.

A patented commercial product for cytodiagnosis, especially for cancer detection and cancer diagnosis, is presented by Koss (1999). PAPNET has been constructed for the purpose of selecting a limited number of cells from cytologic preparations for display on a high resolution television monitor. Digitized images, representing abnormal cells from cervical smears are fed into an ANN circuit. The machine showed a sensitivity of 97% for abnormal smears. The ANN based devices are interactive and do not offer an automated verdict, leaving the diagnosis to trained humans.

Further applications of ANN in medical image analysis are listed in Table 4.

A proposal for the segmentation of images based on active contours is presented by Vilarino et al. (1998). The application of cellular neural networks (CNN) (Chua & Yang, 1988) operates by means of active contours. The CNNs are defined as a n-dimensional array of dynamic processing elements called cells with local iterations between them. The CNN allows for a continuous treatment of the contour and leads to greater precision in the adaptation implemented in the CNN.

An alternative approach for image analysis in the context of recognizing lymphocytes in tissue sections is suggested by Nattkemper et al. (2001). After data reduction of digitized images by means of principal component analysis, local linear maps (LLM) were applied for automatic quantization of fluorescent lymphocytes in tissue section. The LLM approach was originally motivated by the Kohonen self-organizing map (SOM) (Kohonen, 1982, 2001) with the intention of obtaining a better map resolution even with a small number of units. The LLM combines supervised and unsupervised learning which differs from MLPs trained with back propagation. The neural cell detection system (NCDS) detected a minimum of 95% and delivered the number, the positions, and the phenotypes of the fluorescent cells once it was trained within 2 minutes. In comparison to human experts and support vector machines (SVM) (Nattkemper et al., 2003), this LLM-based high-throughput screening approach is much faster and achieves the best recognition rate. A further advantage of LLM can be seen in its robustness because, for micrographs of varying quality, it is more resistant to variations in the image domain.

Table 4. Applications of ANNs in medical image analysis (? = not specified in reference)

Authors	Objective	Input	Output	Type of ANN	Results /remarks
Nattkemper et al. (2001)	Image analysis Lymphocytes in tissue sections	6 dim feature vector extracted by PCA	Combined supervised and unsupervised	Local linear map (LLM)	Detected 95% of the cells Experts detected only 80% The trained system evaluates an image in 2 min calculating
Nattkemper et al. (2003)	Microscopic analysis of lymphocytes	658x517 pixel micrographs PCA six-eigenvectors	dto.	1) SVM 2) LLM	ANNs classified microscopy data with satisfactory results
Pizzi et al. (1995)	Alzheimer's diseased tissue	1) Infrared spectra (IS) 2) PCA of infrared spectra	Classification 2 groups 5 groups	1) LDA 2) MLP	PCA of IS, 2 groups: 98% PCA of IS, 2 groups 100% Only IS always provided poorer results
Tjoa and Krishnan (2003)	Colon status from endoscopic images	Texture features, texture spectra, colon features, PCA	Normal abnormal	MLP (?/5-25/2)	Texture and color: 97.7% Texture: 96.6% Color: 90.5%
Vilarino et al. (1998)	Images, e.g., computational tomography (CT)	Images (with energy information, i.e. different gray scales)	Contours in images	Discrete-time cellular neural network (DTCNN)	(automatic) Detection of contours in images for segmentation
Zhou et al. (2002)	Identification of Lung cancer cells	Images of the specimen of needle biopsis	1) Normal cell 2) Cancer cell a) adenocarcinoma, b) squamous cell c) small cell c. d) large cell c. e) normal	ANN-ensembles	Automatic pathological diagnosis procedure named Neural Ensemble-based Detection (NED) is proposed

The importance of data preprocessing in a similar context is rationale in the investigation of Pizzi et al. (1995). ANN classification methods were applied to the infrared spectra of histopathologically confirmed Alzheimer's-diseased and control brain tissue. When data were preprocessed with PCA, the ANNs outperformed their linear discriminant counterparts: 100% vs. 98% correct classifications. Only one of the three selected ANN architectures produced comparable results when the original spectra were used.

Providing assistance for the physician in detecting the colon status from colonoscopic images was intended by the development of an ANN model by Tjoa and Krishnan (2003). Schemes were developed to extract texture features from the texture spectra in the chromatic and achromatic domains, and color features for a selected region of interest from each color component histogram of the colonoscopic images. Similarly to the previous investigations, the features were first reduced in size by means of PCA before they were evaluated with back

Figure 1. A classifier ensemble of neural networks

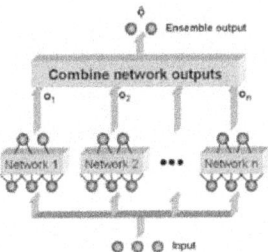

propagation ANN. Using texture and color features with PCA led to an average classification accuracy of 97.7%, and classification only by means of texture (96.9%) or color (90.5%) features were outperformed.

An ensemble of artificial neural networks was applied by Zhou et al. (2002) for the identification of lung cancer cells in the images of the specimens of needle biopsies. Neural network ensembles (Figure 1) were proposed by Hansen and Salamon (1990) for improving the performance and training of neural networks for classification. Cross validation is used as a tool for optimizing network parameters and architectures, where remaining residual generalization errors can be reduced by invoking ensembles of similar networks (Islam et al., 2003; Krogh & Vedelsby, 1995) The comparison of single neural networks and ensembles of neural networks showed a clear decrease in the error rate from 45.5% down to 13.6% on average.

MRI

Within the area of image analysis, a comprehensive amount of publications are focused on Magnetic Resonance Imaging (MRI) and functional Magnetic Resonance Imaging (fMRI) (Table 5). The imaging methods can lead to automated techniques to identify and quantify cortical regions of the brain. Hall et al. (1992) compare segmentation techniques for MRI on the basis of pixel and feature data. Segmentation methods for MRI data are developed to enhance tumor/edema boundary detection, for surgery simulation and for radiation treatment planning. Similar results are provided by supervised (forward cascade

Table 5. Applications of ANNs in medical image analysis: MRI images

Authors	Objective	Input	Output	Type of ANN	Results/remarks
Dimitriadou et al. (2004)	fMRI comparison of clustering methods	fMRI image data	Tissue Classification	Hierarchical, crisp (neural gas, self-organizing maps, hard competitive learning, k-means, maximium and minimum distance, CLARA) and fuzzy (c-means, fuzzy competitive learning)	Neural gas method seems to be the best choice for fMRI Cluster analysis, neural gas, and the k-means algorithm perform significantly better than all others
Gelenbe et al. (1996)	Volumetric Magnet Resonance Imaging	5x5 Blocks of pixels of the MRI with their grey level	A finite set of M regions $R_1, ..., R_M$ of the MRI which are wished to be identified	Recurrent pulsed random network (RPRN)	Results are similar to a human expert carrying out manual volumetric analysis of brain MR images
Hall et al. (1992)	Magnet resonance images	MRI Data (256x256 pixel with three features: T1, T2,) leading to a 65536x3 matrix for each image	Up to seven classes of (MR) tissue, e.g., white or grey matter or edema	1) Fuzzy c-means algorithms (unsupervised) 2) approximate fuzzy c-means (unsupervised) 3) FF cascade correlation NN (supervised)	Supervised and unsupervised segmentation techniques provide similar results
Lai and Fang (2000)	MR images	1) Wavelet histogram features 2) spatial statistical features	Classifying into multiple clusters	One hierarchical NN (RBF) for clustering and a number of estimating networks	Automatic adjustment of display window width and center for a wide range of magnetic resonance (MR) images
Reddick et al. (1997)	Multispectral Magnetic Resonance Images	1) Input vector of the non-normalized T1, T2, and PD signal intensities for a single pixel within the region of interest in MRI 2) Three components of weight vector associated with each neuron of the SOM	1) Nine levels of segmented images 2) Classification of MRI pixel into seven classes: white, white/grey, grey, grey/CSF, CSF, other, Background	1) 3x3 SOM for segmentation 2) MLP (3/7/7) for classification	ICC (r_i) of 0.91, 0.95, and 0.98 for white matter, gray matter, and ventricular cerebrospinal fluid (CSF), respectively
Wismuller et al. (2004)	fMRI	Five slices with 100 images Resolution 3x3x4mm	Tissue Classification	1) Neural gas (NG) network 2) SOM 3) Fuzzy clustering based on deterministic annealing	Neural gas and fuzzy clustering outperformed KSOM NG outperformed with respect to quantization error KSOM outperformed with respect to computational expense

correlation neural network) and unsupervised (fuzzy algorithms) segmentation techniques.

Lai and Fang (2000) present a hierarchical neural network-based algorithm for robust and accurate display-window parameter estimation. Instead of image pixels, wavelet histogram features and spatial statistical features are extracted from the images and combined into an input vector. The hierarchical neural networks consist of a competitive layer neural network for clustering two radial basis function networks, a bimodal linear estimator for each subclass, and a data fusion process using estimates from both estimators to compute the final display parameters. The algorithm was tested on a wide range of MR images and displayed satisfactory results.

A geometric recurrent pulsed random network for extracting precise morphometric information from MRI scans is presented by Gelenbe et al. (1996). The network is composed of several layers with internal interneural interaction and recurrency in each individual layer. Correct classification of 98.4% was observed, based on 5x5 pixel matrices for input data.

A hybrid-neural-network method for automated segmentation and classification of multispectral MRI of brain is demonstrated by Reddick et al. (1997). The automated process uses Kohonen's self organizing ANN for segmentation and an MLP back propagation network for classification for distinguishing different tissue types. An intraclass correlation of the automated segmentation and classification of tissues with the standard radiologist identification led to coefficients of $r = 0.91$ (white matter), $r = 0.95$ for gray matter, and 0.98 for ventricular cerebrospinal fluid. The fully automated procedure produced reliable MR image segmentation and classification while eliminating intra- and inter-observer variability.

FMRI based on blood oxygenation-level-dependent signal changes allows assessment of brain activity via local hemodynamic variations over time (Ogawa et al., 1992, 1993).

An alternative approach for fMRI analysis, based on unsupervised clustering, is suggested by Wismuller et al. (2004). The proposed neural gas (Martinetz et al., 1993) is a neuronal clustering algorithm that solves several points of weakness in classical Kohonen nets. One problem in clustering unknown data by means of Kohonen nets is the advanced determination of the nets' dimensions. When the choice does not fit with the dimensionality of the data, topological defects may occur that can lead to deficient mapping. In contrast, the neural gas has no predefined topology which determines the neighborhood relation between the neurons. The neighborhood in the neural gas (Figure 2) is exclusively determined by the relation of the weights of the neurons in the input data space. The reference vectors are moving "free" in the data space. Wismuller et al. (2004) analyzed fMRI data from subjects performing a visual task. Five slices with 100 images were acquired. The clustering results were evaluated by assessment of cluster assignment maps, task-related activation maps, and associated time courses. The major findings were that neural gas and fuzzy clustering outperformed Kohonen's map in terms of identifying signal components with high correlation to the fMRI stimulus. The neural gas outperformed the two other

Figure 2. Growing neural gas (from Fritzke, 1997)

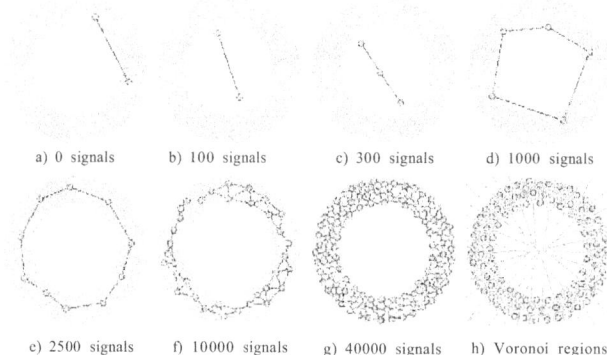

methods regarding the quantization error, and Kohonen's map outperformed the two other methods in terms of computational expense.

Similarly, Gelenbe et al. (1996) compared several fMRI cluster analysis techniques. The clustering algorithms used were hierarchical, crisp (neural gas, SOM, hard competitive learning, k-means, maximum distance, CLARA) and fuzzy (c-means, fuzzy competitive learning). The results clearly showed that the neural gas and the k-means algorithm perform significantly better than all the other methods using their set-up. Overall the neural gas method seems to be the best choice for fMRI cluster analysis, given its true positives while minimizing false positives and showing stable results.

Neuromuscular Control

Low Back Pain

Besides categorizing groups with common degrees of impairment during gait (cf. Chapter X), one of the most disabling orthopaedic problems is most often subject to classification tasks with ANNs: low back pain and trunk motion. Selected publications are listed in Table 6.

Bishop et al. (1997) analyzed several forms of MLPs in assigning sensed low-back pain during a set of trunk motions to selected kinematic parameters that were collected with a tri-axial goniometer. In comparison to linear classifiers, the ANN classifier produced superior results with up to 85% accuracy on test data. Despite the dependence of the system on the low-back classification, the authors claim to have found a system that could markedly improve the management of lower back pain in the individual patient.

With a similar goal of classifying the relationship between pain and vertebral motion, Dickey et al. (2002) collected data of vertebral motions of the lumbar

Table 6. Applications of ANNs in neuromuscular control/orthopaedics— low back pain and trunk motion (? = not specified in reference)

Authors	Objective	Input	Output	Type of ANN	Results /remarks
Bishop et al. (1997)	Low back pain	Tri-axial goniometer data	Low back pain	MLP (?/?/?) (RBF)	85% correct; Compared with Quebec Task Force pain classification
Dickey et al. (2002)	Low back pain	Kinematic motion parameters derived from percutaneous intra-pedicle screws L4 L5 S1	Level of pain (0-10)	MLP (32/10/1) Linear Discriminant Analysis (LDA)	MLP train and test: R^2= 0.997 LDA: train r^2=0.5 and test r^2=0.14
Gioftsos and Grieve (1996)	Chronic low back pain	242 variables Forces + pressure at feet, knee, hip, and lumbar movements	Three classes of subjects (Healthy -H, one previous back-pain episode at least 1 year before experiment -M, subjects with chronic low back-pain problems -P)	MLP (242/20/3) classification	86% were diagnosed correctly More successful than physiotherapists
Hallner and Hasenbring (2004)	Psychosocial risk factor and low back pain	3 Parameters a) Depression b) Suppressive behavior c) Thoughts of suppression	Pain intensity after 6 months	MLP (3/3/1)	Correct classification: 83.1%, Sensitivity: 73% Specificity: 97%
Langdell and Mason (1999)	Shapes of spines	Ratio of width to height of the five vertebrae in the lumbar region of the spine	Classification exposed unexposed	RBF Combined with SOMs	
Mann and Brown (1991)	Low back pain	Pain drawings	a) Benign back pain b) Herniation of the nucleus Pulposus c) Spinal stenosis d) Serious underlying disorders e) Psychogenic regional pain disturbance	1) MLP (?/?/5) 2) Traditional Statistics 3) Human experts	All provide comparable results with small advantages to MLPs
Nussbaum and Chaffin (1997)	Trunk motion	Surface EMGs of 7 lumbar muscles Moment magnitudes	Classification	Two layer competitive	Majority responders Minority responders

Table 6. Applications of ANNs in neuromuscular control/orthopaedics—low back pain and trunk motion (? = not specified in reference) (cont.)

Nussbaum et al. (1995)	Trunk motion	Four parameters of external moments	2x4 moment EMG patterns left and right, m. erector spinae, m. rectus abdominis, m. external oblique, m. latissimus dorsi	1) MLP (4/5-20/8) 2) Minimum intensity compression 3) sum cubed intensities	1) $r^2 = 0.83$ 2) $r^2 = 0.65$ 3) $r^2 = 0.65$
Nussbaum et al. (1997b)	Trunk motion simulation	Six magnitudes of external loading	Sagittal, frontal, and axial moments	MLP (6/4-7/10/3)	$R^2 = 0.4$-0.9 with experimental EMG data
Oliver and Atsma (1996)	Back pain and trunk motions Paraspinal power spectra	Surface EMG erector spinae L4-5 power spectra	No back pain Chronic back pain	MLP (300/1,51,10,15/2)	Specificity: 79% Sensitivity: 80% Results highly dependent on clinician correctly labelling
Sanders and Mann (2000)	Pain drawings low back pain	Nature and region of low back pain	a) Spinal stenosis b) Herniated disk c) Underlying disorders d) Benign disorder e) Psychogenic	1) MLP (378/?/5) 2) Linear Discriminant Analysis	Classification results are the same as was achieved by discriminant analysis of low back pain expert physicians

spine by means of percutaneous intra-pedicle screws. The levels of pain, together with parameters of kinematic data, were recorded as the subjects performed a battery of trunk motions similar to Bishop et al. (1997). In contrast to the linear discriminant analysis, ($r^2=0.514$), the non-linear trained ANN displayed a strong relationship between observed and predicted pain ($r^2=0.997$).

Gioftsos and Grieve (1996) present ANNs as an additional tool in the assessment and possible diagnosis of pathological movements. Forces and centers of pressure at the feet and knees, plus hip and lumbar movements during sit-to-stand maneuvers provided input for a three-layered feedforward MLP with sigmoidal transfer functions. Subjects (31 out of 36) were correctly classified into one of three categories. The ANNs outperformed the assessment rate of nine experienced physiotherapists (56%) who assessed the patterns of movement by watching the videotaped sit-stand and stand-sit maneuvers in randomized order. Overall, the ANNs were found to have satisfactory accuracy in the recognition of pathological patterns of movement.

A more patient-oriented approach of dealing with low back pain is followed by Mann and Brown (1991) and Sanders and Mann (2000). The research intended to make patients pain drawings a more useful tool. These drawings are often used in order to get a first impression of a patient's low back pain location. Classifying patients pain descriptions, that were previously transformed into discrete numeric data in the form of a two dimensional pattern, formed the input data to the ANNs. The descriptions were topographical pain representations from patient drawings, following dermatomal mappings. With the obtained classification sensitivity of 49% achieved by Sanders and Mann (2000) for five groups, the results were approximately as good as an expert physician and discriminant analysis.

The goal of Oliver and Atsma (1996) was to automatically classify normal and chronic back pain diagnostic groups on the basis of electromyogram EMG power spectra. From 1 to 15 units for the hidden layer within a three layer MLP were tested for best specificity and sensitivity, ending up with five units. The weights in the trained MLPs were utilized in order to reduce the number of inputs and optimize the preprocessing of data. Nevertheless, all the techniques seem to be "dependent on the clinician correctly labeling each subject used in training" (Oliver & Atsma, 1996, p. 423).

A more interdisciplinary approach to low back pain is pursued by Hallner and Hasenbring (2004). Instead of applying ANNs to input-output data that follow in their internal logic classical assumptions as in traditional medicine, Hallner and Hasenbring (2004) modeled the relationship between psychosocial factors and low back pain with remarkable success. The pain intensity after a 6-month hospitalization was classified on the basis of 3 psychosocial variables correctly in 83.1%, with a sensitivity of 73% and a specificity of 97%. In comparison, the results of the linear discriminant analytical approach leads to a sensitivity of 78% and a specificity of 81%.

Trunk Motion

Nussbaum et al. (1995) assembled a three-layer network in the attempt to reconstruct an EMG of four lumbar muscles from moment magnitudes applied over a shoulder harness in upright posture. The model predictions were more correlated with experimental data than predictions made by using two optimization based methods. Sensitivity analyses showed that the choice of specific network parameters was not critical except at extreme values to those parameters. Variation of hidden units revealed that at least a minimum of hidden neurons is required for reducing the error below a certain criterion level.

A simple classification tool in the form of two layered competitive ANN was developed by Nussbaum and Chaffin (1997) in order to classify lumbar EMG patterns during static-moment loading. The applied competition algorithm was originally introduced by Rumelhart and Zipser (1985) for binary data. The competitive ANN consisted of 7 input and 10 output neurons which followed "the winner takes all" algorithm. Different combinations of magnitudes and directions were applied to the subjects via masses attached to a shoulder harness. They were able to categorize the subjects based on how their muscle responses were classified. The ANN classifier found distinct clusters of two groups of response patterns, whereby the muscle activity of subjects categorized as majority-type responders were in better correspondence with optimization-based predicted forces.

An ANN for the simulation of lumbar muscle response to static-moment loads was created by Nussbaum et al. (1997). Based on an abstract representation of a motor control system in which muscle activity is driven primarily to maintain equilibrium, a 4-layered feed forward and fully interconnected MLP was employed. The input layer consisted of six neurons representing the magnitudes of external static moments about the lower lumbar spine. The first hidden layer contained a variable number of neurons and was used for the development of internal representations of the moment loads. The second hidden layer contained 10 units corresponding to the bilateral pairs of torso muscles that developed the main reactive moments of the torso. Assumptions regarding the moment generating capacity of muscles and competitive interactions between muscles were employed and enabled the prediction of realistic patterns of muscle activity upon comparison with experimental normalized EMG data sets. Nussbaum suggested that a motor recruitment plan can be mimicked with relatively simple systems, and competition between responsive muscles may be intrinsic to the learning process. Alternative patterns and differing magnitudes of co-contractile activity were achieved by varying competition parameters with and between units.

Langdell and Mason (1999) applied radial basis function (RBF) networks for the classification of spinal measurements on a variety of male workers. Input variables were several measures of the lumbar spine derived from X-ray photographs. The RBF network training algorithm was tested and found to classify spinal measurements to an accuracy of 80.1%.

Neural Control, Bone Strength, Arthritis, Rehabilitation, and the Like

Further research on neurological, orthopaedic, and related fields are listed in Table 7. Babiloni et al. (2000) tested ANNs to verify its capacity to select different classes of single trials based on the spatial information in electroencephalographic activity related to voluntary unilateral finger movements. In order to reduce head volume conductor effects and to model the response of the primary sensory-motor cortex, the movement related potentials were surface Laplace transformed. To find the appropriate architecture, three three-layered and three four-layered ANNs were evaluated. The output units

Table 7. Applications of ANNs in neuro muscular control/orthopaedics— miscellaneous (? = not specified in reference)

Authors	Objective	Input	Output	Type of ANN	Results/remarks
Babiloni et al. (2000)	EEG—finger movement	52 amplitude values of Laplace transform	Classification 0-0 bilateral single trials 1-1 contralateral single trials 0-1, 1-0 spatially incoherent single trials	2 MLPs (52/?/2) (52/?/?/2)	Best results, when 4 input signals were applied
Davoodi et al. (2001)	Arm forces in paraplegia during stand-up movement	Ankle, knee, hip positions	Arm forces	MLP (14-24/0-8/3)	Personal strategies in controlling arm
Perl (2004)	Rehabilitation process	Weekly records of attributes	Characteristic Rehabilitation process	DyCON	Individual rehabilitation processes
Shan et al. (2004)	Sensory-motor-degradation assessment	26 parameters: body weight, height, COP-parameters (length, maximum excursion, min-max velocity, etc.	Age Faller/nonfaller	MLP (26/60/2)	Tai Chi causes seniors to be 4.91 years younger in their sensory-motor age than in their chronological age
Wigderowitz et al. (2000)	Fracture risk Bone strength from cancellous structure (osteoporosis)	Digitized x-ray image characteristics	Load at fracture	MLP (3/1-10/1-10/1)	91% correct; image data superior to x-ray and bone density
Wyns et al. (2004)	Rheumatoid arthritis	14 histological features 10 var (0-3) 4 var 0,1	Classification a) Rheumatoid arthritis (RA) b) Spondyloarthopathy (SPA) c) other	SOM 15x15 Kohonen combined with case-based reasoning (CBR)	Accuracy: RA: 92.9% SPA: 75% Other: 66% Overall: 84% Global accuracy (including errors): 75.6%

coded the classes to be used for single trial classification: 0-0 for the class of the bilateral single trials, 1-1 for the class of the contralateral single trials, and 0-1 and 1-0 for the class of the spatially incoherent single trials. Babiloni et al. (2000) obtained percentages of correct classification from 64% to 84%. Applications of this research are seen in the rapid evaluation of impairment and recovery of cortical motor areas in patients with unilateral cerebral hemisphere damage.

Developing ANN models capable of cloning the personal strategies of paraplegics to control their arms during standing up was the aim of the study of Davoodi et al. (2001). The standing up of paraplegics was supported by activation of paralyzed leg muscles by means of a functional electric stimulation (FES) controller. ANN models were developed to predict voluntary arm forces from measured angular positions of the ankle, knee, and hip joint during FES-assisted standing up in paraplegia. The comparison of the individual models showed clear similarities among the voluntary controls adopted by different subjects although each subject developed his/her own individual strategy to control arm forces, which were consistent from trial to trial.

An approach suggested by Perl (2004) copes with some major disadvantages of Kohonen feature maps, like very high demands on the training data, and, once finished, training cannot be started or continued again. The DyCoN (i.e., dynamically controlled network) allows for individual adaptation of the neurons to the learning content and so enables continuous learning as well as learning in separate steps. A DyCoN first can be prepared using Monte-Carlo-generated data, then this reference network can be specifically labeled using original data. The net can be interpreted semantically, e.g., by marking areas of good or bad conditions during a rehabilitation process. In order to diagnose successful and unsuccessful rehabilitation on the basis of small data sets, DyCoN has been applied in practice.

Shan et al. (2004) present the application of a three-layered MLP for assessing sensory-motor degradation. On the basis of 26 input parameters of body weight, height and parameters obtained from the center of pressure (COP), which was measured during standing with open and closed eyes, the MLP was trained. Two output neurons served for predicting the sensory-motor age and fall probability. The ANN technology with COP data are considered as a feasible tool in the exploration of sensory-motor degradation for evaluating the risk in falling with increasing age. However, practicing activities like Tai Chi slowed down the effect of sensory-motor aging.

The rationale of the investigation of Wigderowitz et al. (2000) was the improvement of non-invasive determination of bone strength obtained from computerized image analysis of radiographs. A number of characteristics of the image, including periodicity and spatial orientation of the trabecular, were derived from unembalmed human distal radii and used as input. The structure of the specimen was tested on compression in a mechanical testing machine. The values of mechanical parameters predicted by the MLP displayed a very high correlation: 0.91 for the load at fracture and 0.93 for the ultimate stress. Both correlations were superior to the correlations obtained with dual-energy X-ray absorptiometry and with the cross-sectional area from CT scans. One advantage of this approach is seen in the property of nonlinearity of ANNs, which enables them to recognize alterations that are not straightforward. Osteoporotic bone may sometimes have thicker trabecular than normal bone, when generalized thinning of trabecular is expected.

Predicting diagnosis in patients with early arthritis by means of self-organizing ANN in combination with case-based reasoning was the subject of Wyns et al.'s (2004) investigation. Two of the most frequent forms of chronic autoimmune arthritis, rheumatoid arthritis (RA) and spondyloarthropathy (SpA) could be classified on the basis of 14 histological features. In combination with the Kohonen feature map and case-based reasoning, an overall accuracy of 75.6% was achieved, whereas statistical tree classification Quest and backpropagation resulted in 50.9% and 54.7% accuracy, respectively.

Prosthesis

Table 8 displays only a few selected publications in the area of applications of ANNs in prosthesis research.

Borrett et al. (2005) included ANNs in evolutionary autonomous agents (EAA) for controlling a robot in order to suggest an alternative approach for controlling movements. EAA are robots or robot simulations that have a controller, which is a dynamical neural network, and its evolution occurs autonomously under the guidance of a fitness-function without the detailed or explicit direction of an external programmer. EAAs provide a system by which development of cognitive structures evolve in an embodied agent constrained only by the nature of the environment and the definition of fitness. They assume no structural characteristics of perception or movement but provide a forum by which sensory-motor structures arise as the organism self-organizes in response to its interaction with the environment.

Feedback Error Learning (FEL) can be regarded as a feedforward neural network structure which, when training, "learns" the inverse dynamics of the controlled plant (Kalanovic et al., 2000). One network was used to support the control of the knee joint; the other network was trained to control the hip joint. The inverse dynamic model was identified within 1,000 repetitions of training.

Table 8. Applications of ANNs in the area of prosthesis research

Authors	Objective	Input	Output	Type of ANN	Results/remarks
Archambeau et al. (2004)	Visual implant prosthesis	Stimulation parameters	Phosphenes (location, area, color, shape, intensity)	Hybrid NN with MLP and RBFN	ANNs outperformed linear statistical models by 25%
Borrett et al. (2005)	Apraxia 2-wheeled robot	Eight infrared proximity sensors	Rotation encoder for each wheel	5 fully connected radial basis function units	Control robot Dynamic network controller embedded in evolutionary algorithms
Kalanovic et al. (2000)	Transfemoral prosthesis control	Desired position and its derivatives of thigh and shank	Total energy	Feedback error learning (FEL) NN with a proportional plus derivative feedback controller	FEL can be regarded as hybrid control because it combines nonparametric identification with parametric modeling and control

Once the networks were trained, they could even control different movements than the ones used for training. FEL was able to adapt to disturbances as well.

Within the framework of the project "Optimisation of the Visual Implantable Prosthesis", Archambeau et al. (2004) propose an optic nerve-based visual prosthesis in order to restore partial vision to the blind. They use artificial neural networks (ANNs) for predicting the features of the visual sensations. This is developed in order to restore partial vision to the blind. Archambeau et al. (2004) propose to use adaptive neural techniques on the basis of the comparison of two non-linear and one linear prediction model. They were able to show that the ANN models provide satisfactory prediction tools and achieve similar prediction accuracies. Moreover, a significant improvement (25%) was gained in comparison to linear statistical methods, suggesting that the biological process is strongly non-linear.

Psychology, Psychiatry, and Sociology

For a long time, applications in the field of psychology and health, psychiatry, and sociology were nearly neglected. A comprehensive review of applications to psychological assessment is provided by Price et al. (2000). A selection of publications is listed in (Table 9).

Berdia and Metz (1998) classify schizophrenic and normal subjects on the basis of a psychological test. They only succeeded when noise was added in the ANN. Zou et al. (1996) suggest and compare two ANNs for assistance in psychiatric diagnosis. Both ANNs were able to distinguish three psychiatric groups more effectively than traditional expert systems.

Different combinations of input variables were taken by Buscema et al. (1998) in order to find the optimal prediction of eating disorders by means of a feedforward network. Starting from only generic variables, ANN provided 86.9% of the prediction precision.

Maurelli and Di Gulio (1998) compared the results of nine classification systems for alcoholics on the basis of five biochemical data and revealed best results with a Metasystem followed by two ANNs.

In the field of sociology and medicine, only two examples about community-acquired pneumonia (Heckerling et al., 2004) and healthcare information (Lloyd-Williams and Williams, 1996) are listed in the lower part of Table 9. A genetic algorithm was used by Heckerling et al. (2004) for optimizing an MLP for the prediction of pneumonia on the basis of sociodemographic, symptom, sign, and

Table 9. Applications of ANN in psychology, psychiatry, and sociology

Authors	Objective	Input	Output	Type of ANN	Results/remarks
Berdia and Metz (1998)	Schizophrenics	Wisconsin card sorting test	Schizophrenic normal	ANN Noise and Gain was varied	Classification only with adding noise possible
Buscema et al. (1998)	Eating disorders	89-124 variables: for example, generic variables, alimentary behavior, eventual treatment, menstrual cycles, weight height, psychodiagnostic tests, etc.	Four classes: a) anorexia nervosa b) nervous bulimia c) binge eating disorders d) psychogenetic eating disorders that are not otherwise specified	MLP (75,86,89,93/2-4)	Dependent on type and number of variables Prediction correctness from 84-100%
Heckerling et al. (2004)	Community acquired pneumonia	Clinical variables	Pneumonia yes/no	MLP (35/0,15/0,15/0,15/ 1)	Genetic algorithms for evaluating optimal number of hidden units
Lloyd-Williams and Williams (1996)	Healthcare information	Health for all (HFA) database of the WHO, e.g., life expectancy at birth, probability of dying before 5 years, etc.	1) Two clusters 2) Six clusters	1) 2x2 KFM 2) 8x2 KFM	Core distinction is found by creation of a classification of European countries according to mortality rates
Maurelli and Di Gulio (1998)	Levels of alcoholism	5 variables of biochemical tests	Light alcoholic Heavy alcoholic	1) Genetic algorithms 2-8) 7 types of ANN 9) Metasystem	Metanet (9) showed best results followed by two ANNs
Zou et al. (1996)	Assist psychiatry diagnosis	Psychiatry diagnosis variables	a) Neurosis b) Schizophrenia c) Normal	1) MLP – BP 2) SOM	Compared to ICD10 1) kappa = 0.94 2) kappa = 0.88 ANN better than traditional expert systems

comorbidity data. The evolved ANNs discriminated pneumonia from other respiratory conditions accurately within a training cohort and within a testing cohort consisting of cases on which the networks had not been trained.

Information from the "health for all" database of the WHO (World Health Organization) was taken for clustering 39 European countries with two self-organizing Kohonen feature maps (KFM) (Lloyd-Williams & Williams, 1996). The resulting clusters exhibited significantly different characteristics with respect to life expectancy, probability of death before the age of five years, infant mortality, standardized death rate (SDR) for diseases of the circulatory system, and SDR for external causes of injury and poisoning. A clear distinction of countries from central and eastern Europe/former Soviet Republics, on the one hand, and countries from northern, western, or southern Europe, on the other, occurred. The 2x2 KFM provided a core distinction, whereas the 8x8 KFM provided more differentiated clusters.

Miscellaneous

Examples of ANN applications in a couple of other medical areas are shown in Table 10 through Table 12. These examples serve as a short overview of the versatile opportunities and diverse possibilities in which ANN can support and take over the medical decision process.

Arle et al. (1999) trained several MLPs for optimizing the prediction of postoperative seizures in epilepsy surgery. The exclusion of several input variables increased the number of correct predictions from 96% up to 98%.

The same approach and type of ANN was applied by Accardo and Pensiero (2002) for classifying three categories of corneal topography. Similar to Berdia and Metz (1998), the classification of glaucoma was enhanced when data were augmented with noise in the model of Henson et al. (1997).

Table 10. Applications of ANN in miscellaneous areas of healthcare (? = not specified in reference)

Authors	Objective	Input	Output	Type of ANN	Results /remarks
Accardo and Pensiero (2002)	Cornea— keratoconus detection from corneal topography	Parameters from corneal topographic maps	1) Normal 2) Keratoconus 3) Other alterations	MLP (9-19/4-55/3-6)	Global sensitivity 87.86%-94.17%
Arle et al. (1999)	Outcome in epilepsy surgery	25 clinical parameters	Number of postoperative seizures	MLP (3-25/7-30/0,7,15/1)	Dependent on type and amount of data 93-98%
Folland et al. (2004)	Tracheal-bronchial breath sounds by respiratory auscultation	15 coefficients of frequency spectra of Tracheal-bronchial breath sounds	14 sound classes Classification	1) Constructive probabilistic neural network (CPNN) 2) MLP (15/?/14) 3) RBFN	CPNN: 97.8% MLP: 77.8% RBFN: 96.2% Experts: 79.3%
Fontenla-Romero et al. (2004)	Sleep apnea	16 Wavelet transform coefficients of thoracic effort signal	Classification a) Obstructive b) Central c) mixed	3 supervised ANN: 1) SCG learning algorithm 2) MSE cost function 3) Bayesian NN	Average 93.8% Best ANN was with Bayesian framework and a cross entropy error function
Henson et al. (1997)	Visual field data in glaucoma	Ophtalmological data	Glaucoma	5x5 Kohonen SOFM	Data were augmented with noise
Huang and Huang (1998)	Sign language recognition	Shape variant hand motion Rotation invariant Fourier descriptor Graph matching Hausdorff distance	15 hand gestures	3D Hopfield Neural Net	91% recognition rate 10 seconds
Koprinska et al. (1996)	Sleep stages classification	15 Parameter, e.g., EEG, Heart Rate, HR Variability, actogram of hands	7 Classes, for example, movement, wakefulness, REM	1) Tree-Based NN (TBNN) 2) MLP	TBNN better than MLP

In the context of breathing, Folland et al. (2004) compared different types of ANNs by means of frequency spectra of bronchial breath sound with clear advantages of constructive probabilistic neural networks and radial basis function networks in comparison to MLPs and expert systems.

Fontenla-Romero et al. (2004) compared three types of supervised ANNs for classifying sleep apnea on the basis of wavelet coefficients of thoracic effort signals. Advantages of tree-based neural nets in comparison to MLPs were found by Koprinska et al. (1996) for the classification of seven sleep stages by means of physiological parameters. A 3D binary Hopfield model served Huang and Huang (1998) in the recognition of 15 hand gestures in sign language with a 91% recognition rate and a recognition time of 10 seconds.

A number of other networks have been developed to diagnose a broad spectrum of further diseases and clinical conditions. Gurgen and Gurgen (2003) developed a model for the diagnosis of diabetes mellitus on the basis of personal and physiological parameters. The assignment of patients to four classes of

Table 11. Applications of ANNs in the miscellaneous fields of healthcare

Authors	Objective	Input	Output	Type of ANN	Results/remarks
Gurgen and Gurgen (2003)	Diabetes mellitus DM With and without ischemic stroke	Personal and physiological parameters PCA reduced to 7	DM With/without	1) MLP 2) KNN	1) 66% correct 2) 68.2% correct
Hayashi et al. (2000)	Diagnosis of hepatobiliary disorders	Sex, 9 biochemical test parameters	4 classes: a) Alcoholic liver damage b) Primary hepatoma c) Liver cirrhosis d) cholelithiasis	MLP (11/5/4)	NN rule extraction High predictive accuracy (90%)
Pesonen (1997)	Acute appendicitis	17 personal and laboratory parameters	Acute appendicitis	1) Discriminant analysis 2) Logistic regression 3) Cluster analysis 4) MLP	1) and 4) showed slightly better results
Pesonen et al. (1998)	Acute abdominal pain	43 parameters from patients with acute abdominal pain	3 classes (number of Leucocytes): Low (<10) Moderate (10-20) High (>20)	1) MLP (43/6/3) 2) LVQ	Diagnostic accuracy: 0.87 Predictive value: 0.56 Missing data
Tafeit et al. (1999)	Body fat Diabetes mellitus	-"-	-"-	1) MLP (15/3/15) 2) Factor Analysis	
Tafeit et al. (2000)	Body fat Diabetes mellitus	15 measures for subcutaneous adipose tissue	Classification	1) MLP (15/2/15) 2) Factor Analysis	Data reduction Comparable results Classifying new subjects MLP superior
Tafeit et al. (2005)	Bodyfat	3 Light pattern values of LIPOMETER	Layer thickness	1) MLP (3/2/1) 2) Nonlinear regression	MLP better than nonlinear regression

Table 12. Applications of ANNs in the miscellaneous fields of healthcare (laboratory medicine and intensive healthcare)

Authors	Objective	Input	Output	Type of ANN	Results /remarks
Futschik et al. (2003)	Knowledge discovery from gene expression data of cancer tissue	100 selected genes from gene matrix data	a) Leukaemia, b) Colon cancer	Evolving Fuzzy Neural Networks (EFuNN)	Average classification accuracy: 90.3-97.2% Rule extraction
Linkens and Vefghi (1997)	Levels of anaesthetic state	6 input nodes (SAP, HR, RR, Age, Weight, Sex)	Classification a) aware b) relaxed c) deep	MLP (6/div./3)	Hidden nodes were analyzed by PCA and Canonical Discriminant Analysis
Lisboa et al. (1998)	NMR spectral classification and metabolite selection for tissue discrimination	28 metabolite variables Data reduction by a) PCA and b) partial least squares (PLS)	Spectral classes	1) LDA 2) Nearest neighbor classification 3) MLP	Data reduction by means of PCA provides worst results
Marble and Healy (1999)	Trauma complications assessment Morbidity outcomes in trauma care	Patient age, prehospital pulse rate, respiratory rate, systolic blood pressure, Glasgow Coma Score, Revised Trauma Score, emergency department temperature, etc.	Sepsis No sepsis	MLP (18/10/4/1)	100% sensitivity 96.5% specificity
Paetz (2003)	Septic shock patients	12 measured laboratory variables	Survived, deceased	Trapezoidal activation functions	Training correct: 74% Test correct: 69% Rule generation
Radivojac et al. (2004)	Protein database	6 protein data sets	10 functional subsets	1) Logist. Reg. 2) Decision tree 3) MLP	ANNs are best for large datasets Log reg. robust to noise and low sample density in a high-dimensional feature space

hepatobiliary disorder by means of biochemical test parameters was the goal of Hayashi et al. (2000). At the same time, the hidden nodes served to extract rules.

Starita and Sperduti (1999) present a system for the diagnosis of diabetic retinopathies with the main emphasis on two complementary aspects: (1) the use of committees of networks for improving the overall accuracy of the classifier and (2) the design of the human computer interface.

Pesonen et al. (1998) and Pesonen (1997) modeled the diagnosis of acute appendicitis and compared the performance of linear and non-linear approaches on the basis of different numbers of parameters as well as with missing data. Four different methods for replacing missing data were compared: substituting means, random values, nearest neighbor, and neural network. Great differences between the substitute values and other methods were found, and only nearest neighbor and neural network correlated on most of the cases. In the neural network method, all possible combinations of missing data value patterns were searched. For each pattern, a separate MLP was trained to estimate the values of the variables in the pattern. The learning vector quantization (LVQ) was used in detecting acute appendicitis diagnosis. The test set of complete data cases resulted in diagnostic accuracy 0.87 and predictive value 0.56. In comparison with previous studies of Pesonen (1997) that were conducted with complete data these results are considered as slightly worse.

Tafeit et al. (1999, 2000, 2005) developed linear and non-linear models for the diagnosis of layer thickness on the basis of light patterns of a lipometer. The light patterns of the lipometer device were fitted to absolute values provided by computed tomography. MLPs provided better fit of lipometer light patterns to absolute subcutaneous adipose tissue layer thickness than non-linear regression analysis.

In the field of laboratory medicine (Table 12), ANNs found several areas of application. Three approaches in genetics (Futschik et al., 2003), NMR spectral analysis (Lisboa et al., 1998), and protein data analysis (Radivojac et al., 2004) are listed exemplarily in Table 12. Lisboa et al. (1998) and Radivojac et al. (2004) compared several linear and non-linear models for classifying protein data sets (Radivojac et al., 2004) and discriminating tissue on the basis of NMR data (Lisboa et al., 1998). Most intriguingly, Lisboa et al. (1998) found the worst results when data were reduced by means of PCA. Radivojac et al. (2004) found best classification results for MLP in a large dataset, but best robustness against noise in low density samples in logistic regression.

Futschik et al. (2003) developed a knowledge discovery system from gene expression data of cancer by means of evolving fuzzy neural networks. Fuzzy logic rules could be extracted from the trained networks and offer knowledge about the classification process in an accessible form.

Graham and Errington (1999) presented a system for supporting time-consuming chromosome analysis. The results indicate that it is the selection of image derived features rather than the accuracy of the measurement taken of those features. Furthermore, it is not the choice of classifier that is critical for optimal performance in this application (Lisboa et al., 1999).

Linkens and Vefghi (1997) developed a model in order to recognize three levels of anaesthetic states of a patient on the basis of six physiological and personal parameters. Thereby, the number of hidden nodes was optimized by means of PCA and Canonical Discriminant Analysis.

Marble and Healy (1999) developed a model for trauma complication assessment by predicting sepsis on the basis of personal and clinical parameters.

The future prediction of septic shock patients is subject to the model of Paetz (2003). The process of generating rules, the basis of trapezoidal activations function, is demonstrated and explained extensively.

Conclusion

Artificial neural nets have played a key role in the past years for many important developments in medicine and healthcare. Despite this development, many future challenges are ahead of us. Promising potential developments are seen in hybrid systems that emerge combining various artificial intelligence tools with improved performance in medical diagnosis and rehabilitative prediction. However, the practical application presupposes much experience for handling artificial neural nets adequately with respect to the chosen type of net to data normalization or to net parameters in order to achieve results that support physicians in their decision process optimally.

References

Abbass, H. A. (2002). An evolutionary artificial neural networks approach for breast cancer diagnosis. *Artificial Intelligence in Medicine, 25*(3), 265-281.

Accardo, P. A., & Pensiero, S. (2002). Neural network-based system for early keratoconus detection from corneal topography. *Journal of Biomedical Informatics, 35*(3), 151-159.

Aizenberg, I., Aizenberg, N., Hiltnerb, J., Moraga, C., & Meyer zu Bexten, E. (2001). Cellular neural networks and computational intelligence in medical image processing. *Image and Vision Computing, 19*(4), 177-183.

Akay, M. (2000). *Nonlinear Biomedical signal processing.* Piscataway, NJ: IEEE Press.

Alonso-Betanzos, A., Mosqueira-Rey, E., Moret-Bonillo, V., & Baldonedo del Ry'o, B. (1999). Applying statistical, uncertainty-based and connectionist approaches to the prediction of fetal outcome: A comparative study. *Artificial Intelligence in Medicine, 17*, 37-57.

Archambeau, C., Delbekeb, J., Veraartb, C., & Verleysena, M. (2004). Prediction of visual perceptions with artificial neural networks in a visual prosthesis for the blind. *Artificial Intelligence in Medicine, 322*, 183-194.

Arle, J. E., Perrine, K., Devinsky, O., & Doyle, W.K. (1999). Neural network analysis of preoperative variables and outcome in epilepsy surgery. *Journal of Neurosurgery, 90*(6), 998-1004.

Azuaje, F., Dubitzky, W., Lopes, P., Black, N., Adamson, K., Wu, X., & White, J.A. (1999). Predicting coronary disease risk based on short-term RR interval measurements: A neural network approach. *Artificial Intelligence in Medicine, 15*, 275-297.

Babiloni, F., Carducci, F., Cerutti, S., Liberati, D., Rossini, P. M., Urbano, A., & Babiloni, C. (2000). Comparison between human and artificial neural network detection of Laplacian-derived electroencephalographic activity related to unilateral voluntary movements. *Computers and Biomedical Research, 33*(1), 59-74.

Baxt, W. G. (1991). Use of an artificial neural network for the diagnosis of myocardial infarction. *Annals of Internal Medicine, 115*, 843-848.

Baxt, W. G., & Skora, J. (1996). Prospective validation of artificial neural network trained to identify acute myocardial infarction. *Lancet, 347*(8993), 12-15.

Benitez, J. M., Castro, J. L., & Requena, I. (1997). Are artificial neural networks black boxes? *IEEE Transactions on Neural Networks, 8*(5), 1157-1164.

Berdia, S., & Metz, J. T. (1998). An artificial neural network stimulating performance of normal subjects and schizophrenics on the Wisconsin card sorting test. *Artificial Intelligence in Medicine, 13*, 123-138.

Bishop, J. B., Szalpski, M., Ananthraman, S., McIntyre, D. R., & Pope, M. H. (1997). Classification of low back pain from dynamic motion characteristics using an artificial neural network. *SPINE, 22*(24), 2991-2998.

Borrett, D. S., Jin, F., & Kwan, H. C. (2005). Evolutionary autonomous agents and the nature of apraxia. *Biomedical Engineering Online, 4*(1), 1. Retrieved from http://www.biomedical-engineering-online.com/content/4/1/1

Buller, D., Buller, A., Innocent, P. R., & Pawlak, W. (1996). Determining and classifying the region of interest in ultrasonic images of the breast using neural networks. *Artificial Intelligence in Medicine, 8*, 53-66.

Buscema, M., Maszetti di Pietralata, M., Salvemini, V., Intragaligi, M., & Indrimi, M. (1998). Application of artificial neural networks to eating disorders. *Substance Use & Missuse, 33*(3), 765-791.

Castro, A., & Miranda, V. (2002, June 24-28). Mapping neural networks into rule sets and making their hidden knowledge explicit application to spatioal load forecasting. *Proceedings of the 14th Power Systems Computation Conference (PSCC'02)*, Sevilla, Spain, Session 20, paper 3 (pp. 1-7).

Chen, D. R., Chang, R. F., & Huang, Y. L. (1999). Computer-aided diagnosis applied to US of solid breast nodules by using neural networks. *Radiology, 213*, 407-412.

Chua, L. O., & Yang, L. (1988). Cellular neural networks: Theory and applications. *IEEE Transactions on Circuit Systems, 35*, 1257-1290.

Cross, S. S., Downs, J., Drezet, P., Ma, Z., & Harrsion, R. F. (1999). Intelligent decision support systems in the cytodiagnosis of breast carcinoma. In P. J. Lisboa, E. C. Ifeachor, & P. S. Szczepaniak (Eds.), *Artificial neural network in biomedicine* (pp. 213-226). London: Springer.

Cunningham, P., Carney, J., & Jacob, S. (2000). Stability problems with artificial neural networks and the ensemble solution. *Artificial Intelligence in Medicine, 20*, 217-225.

Davoodi, R., Kamnik, R., Andrews, B., & Bajd, T. (2001). Predicting the voluntary arm forces in FES-assisted standing up using neural networks. *Biological Cybernetics, 85*(2), 133-43.

Delen, D., Walker, G., & Kadam, A. (2004). Predicting breast cancer survivability: A comparison of three data mining methods. *Artificial Intelligence in Medicine*. Retrieved September 23, 2005, from http://www.intl.elsevierhealth.com/journals/aiim

Dellepiane, S. G. (1999). The importance of features and primitives for multi-dimensional/multi-channel image processing. In P. J. Lisboa, E. C. Ifeachor, & P. S. Szczepaniak (Eds.), *Artificial neural network in biomedicine* (pp. 267-282). London: Springer.

Dickey, J. P., Pierrynowski, M. R., Bednar, D. A., & Yang, S. X. (2002). Relationship between pain and vertebral motion in chronic low-back pain subjects. *Clinical Biomechanics, 17*, 345-352.

Dimitriadou, E., Barth, M., Windischberger, C., Hornika, K., & Moser, E. (2004). A quantitative comparison of functional cluster analysis. *Artificial Intelligence in Medicine, 31*, 57-71.

Dorffner, G., & Porenta, G. (1994). On using feedforward neural networks for clinical diagnostic tasks. *Artificial Intelligence in Medicine, 6*, 417-435.

Downs, J., Harrison, R. F., Kennedy, R. L., & Cross, S. S. (1996). Application of the fuzzy ARTMAP neural network model to medical pattern classification tasks. *Artificial Intelligence in Medicine, 8*, 403-428.

Duch, W., Adamczak, R., & Grabczewski, K. (2001). A new methodology of extraction, optimization and application of crisp and fuzzy logical rules. *IEEE Transactions on Neural Networks, 12*, 277-306.

Egmont-Petersen, M., de Ridder, D., & Handels, H. (2001). Image processing with neural networks: A review. *Pattern Recognition, 35*, 2279-2301.

Fogel, D. B., Wasson, E. C., Boughton, E. M., & Porto, V. W. (1998). Evolving artificial neural networks for screening features from mammograms. *Artificial Intelligence in Medicine, 14*, 317-326.

Folland, R., Hines, E., Dutta, R., Boillot, P., & Morgan, D. (2004). Comparison of neural network predictors in the classification of tracheal-bronchial breath sounds by respiratory auscultation. *Artificial Intelligence in Medicine, 31*, 211-220.

Fontenla-Romero, O., Guijarro-Berdinas, B., Alonso-Betanzos, A., & Moret-Bonillo, V. (2004). A new method for sleep apnea classification using wavelets and feedforward neural networks. *Artificial Intelligence in Medicine.* Retrieved September 25, 2005, from http://www.intl.elsevierhealth.com/journals/aim

Fritzke, B. (1997). *Some competitive learning methods.* Retrieved September 23, 2005, from http://www.neuroinformatik.ruhr-uni-bochum.de/ini/VDM/research/gsn/JavaPaper/t.html

Futschik, M. E., Reeve, A., & Kasabov, N. (2003). Evolving connectionist systems for knowledge discovery from gene expression data of cancer tissue. *Artificial Intelligence in Medicine, 28*, 165-189.

Gelenbe, E., Feng, Y., & Krishnan, K. R. (1996). Neural network methods for volumetric magnetic resonance imaging of the human brain. *Proceedings of the IEEE, 84*(10), 1488-1496.

Gioftsos, G., & Grieve, D. W. (1996). The use of artificial neural networks to identify patients with chronic low-back pain conditions from patterns of sit-to-stand manoeuvres. *Clinical Biomechanics, 11*(5), 275-280.

Gomez-Ruiz, J. A., Jerez-Aragones, J. M., Munoz-Perez, J., & Alba-Canejo, E. (2004). A neural network based model for prognosis of early breast cancer. *Applied Intelligence, 20*, 231-238.

Graham, J., & Errington, P. A. (1999). Classification of chromosomes: A comparative study of neural network and statistical approaches. In P. J. Lisboa, E. C. Ifeachor, & P. S. Szczepaniak (Eds.), *Artificial neural network in biomedicine* (pp. 249-265). London: Springer.

Gurgen, F. (1999). Neural-network-based decision making in diagnostic applications. *IEEE Engineering in Medicine and Biology, 18*(4), 89-93.

Gurgen, F., Guler, N., & Varol, F. (2001). Antenatal fetal risk assessment using neurofuzzy technique. *IEEE Engineering in Medicine and Biology, 20*(6), 165-169.

Gurgen, F., & Gurgen, N. (2003). Intelligent data analysis to interpret major risk factors for diabetic patients with and without ischemic stroke in a small population. *Biomedical Engineering Online, 2*(1), 5. Retrieved from http://www.biomedical-engineering-online.com/content/2/1/5

Gurgen, F., Onal, E., & Varol, F. G. (1997). IUGR detection by ultrasonographic examinations using neural networks. *IEEE Engineering in Medicine and Biology, 16*(3), 55-58.

Gürgen, F. S., Sihmanoglu, M., & Varol, F. G. (1995). The assessment of LH surge for predicting ovulation time using clinical, hormonal, and ultrasonic indices in infertile women with an ensemble of neural networks. *Computers in Biology and Medicine, 25*(4), 405-413.

Hall, L. O., Bensaid, A. M., Clarke, L. P., Velthuizen, R. P., Silbiger, M. S., & Bezdek, J. C. (1992). A comparison of neural network and fuzzy clustering techniques in segmenting magnetic resonance images of the brain. *IEEE Transactions on Neural Networks, 3*(2), 672-682.

Hallner, D., & Hasenbring, M. (2004). Classification of psychosocial risk factors (yellow flags) for the development of chronic low back and leg pain using artificial neural network. *Neuroscience Letters, 361*(1-3), 151-154.

Hammer, B., Rechtien, A., Strickert, M., & Villmann, T. (2002). Rule extraction from self-organizing maps. In J. R. Dorronsoro (Ed.), *Artificial Neural Networks; ICANN 2002.* Berlin: Springer.

Hammer, B., Rechtien, A., Strickert, M., & Villmann, T. (2003). *Vector quantization with rule extraction for mixed domain data* (Internal Report). Osnabrück, Germany: University of Osnabrück.

Hansen, L., & Salamon, P. (1990). Neural network ensembles. *IEEE Transactions on Pattern Analysis and Machine Intelligence, 12*(10), 993-1001.

Hayashi, Y., Seiono, R., & Yoshida, K. (2000). A comparison between two neural network rule extraction techniques for the diagnosis of hepatobiliary disorders. *Artificial Intelligence in Medicine, 20*, 205-216.

Heckerling, P. S., Gerber, B. S., Tapec, T. G., & Wigton, R. S. (2004). Use of genetic algorithms for neural networks to predict community-acquired pneumonia. *Artificial Intelligence in Medicine, 30*, 71-84.

Henson, D. B., Spenceley, S. E., & Bull, D. R. (1997). Artificial neural network analysis of noisy visual field data in glaucoma. *Artificial Intelligence in Medicine, 10*, 99-113.

Huang, C. L., & Huang, W. Y. (1998). Sign language recognition using model-based tracking and a 3D Hopfield neural network. *Machine Vision and Applications, 10*, 292-307.

Islam, M., Yao, X., & Murase, K. (2003). A constructive algorithm for training cooperative neural network ensembles. *IEEE Transactions on Neural Networks, 14*(4), 820-834.

Jang, J. S. R., & Sun, C. T. (1993). Functional equivalence between radial basis function networks and fuzzy inference systems. *IEEE Transactions on Neural Networks, 4*(1), 156-159.

Jerez-Aragones, J. M., Gomez-Ruiz, J. A., Ramos-Jimenez, G., Munoz-Perez, J., & Alba-Canejo, E. (2003). A combined neural network and decision trees model for prognosis of breast cancer relapse. *Artificial Intelligence in Medicine, 27*(1), 45-63.

Kalanovic, V. D., Popovic, D., & Skaug, N. T. (2000). Feedback error learning neural network for trans-femoral prosthesis. *IEEE Transactions on Rehabilitation Engineering, 8*(1), 71-80.

Kennedy, R. L., Harrison, R. F., Burton, A. M., Fraser, H. S., Hamer, W. G., MacArthur, D., McAllum, R., & Steedman, D. J. (1997). An artificial neural network system for diagnosis of acute myocardial infarction (AMI) in the accident and emergency department: Evaluation and comparison with serum myoglobin measurements. *Computational Methods and Programs in Biomedicine, 52*(2), 93-103.

Kohonen, T. (1982). Self-organized formation of topological correct feature maps. *Biological Cybernetics, 43*, 59-69.

Kohonen, T. (2001). *Self-organizing maps* (3rd ed.). Berlin: Springer.

Koprinska, I., Pfurtscheller, G., & Flotzinger, D. (1996). Sleep classification in infants by decision tree-based neural networks. *Artificial Intelligence in Medicine, 8*, 387-401.

Koss, L.G. (1999). The application of PAPNET to diagnostic cytology. In P. J. Lisboa, E. C. Ifeachor, & P. S. Szczepaniak (Eds.), *Artificial neural network in biomedicine* (pp. 51-67). London: Springer.

Kovalerchuk, B., Triantaphyllou, E., Ruiz, J. F., Torvik, V. I., & Vityaev, E. (2000). The reliability issue of computer-aided breast cancer diagnosis. *Computers in Biomedical Research, 33*(4), 296-313.

Krogh, A., & Vedelsby, J. (1995). Neural network ensembles, cross validation, and active learning. In G. Tesauro, D. S. Touretzky, & T. K. Leen (Eds.), *Advances in Neural Information Processing Systems 7* (pp. 231-238). Cambridge, MA: MIT Press.

Kukar, M., Kononenko, I., Groselj, C., Kralj, K., & Fettich, J. (1999). Analysing and improving the diagnosis of ischaemic heart disease with machine learning. *Artificial Intelligence in Medicine, 16*, 25-50.

Lai, S. H., & Fang, M. (2000). A hierarchical neural network algorithm for robust and automatic windowing of MRimages. *Artificial Intelligence in Medicine, 19*, 97-119.

Langdell, S. J., & Mason, J. C. (1999). Classifying spinal measurements using a radial basis function network. In P. J. Lisboa, E. C. Ifeachor, & P. S. Szczepaniak (Eds.), *Artificial neural network in biomedicine* (pp. 93-104). London: Springer.

Linkens, D. A., & Vefghi, L. (1997). Recognition of patient anaesthetic levels: Neural network systems, principal components analysis and canonical discriminant variates. *Artificial Intelligence in Medicine, 11*, 155-173.

Lisboa, P. J. G., Ifeachor, E. C., & Szczepaniak, P. S. (1999). *Artificial neural networks in biomedicine*. London: Springer.

Lisboa, P. J., Kirby, S. P., Vellido, A., Lee, Y. Y., & El-Dedery, W. (1998). Assessment of statistical and neural networks methods in NMR spectral classification and metabolite selection. *NMR Biomedicine, 11*(4-5), 225-34.

Lisboa, P. J., Wong, H., Harris, P., & Swindell, R. (2003). A Bayesian neural network approach for modelling censored data with an application to prognosis after surgery for breast cancer. *Artificial Intelligence in Medicine, 28*, 1-25.

Lloyd-Williams, M., & Williams, T. S. (1996). A neural network approach to analyzing health care information. *Top Health Information Management, 17*(2), 26-33.

Mann, N. H., & Brown, M. D. (1991). Artificial intelligence in the diagnosis of low back pain. *The Orthopedic Clinics of North America, 22*(2), 302-314.

Marble, R. P., & Healy, J. C. (1999). A neural network approach to the diagnosis of morbidity outcomes in trauma care. *Artificial Intelligence in Medicine, 15*, 299-307.

Markey, M. K., Lo, J. Y., Tourassi, G. D., & Floyd,C.E., Jr. (2003). Self-organizing map for cluster analysis of a breast cancer database. *Artificial Intelligence in Medicine, 27*, 113-127.

Markowska-Kaczmar, U., & Trelak, W. (2003, April 23-25). Extraction of fuzzy rules from trained neural network using evolutionary algorithm. *ESANN 2003 Proceedings*, Bruges, Belgium (pp. 149-154).

Martinetz, T. M., Berkovich, S., & Schulten, K. (1993). Neural gas network for vector quantization and its application to time series prediction. *IEEE Transactions on Neural Networks, 4*(4), 558-569.

Maurelli, G., & Di Gulio, M. (1998). Artificial neural networks for the identification of the differences between "light" and "heavy" alcoholics, starting from five nonlinear biological variables. *Substance Use & Missuse, 33*(3), 693-708.

Miller, A. S., Blott, B. H., & Hames, T. K. (1992). Review of neural network applications in medical imaging and signal processing. *Medical & Biolocigal Engineering & Computing, 30*, 449-464.

Mobley, B. A., Schechter, E., Moore, W. E., McKee, P. A., & Eichner, J. E. (2000). Predictions of coronary artery stenosis by artificial neural network. *Artificial Intelligence in Medicine, 18*, 187-203.

Mobley, B. A., Schechter, E., Moore, W. E., McKeed, P. A., & Eichnere, J. E. (2004). Neural network predictions of significant coronary artery stenosis in men. *Artificial Intelligence in Medicine.* Retrieved September 23, 2005, from http://www.intl.elsevierhealth.com/journals/aiim

Nattkemper, T. W. (2004). Multivariate image analysis. *Journal of Biomedical Informatics, 37*(5), 380-391.

Nattkemper, T. W., Ritter, H., & Schubert, W. (2001). A neural classifier enabling high-throughput topological analysis of lymphocytes in tissue sections. *IEEE Transactions Informatics Technology Biomedicine, 5*(2), 138-149.

Nattkemper, T. W., Twellmann, T., Ritter, H., & Schubert, W. (2003). Human vs. machine: Evaluation of fluorescence micrographs. *Computers in Biology and Medicine, 33*(1), 31-43.

Nussbaum, M. A., & Chaffin, D. B. (1997). Pattern classification reveals intersubject group differences in lumbar muscle recruitment during static loading. *Clinical Biomechanics, 12*(2), 97-106.

Nussbaum, M. A., Chaffin, D. B., & Martin, B. J. (1995). A back propagation neural network model of lumbar muscle recruitment during moderate static exertions. *Journal of Biomechanics, 28*(9), 1015-1024.

Nussbaum, M. A., Martin, B. J., & Chaffin, D. B. (1997). A neural network model for simulation of torso muscle coordination. *Journal of Biomechanics, 30*(3), 251-258.

Ogawa, S., Menon, R. S., Tank, D. W., Kim, S. G., Merkle, H., Ellermann, J. M., & Ugurbil, K. (1993). Functional brain mapping by blood oxygenation level-depenent contrast magnetic resonance imaging. A comparison of signal characteristics with a biophysical model. *Biophysics, 64*(3), 803-812.

Ogawa, S., Tank, D. W., Menon, R. S., Ellermann, J. M., Kim, S. G., Merkle, H., & Ugurbil, K. (1992). Intrinsic signal changes accompanying sensory stimulation: Functional brain mapping with magnetic resonance imaging. *Proceedings of the National Academy of Sciences USA, 89*(13), 5951-5955.

Oliver, C. W., & Atsma, W. J. (1996). Artificial intelligence of paraspinal power spectra. *Clinical Biomechanics, 11*(7), 422-424.

Ossen, A., Zamzow, T., Oswald, H., & Fleck, E. (1994). Segmentation of medical images using neural network classifiers. In E.C. Ifeachor & K. Rosen (Eds.), *Proceedings of the International Conference on Neural Networks and Expert Systems in Medicine and Healthcare,* Plymouth, UK (pp. 427-432).

Paetz, J. (2003). Knowledge-based approach to septic shock patient data using a neural network with trapezoidal activation functions. *Artificial Intelligence in Medicine, 28*, 207-230.

Papadopulos, A., Foriadis, D. I., & Likas, A. (2002). An automatic microcalcification detection system based on a hybrid neural network classifier. *Artificial Intelligence in Medicine, 25*(2), 149-167.

Papadopulos, A., Foriadis, D. I., & Likas, A. (2004). Characterization of clustered microcalcifications in digitized mammograms using neural networks and support vector machines. *Artificial Intelligence in Medicine.* Retrieved September 23, 2005, from http://www.intl.elsevierhealth.com/journals/aiim

Parkin, D. M., Bray, F., Ferlay, J., & Pisani, P. (2001). Estimating the world cancer burden: Globocan 2000. *International Journal for Cancer, 94*(2), 153-156.

Perl, J. (2004). Artificial neural networks in motor control research. *Clinical Biomechanics, 19*, 873-875.

Pesonen, E. (1997). Is neural network better than statistical methods in diagnosis of acute appendicitis. In C. Pappas, N. Maglaveras, & J. P. Scherrer (Eds.), *Medical informatics Eruope '97* (pp. 377-381). Amsterdam: IOS Press.

Pesonen, E., Eskelinen, M., & Juhola, M. (1998). Treatment of missing data values in a neural network based decision support system for acute abdominal pain. *Artificial Intelligence in Medicine, 13*, 139-146.

Pisani, P., Parkin, D. M., & Ferlay, J. (1999). Estimates of the worldwide incidence of 25 major cancers in 1990. *International Journal for Cancer, 80*(6), 827-841.

Pizzi, N., Choo, L. P., Mansfield, J., Jackson, M., Halliday, W. C., Mantsch, H. H., & Somorjai, R. L. (1995). Neural network classification of infrared spectra of control and Alzheimer's diseased tissue. *Artificial Intelligence in Medicine, 7*, 67-79.

Price, R. K., Spitznagel, E. L., Downey, T. J., Meyer, D. J., Risk, N. K., & el-Ghazzawy, O. G. (2000). Applying artificial neural network models to clinical decision making. *Psychological Assessment, 12*(1), 40-51.

Radivojac, P., Chawla, N. V., Dunker, A. K., & Obradovic, Z. (2004). Classification and knowledge discovery in protein databases. *Journal of Biomedical Informatics, 37*(4), 224-239.

Reddick, W. E., Glass, J. O., Cook, E. N., Elkin, T. D., & Deaton, R. J. (1997). Automated segmentation and classification of multispectral magnetic resonance images of brain using artificial neural networks. *IEEE Transactions on Medical Imaging, 16*(6), 911-918.

Ronco, A. L. (1999). Use of artificial neural networks in modeling associations of discriminant factors: Towards an intelligent selective breast cancer screening. *Artificial Intelligence in Medicine, 16*, 299-309.

Rumelhart, D. E., & Zipser, D. (1985). Feature discovery by competitive learning. *Cognitive Science, 9*, 75-112.

Sanders, N. W., & Mann, N. H. (2000). Automated scoring of patient pain drawings using artificial neural networks: Efforts toward a low back pain triage application. *Computers in Biology and Medicine, 30*, 287-298.

Setiono, R. (1996). Extracting rules from pruned neural networks for breast cancer diagnosis. *Artificial Intelligence in Medicine, 8*, 37-51.

Setiono, R. (2000). Generating concise and accurate classification rules for breast cancer diagnosis. *Artificial Intelligence in Medicine, 18*, 205-219.

Shan, G., Daniels, D., & Gu, R. (2004). Artificial neural networks and center-of-pressure modeling: A practical method for sensorimotor-degradation assessment. *Journal of Aging and Physical Activity, 11*, 75-89.

Shortliffe, E. H., & Buchanan, B. G. (1975). A model of inexact reasoning in medicine. *Mathematical Bioscience, 23*, 351-379.

Starita, A., & Sperduti, A. (1999). A neural-based system for the automatic classification and follow-up of diabetic retinopathies. In P. J. Lisboa, E. C. Ifeachor, & P. S. Szczepaniak (Eds.), *Artificial neural network in biomedicine* (pp. 233-246). London: Springer.

Tafeit, E., Moller, R., Sudi, K., & Reibnegger, G. (1999). The determination of three subcutaneuos adipose tissue compartments in non insulin-dependent diabetes mellitus women with artificial neural networks and factor analysis. *Artificial Intelligence in Medicine, 17*(2), 181-193.

Tafeit, E., Moller, R., Sudi, K., & Reibnegger, G. (2000). Artificial neural networks compared to factor analysis for low dimensional classification of high-dimensional body fat topography data of healthy and diabetic subjects. *Computational Biomedical Research, 33*(5), 365-374.

Tafeit, E., Moller, R., Sudi, K., & Reibnegger, G. (2005). Artificial neural networks as a method to improve the precision of subcutaneus adipose tissue thickness measurements by means of the optical device LIPOMETER. *Computational Biomedical Research, 30*(6), 355-365.

Tickle, A. B., Andrews, R., Golea, M., & Diederich, J. (1998). The truth will come to light: Directions and challenges in extracting the knowledge embedded within trained artificial neural networks. *IEEE Transactions on Neural Networks, 9*(6), 1057-1068.

Tjoa, M. P., & Krishnan, S. M. (2003). Feature extraction for the analysis of colon status from the endoscopic images. *Biomedical Engineering Online, 2*(9).

Ulbricht, C., Dorffner, G., & Lee, A. (1998). Neural networks for recognizing patterns in cardiotocograms. *Artificial Intelligence in Medicine, 12*, 271-284.

Vilarino, D. L., Brea, V. M., Cabello, D., & Pardo, J. M. (1998). Discrete-time CNN for image segmentation by active contours. *Pattern Recognition Letters, 19*, 721-734.

Wigderowitz, C. A., Paterson, C. R., Dashti, H., McGurty, D., & Rowley, D. I. (2000). Prediction of bone strength from cancellous structure of the distal radius: Can we improve on DXA? *Osteoporosis International, 11*(10), 840-846.

Wismuller, A., Meyer-Base, A., Lange, O., Auer, D., Reiser, M. F., & Sumners, D. (2004). Model-free functional MRI analysis based on unsupervised clustering. *Journal of Biomedical Informatics, 37*(1), 10-18.

Wyns, B., Sette, S., Boullart, L., Baeten, D., Hoffman, I. E. A., & De Keyser, F. (2004). Prediction of diagnosis in patients with early arthritis using a combined Kohonen mapping and instance-based evaluation criterion. *Artificial Intelligence in Medicine, 31*, 45-55.

Zhou, Z. H., Jiang, Y., Yang, Y. B., & Chen, S. F. (2002). Lung cancer cell identification based on artificial neural network ensembles. *Artificial Intelligence in Medicine, 24*(1), 25-36.

Zou, Y., Shen, Y., Shu, L., Wang, Y., Feng, F., Xu, K., Ou, Y., Song, Y., Zhong, Y., Wang, M., & Liu, W. (1996). Artificial neural network to assist psychiatric diagnosis. *British Journal of Psychiatry, 169*(1), 64-67.

Section II

Electrocardiography

Chapter III

The Role of Neural Networks in Computerized Classification of the Electrocardiogram

Chris D. Nugent, University of Ulster at Jordanstown, Northern Ireland

Dewar D. Finlay, University of Ulster at Jordanstown, Northern Ireland

Mark P. Donnelly, University of Ulster at Jordanstown, Northern Ireland

Norman D. Black, University of Ulster at Jordanstown, Northern Ireland

Abstract

Electrical forces generated by the heart are transmitted to the skin through the body's tissues. These forces can be recorded on the body's surface and are represented as an electrocardiogram (ECG). The ECG can be used to detect many cardiac abnormalities. Traditionally, ECG classification algorithms have used rule based techniques in an effort to model the thought and reasoning process of the human expert. However, the definition of an ultimate rule set for cardiac diagnosis has remained somewhat elusive, and much research effort has been directed at data driven techniques. Neural networks have emerged as a strong contender as the highly non-linear and chaotic nature of the ECG represents a well-suited application for this technique. This study presents an overview of the application of neural networks in the field of ECG classification, and, in addition, some preliminary results of adaptations of conventional neural classifiers are presented. From this work, it is possible to highlight issues that will affect the acceptance of this technique and, in addition, identify challenges faced for the future. The challenges can be found in the intelligent processing of larger amounts of ECG information which may be generated from recording techniques such as body surface potential mapping.

Introduction

Recent figures published by the World Health Organization state that an estimated 17 million people die from cardiovascular disease (CVD) each year (World Health Organization, 2004). This illustrates that CVD is a major cause for concern and warrants further consideration as to how these figures can be reduced in the future. It has been suggested (Andresen et al., 2002) that many deaths could be prevented if new techniques could be established for the early diagnosis of potentially fatal heart conditions.

The heart, though the strongest muscle in the body, is vulnerable to failure and attack from a variety of factors, many of which can now be prevented and treated. There are several types of CVD, namely stroke, coronary, hypertensive, inflammatory, and rheumatic, with the majority of fatalities attributed to stroke (6 million/annum) and coronary heart disease (7 million/annum) (World Health Organization, 2004). Risk factors attributing to CVD include high blood pressure, tobacco use, high cholesterol, alcohol, and obesity to name but a few. It should be noted that more than 60% of the global burden of CVD occurs in the developing countries where medication, early diagnosis, and basic living standards are not provided (World Health Organization, 2004). The figures presented illustrate the urgent need for new methods for the prevention, detection, and treatment of CVD around the world.

Prevention of CVD is directly related to preventing the triggers that cause the disease, such as excess amounts of stress, depression, and cholesterol. Therefore, prevention is the onus of individuals and, as such, very little can be performed by staff in the clinical domain.

On the other hand, much focus has been devoted toward the detection of CVD over the past decades using the electrocardiogram (ECG) with the aim of providing individuals with clinical support. The relationships between the mechanical and electrical operations of the heart permit a diagnosis of the condition of the heart muscle to be made based on the electrical signals measured. A normal ECG pattern is made up of several waves and peaks that occur rhythmically during each cardiac cycle (Hole, 1998). When a patient is admitted to a hospital with chest pain, an ECG is taken and the readings are then examined by a cardiologist who looks for irregular waves and peaks in the recording. Based on the cardiologist's experience and expert knowledge, a diagnosis can be made.

Today, effective and relatively inexpensive medication is available for treatment of almost all types of CVD. Advances in surgical methods have led to safer operation procedures such as bypass surgery, and devices such as pacemakers and prosthetic valves, have been developed to simulate or replace damaged areas of the heart. Clinical developments in other areas, too, have led to a wide array of interventions that can often make surgery unnecessary (World Health Organization, 2004).

This chapter will look to examine, more extensively, the methods used to support detection of CVD and more explicitly for the recording of and classification of the different types of CVD. Specifically, this will involve a discussion of the standard 12-lead ECG and a description of an alternative approach to measuring heart activity known as body surface potential mapping (BSPM). Computerized classification of CVD will be addressed, and, in particular, an artificial intelligence (AI) approach, known as artificial neural networks (ANNs/NNs) will be explained to highlight potential and challenges in this area. In particular, details of successful studies of NNs will be given along with an insight into emerging adaptations of this technique in the area of 12-lead ECG classification. The computational lessons learned from the application of NNs to 12-lead ECG classification will then be considered with the aim of transferring this knowledge into BSPM classification where more clinical information is potentially available, and, hence, improved automated clinical support should be possible.

Electrocardiogram
Recording Techniques

From a physiological perspective, the heart can be viewed as a hollow cone-shaped muscular pump which is divided into four chambers (Hole, 1998). The upper chambers are called the atria, and the lower chambers are called the ventricles. The heart is only about the size of a human fist; however, it is the strongest muscle in the human body. The reason for this may be that a heart will beat somewhere in the region of two and a half billion times in a 70-year lifetime.

The function of the heart can be described as two parallel operations: the left side of the heart, made up of the left atrium and left ventricle, receives oxygenated blood from the lungs and pumps it around the body. Concurrently, the right side of the heart receives deoxygenated blood from the body and pumps it through the lungs. The chambers operate in a coordinated fashion, whereby the atrial walls contract while the ventricular walls relax and vice versa (Hubbard & Mechan, 1997). Such a cycle of events constitutes a complete heartbeat or cardiac cycle. In the heart, contractions of the muscle mass are initiated by a self-stimulating impulse located in the right atrium. It is this electrical charge spreading throughout the heart, known as *depolarization*, that causes the muscles to contract and the heart to beat (Guyton & Hall, 2000).

Generally, non-invasive acquisition of information about the heart's condition is achieved by placing electrodes, connected to some sort of recording apparatus, on the subject's skin. These electrodes sense the heart's electrical activity as it is projected, from the heart onto the body's surface. The recorded activity at each electrode site can be represented as a scalar trace plotted with respect to time; this is illustrated in Figure 1 where a single heart beat is depicted. Analysis of the recorded electrical signals can provide substantial information about the presence or absence of any disease or abnormality. Various differing recording techniques have been developed based on this principle, the main difference usually being in the configuration of the electrodes used (number and position) and the duration of the recording. The rationale for the selection of a specific recording technique is based upon the cardiac dysfunction that is suspected; in some cases, a subject may be monitored for a few seconds using several electrodes; in other cases, a subject may be monitored for several hours or even days, using fewer electrodes.

Although representation of an ECG recording as a scalar trace has been briefly mentioned and illustrated in Figure 1, several other techniques for cardiac

Figure 1. Scalar waveform representing the electrical activity recorded on the body's surface over the duration of one heart beat. The various components of the waveform are labelled P, Q, R, S, and T.

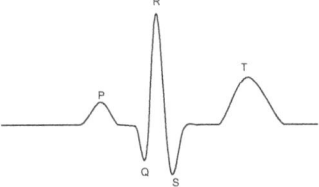

electrical representation, usually closely linked to the recording technique, exist. In the following sections, several recording techniques and the associated representation techniques shall be discussed.

Ambulatory ECG Recordings

In this approach, a small number of electrodes are placed on the patient's chest, usually providing two to three channels of ECG data (Kowey & Kocovic, 2003). A compact device, worn by the patient around the waist or neck, stores the recorded data, which are typically sampled over a period of 24-48 hours. As the name suggests, this type of recording attempts to capture information on the heart's condition while the patient is moving (ambulatory) or is carrying out every day tasks. In some cases, patients are asked to keep a brief log of their activity for the duration of the recording; this can later be correlated with the acquired ECG data, providing further diagnostic information about the heart's operation under certain conditions. In the analysis of ambulatory ECG data, a clinical expert will primarily look at the variations in heart rate over time and in addition try to identify any aberrant waveforms which may have occurred during the recording period.

Resting ECG

Although ambulatory ECGs provide useful diagnostic information for certain diseases, in some cases, it is of more use to record the heart's activity for a shorter time at more sites on the torso. In the "resting ECG" approach, an increased number of electrodes (five plus) are used to gain a more detailed insight into the heart's operation over a shorter period (less than one minute). The resting ECG can provide detailed information about abnormalities such as enlargement of the heart muscle, electrical conduction defects, insufficient blood flow, and death of the heart muscle due to a clot (myocardial infarction).

12-Lead ECG

The 12-lead ECG remains one of the most widely used tools to non-invasively assess cardiac disease state and function (Lux, 2000). In this approach, nine surface electrodes are used to acquire 12 channels of electrocardiographic information, usually for just long enough to record a few heart cycles or beats (10-15 seconds), as shown in Figure 2. The recorded information is represented as 12 scalar traces depicting the heart's electrical activity at the various sample

Figure 2. Typical example of 12-lead ECG recording attained through nine surface electrodes. Information is displayed as a series of 12 scalar traces for which morphology can be interpreted to determine presence of cardiac abnormality.

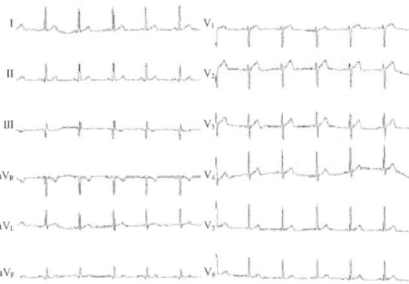

sites. Interpretation of the 12-lead ECG is based upon examination of the shape and size, or amplitude and duration, of the various components of each scalar trace. The increased number of sample sites, six of which are on the chest close to the heart, allows an expert to not only determine the presence of disease, but also the chambers or areas of the heart that are affected.

It is well established (Guyton & Hall, 2000; Lux, 1993, 2000, 2002a, 2002b), however, that the 12-lead ECG does not provide a complete picture of the heart. As many as 50% of patients do not receive the benefits of early treatment for acute myocardial infarction (AMI) due to the inability to detect abnormalities in the ECG at the time of presentation (Maynard et al., 2003; Menown et al., 2000).

Body Surface Potential Mapping (BSPM)

Unlike the 12-lead ECG, where information is recorded from nine sites, BSPM aims to capture the electrical activity of the heart as reflected on the entire surface of the torso (Taccardi et al., 1998). To achieve this, as many as 200 electrodes can be used, providing significantly enhanced spatial resolution over that of the traditional 12-lead ECG approach. This increased spatial resolution provides more diagnostic information, particularly with respect to the exact location of disease within the heart.

Figure 3. Schematic representation of the 192-electrode array. The diagram represents an unrolled cylindrical matrix, with the middle region corresponding with the anterior torso and the left and right regions corresponding with the posterior.

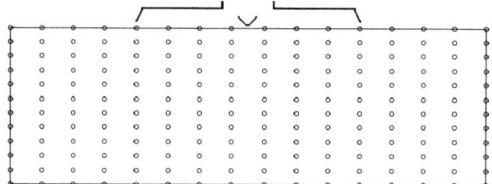

Figure 4. QRS isointegral map calculated from data recorded from a normal patient. Electrode sites highlighted with circles illustrate regions of negative polarity, plus signs illustrate regions of positive polarity. Isolines are plotted at 5mVms intervals.

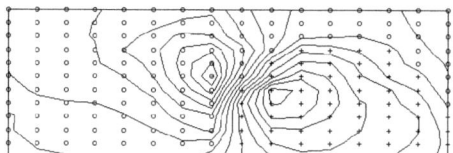

Although the recorded information can be represented as a number of scalar traces, the favored technique is to plot contour maps of the torso. Usually, BSPMs are represented as *isopotential* maps, in which points of equal electrical potential are connected by contour lines, or *isointegral* maps, where a section of the heart beat is integrated and the resulting values plotted on a contour map (Horwitz, 1995). Figure 3 illustrates a schematic of electrode array representation, and Figure 4 illustrates a QRS isointegral map recorded from a normal patient using a 192-electrode array.

Interpretation of BSPMs is primarily a pattern recognition task, as the clinical experts will base their diagnoses on the location and trajectory of maxima and minima on presented maps. Although BSPM has not seen much utilization beyond the research laboratory, its diagnostic superiority over traditional techniques is well recognized.

Figure 5. General overview of stages involved in the computerized processing of the ECG. The overall process can be decomposed into stages of beat detection, feature extraction, and classification. An optional stage of feature selection has also been included.

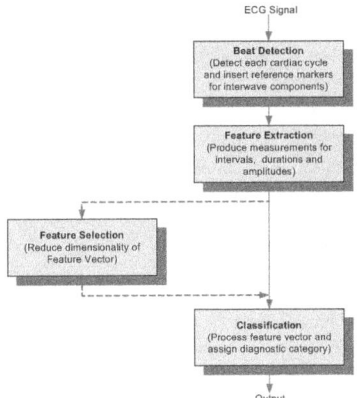

Computerized Processing of the ECG

Computerized processing of the ECG normally consists of three sequential processing stages: beat detection, feature extraction/selection, and classification (Figure 5). Beat detection aims to provide reliable detection of each cardiac cycle in each recording lead and, in addition, locate the temporal location of the reference points for each of the interwave components within each cardiac cycle. The reference markers identified during beat detection are processed by the feature extraction stage to produce measurements of interwave intervals, durations, and amplitudes. Collectively, these measurements can be referred to as the *feature vector*. The feature vector may undergo a further stage of processing prior to classification, when Feature Selection techniques may be employed to reduce the dimensionality of the feature vector, selecting features to maximize the divergence between pattern classes, while still maintaining sufficient information to permit discrimination. The final stage of computerized processing, Classification, processes the feature vector and, based on the information it contains, a classification is made to one of the possible diagnostic categories.

With regard to beat detection techniques, approaches adopted may be considered to have reached their limit in pushing forward the accuracy of automated analysis (Rowlandson, 1990). Nevertheless, accurate detection at this stage is of paramount importance, and errors made may be propagated through to the overall classification result. It is still an active area of research, especially for the detection of specific cardiac anomalies and application of new and evolving signal processing techniques.

Although standards exist which define the exact location from which interwave measurements should be calculated, feature extraction processes are faced with the issue of identifying the most relevant parameters which will aid in the overall diagnostic process from the hundreds that are available. In the computerized ECG domain, no standard set of features has been agreed upon (Kors & van Bemmel, 1990); hence, feature vectors are usually initially dictated in terms of their formation by medical guidance. In an effort to improve the overall classification process, Feature Selection techniques can be employed. These have been shown to be capable of reducing the dimensionality of the feature vector without any loss of classification accuracy.

From a classification perspective, it is clear that there is still room for improvement in the computational approaches. Results from the Common Standards for Quantitative Electrocardiography (CSE) study have shown that the human approach still has the ability to outperform the computerized approach (Willems et al., 1992). From a historical perspective, computational approaches have been based on either deterministic (rule-based) approaches or multivariate statistical approaches. Comparisons between these two have shown advantages and disadvantages of each (Nugent et al., 1999). Flexibility in adding new rules to deterministically based approaches, along with the ability to clearly explain why a specific diagnosis has been made, are seen to be advantages of the deterministic approach. On the other hand, considering rules are provided by human experts and a set of standard rules does not exist, statistical approaches offer the advantage of non-human bias in their design and adaptability to a given training dataset or population.

Over the past two decades, NNs have been an increasingly popular choice in the field of computerized ECG classification. Some feel that this may be attributed to advances made in NN training algorithms during the 1980s providing NNs with the ability to offer comparable levels of classification to existing approaches, with short developmental times (Bortolan & Willems, 1993; Yang et al., 1993). Nevertheless, it has been reported that, within the computerized ECG classification domain, researchers have moved from traditional approaches to adopt NNs (Bortolan et al., 1996).

Studies comparing the classification performance of NNs with rule-based and statistical approaches have reported their successful implementation. Nevertheless, there is a danger that NNs may be treated as a black box approach and, as such, lead to the possibility for their generalisation abilities to be overlooked and not fully appreciated. The following section provides exemplars of NN usage in computerized processing of the ECG and identifies how careful consideration of the NN and the structure of the underlying data can offer improved performance in the area.

NNs in ECG Processing

NNs have gained most interest and success in their application to classification of the 12-lead ECG. As previously mentioned, this is largely attributed to the fact that no widely accepted rule set exists for the computerized classification of the 12-lead ECG, although it is the most widely accepted clinical technique to non-invasively record electrical cardiac activity from a subject. Provided sufficient data are available, a NN can be designed and trained with the ability to classify a 12-lead ECG into one of a possible number of diagnostic classes with little to no clinical input. To date, NNs have been employed by researchers to classify various forms of heart disease. These include myocardial infarction, generally referred to as heart attack; cardiac hypertrophy, where the myocardium thickens due to increased pressure; and other common conduction defects such as bundle branch blockage. NNs have also been used to diagnose some of the early signs of problematic heart conditions, namely Ischemia, so that earlier treatments can be administered.

Within this domain, the most common approach has been the usage of the multi-layered perceptron (MLP) trained with backpropagation (BP). In the most general case, the feature vector produced following the stages of feature extraction and/or feature selection is used as input to the network. The n output nodes of the network are representative of the n diagnostic classes under investigation, and a data set, preferably clinically validated on non-electrocardiographic data, is used for the purpose of testing and training. Figure 6 shows the general usage of an MLP as an ECG classifier. As with the application of NNs in any domain, careful consideration of the network's design parameters must be taken into consideration and have been shown to provide improved performance if established appropriately. Typical (but not exclusive) areas for consideration during design include the number of nodes in the hidden layer, the number of hidden layers and variation of the constants within the BP training algorithm such as the learning constant, and the momentum term.

It has been the success of the MLP (used in this configuration) that has resulted in the establishment of its potential and warranted further investigations of its use as a means of computerized classification of the ECG and a way to further increase the overall diagnostic performance. In a study conducted by Bortolan and Willems (1993), an MLP was used to classify 12-lead ECGs. The NN approach was compared with linear discriminant analysis (LDA) and logistic discriminant analysis (LOG) using a dataset of 3,253 12-lead ECGs. Summary results from the study indicated performance levels following testing of 70.3% for the best NN in comparison with 67.0% and 66.3% for the statistical

Figure 6. General usage of an MLP used to classify a 12-lead ECG following stages of beat detection, feature extraction, and feature selection. The number of input nodes in the MLP is dictated by the number of features selected; the number of diagnostic categories dictates the number of nodes present in the output layer.

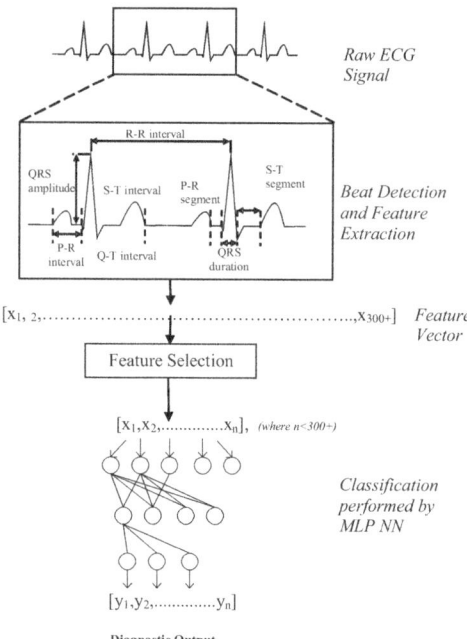

approaches, respectively. In an early study in the diagnosis of atrial fibrillation by Yang et al. (1993) investigating the performance of NNs in comparison to deterministic approaches, the former yielded superior results. Silipo and Bortolan (1997) reported comparable results when comparing MLP based 12-lead ECG classifiers with conventional statistical approaches of LDA and LOG. Average sensitivities of 64% for the NN approach were attained following testing in comparison with 63% for both the LDA and LOG approaches. Baxt et al. (2002) used MLPs to detect the presence of AMI for patients who had reported anterior chest pains. In addition to ECG information, other clinical information, such as patient histories, results from physical examinations, and chemical cardiac markers, were used as input to the NN. The MLP achieved a sensitivity of 94% following testing in comparison with a sensitivity of 77.3% for a Logistic Regression approach. What is apparent with all of these approaches (and others which have not been described here) is that the use of the MLP NN did not require the definition of any statistical properties, did not require any *a priori* hypothesis relating to the input population, and, in some cases were able to provide comparable results in comparison with conventional techniques which may have taken significantly longer to produce (Yang et al., 1993).

Decomposition of Classification Region

Based on the success of the MLP in comparison with conventional statistical approaches, the potential of NNs can be further enhanced by careful consideration of the elements of the classification problem itself (Nugent et al., 2000). Consider N labeled samples $x = [x_1,...,x_N]$ R^N where x is an N-dimensional feature vector, drawn from an underlying distribution $s(x)$, with class label l. For M class classification problems, the associated class for x may be expressed as j {1,.... } where M is the total number of classes, and the class label is l {0,1} . Thus, the j-th element is 1 if x belongs to class j, and the rest of the elements of l are zero.

In the conventional classifier for an M class problem with an unknown pattern x, drawn from $s(x)$, the classifier performs the function $u:R^N$ {0,1} , hence, mapping the unknown pattern to the most likely available diagnostic class. Considering a hypothetical case of decision regions created in the n-dimensional space spanned by the input variables, the conceptual ability of the classification function of a multi-output classifier, segregating between the specified classes, may be considered. An M class classification problem can be accommodated by a family of bigroup classifiers. Each individual bigroup classifier can perform a specific and unique classification function determining if the unknown pattern x belongs to a specific predefined class, or if it belongs to one of the other remaining classes. By considering a family of such bigroup classifiers, each specifically devoted to a different individual class with their outputs combined, a framework may be established to classify an unknown pattern x into one of a possible number of diagnostic classes. In this sense, the same M class classification problem, as accommodated by a multi-output classifier, can be accommodated by a framework of bigroup classifiers, where M is problem specific.

Assuming a predefined space encompassing M classes, M-1 bigroup classifiers are required. Each bigroup classifier can be considered as having a range space $A = \overset{M}{\underset{i=1}{U}} A_i$, where $A_i \mid A_j = 0$, $i \ne j$. Each individual bigroup classifier may be considered to perform the function $BG_i : R^N \quad A_i, 1 \quad i \quad M - 1$, where $BG_i(x)$ equals 1 if x belongs to class i and zero otherwise. For $i = M$ and $\quad , \quad ^1$ 0 provided $BG_i(x) = 0$ for $1 \quad i \quad -1$, $x \quad R^N$ (Nugent et al., 2000).

Decomposition of the classification problem into a number of bigroup classification problems offers a number of practical advantages. From the clinical perspective, it is possible to reduce the complexity of the feature selection problem to one where only discriminating features between one class and the remaining classes are required. This will result in the generation of smaller feature vectors in comparison with a single feature vector produced during Feature Selection for multi-classification problems. Such smaller versions of the feature vector offer the potential to offer enhanced discriminatory capabilities. From a NN perspective, smaller feature vectors reduce the complexity of the NN itself—a significant computational gain. By reducing the complexity of the NN, the potential to offer improved generalization abilities is increased.

Studies employing a family of bigroup NNs in contrast to a multi-output NN in 12-lead ECG classification have shown initial gains in performance (Nugent et al., 2000). In this study, six diagnostic classes identifiable by the 12-lead ECG were considered: Inferior, anterior and combined myocardial infarction, left ventricular hypertrophy, a combination of myocardial infarctions and left ventricular hypertrophy, and normals. A framework of bigroup NNs were developed to accommodate classification of 12-lead ECG recordings into one of the aforementioned categories. The framework consisted of five bigroup NNs. When all networks have a zero output, this was considered to be indicative of a normal 12-lead ECG. Each of the bigroup NNs were generated from MLPs with one hidden layer and a single node in the output layer. For comparative purposes, a single two-layered MLP with six nodes in the output layer was generated. Results following testing of the framework of bigroup NNs and the conventional MLP with six output nodes achieved correct classification results in the region of 80% and 68%, respectively, hence, further supporting the rationale of such an approach.

Challenges for 12-Lead ECG Classification and NNs

One of the common extensions to MLP usage has been the combination of multiple MLPs trained and tested on the same dataset. This exploits the varying generalization abilities of NNs which are inherently caused by the randomization of the network's weights as part of the BP training process, and the inability of the training algorithm to ensure a global minimum is reached. Combination in this manner produces one overall classification output which offers an underpinning combination of the strengths of all of the classifiers involved. Research in this area stems from the machine learning domain through the usage of classifier ensembles, where the goal is to produce a combination of a number of classification models which provides an overall classification performance, superior to any of the classifiers in isolation. Evidence has shown that this approach can provide improved overall classification results (Kuncheva & Whitaker, 2003).

Studies have already shown how overall classification performance can be enhanced by simply combining the output of multiple MLPs trained on the same data; the only difference is related to the randomization of the weights of the network during the process of training (Bortolan et al., 1996). This concept can be further extended by considering ensembles of NNs with differing topologies, trained with different portions of the training data. In this sense, individual classifiers can be specifically designed to classify specific regions of interest within the classification space.

Given that a NN can represent highly nonlinear relations and no optimal classification rule set exists for ECG classification, NNs are appealing solutions within this domain. Results have shown that NNs can achieve similar or better results than statistical or deterministic approaches. This provides us with a hypothesis that NNs can address certain problems better than their conventional counterparts, but may not necessarily be the optimal solution for the entire 12-lead ECG classification process. Identification of specific elements or classification regions, which exhibit low automated classification success or have little clinical understanding, may be where we will expect to see NNs excelling. Already, studies have shown that NNs in conjunction with other classification models (either deterministic or statistical) have provided improved overall classification results (Nugent et al., 2000). The challenge is now to assess where the NN offers improved performance in comparison to other approaches, use the ability of the NN to address this specific problem, and embed the solution into the overall automated classification process.

Challenges in Body Surface Mapping

Although BSPM is widely recognized for its diagnostic superiority over traditional 12-lead ECG techniques, its clinical application, outside of the research arena, has been limited. Many factors contribute to this lack of uptake:

- *Cost:* Increasing the number of recording channels adds complexity to the acquisition system inevitably raising cost. Additionally, as the number of recording sites increase, the electrode (consumable) cost per patient recording increases.
- *Lack of standards:* There is great debate about the number and position of electrodes required to adequately sample cardiac events, and no standard electrode system has ever been agreed on.
- *Clinical impracticalities:* Rapid and accurate application of large numbers of electrodes (30+) is often difficult, especially in emergency situations.
- *Interpretation:* Mainly due to the lack of standards already mentioned, there is no well established rule set for interpretation and classification of BSPMs.

Application of Computers in BSPM

Although the aforementioned issues have had a significant impact on the clinical uptake of BSPM, the increased prevalence in computing power has allowed much ground to be gained. The fundamental need for computers is more evident in BSPM than in most electrocardiographic techniques. This is mainly due to the computational intensity of the recording and representation (map drawing) process. Aside from the mandatory need for automated processing, investigators have utilized computers to uncover information about the significance of the data that are being recorded.

Selection of Optimal Recording Sites

One of the key issues with BSPM is the selection of optimal recording sites on the torso. It is well appreciated that although increasing the number of recording sites improves diagnostic accuracy, recording the ECG using excessive numbers of electrodes (100+) results in significant redundancy as a correlation exists between recording sites on the torso.

Early investigators used numerical techniques to mine for information in the recorded maps with the aim of eliminating redundancy. The classical techniques included looking for the sites that exhibited the most diagnostically significant information, based on discriminant ability (Kornreich et al., 1985), and selecting sites that allowed accurate reconstruction of the ECG at locations that were not sampled, based on correlation (Barr et al., 1971; Lux et al., 1978). Although the rationale used is similar, recent studies have employed more contemporary techniques. One such study was conducted by Lopez (2003) who developed a classifier framework based on "lead experts." Each of these lead experts was based on an MLP classifier whose discrete classification accuracy could provide an indication of the performance of each recording site. In this study, performance of each recording site was considered as a measure of discriminatory significance of the site itself. Hence, by ranking the sites by performance, it was possible to select the top n sites in terms of their discriminatory powers.

Classification of BSPM Data

The process of computerized classification, as described in the preceding sections, is somewhat more complicated for BSPMs. The main reason for this is the high dimensionality of the recorded data, as even in more "practical" lead systems, as many as 32 recording sites can be utilized (Lux et al., 1979). The key challenge is therefore the realization of a mechanism to adequately reduce the number of features presented for classification. Once this has been achieved, experiences gained within the processing of the 12-lead ECG can be exploited.

The most obvious method of reducing the dimensionality of the dataset is to select the features that are deemed most suitable in providing discriminatory information; the features that are deemed irrelevant can be left out. This is similar if not identical to the rationale that can be adopted in defining optimal limited lead systems. A method, similar to that previously mentioned, proposed by Lopez (2003), can be used to select the features that are highly ranked in terms of diagnostic significance.

Alternatively, dimensionality can be reduced by subjecting the recorded data to a mathematical transformation. Principal component analysis (PCA) has emerged as a favored technique in this approach. Here, the basis functions, that can be used to represent the original data, are derived from the original data itself, resulting in an efficient representation using fewer basis functions (Lux, 2003). This is in contrast to similar techniques such as the Fourier series where the basis functions are derived from sine waves. This strategy was adopted by Sun et al. (1988) who used a feedforward architecture with one hidden layer to assess the classification performance of feature sets transformed from 219 lead QRS isointegral maps using only a limited number of principal components (6-15). This study concluded that only ten expansion coefficients were needed to obtain an 82% classification accuracy, evaluated using the cross validation method in separating patients with myocardial ischemia from normal.

Trends in BSPM Classification

The diagnostic content of the BSPM approach from a clinical perspective is significantly superior in comparison with the other approaches currently available. There does, however, remain a number of potential barriers in the development of NN based classifiers for BSPM data; the most significant of these is the associated high dimensionality coupled with the lack of clinical guidance to assist and complement development. Developers have also been constrained by the lack and diversity of experimental datasets available in this domain. For these reasons, the application of NNs is nowhere near as apparent as in the more conventional 12-lead approach. If we learn from the experiences gained within the application of NNs to 12-lead ECG classification, we can begin to address the problem by decomposing the process into a number of sequential processing steps and address the overall classification as a series of smaller and more specific areas of interest.

Conclusion

NNs have been widely used as a means to perform automated ECG classification. With such an approach, the digitized information recorded from a patient's torso can be analyzed, and a suggested categorization to one of a possible number of diagnostic classes can be made.

The most widely used and clinically accepted recording technique is the 12-lead ECG. This area has received much interest, and results using MLP NNs have shown that improved performance can be gained in comparison with deterministic and statistical approaches. The future potential success of NNs in this area can be related to the careful consideration and design of the architecture and application of the NN itself. This is a well known and appreciated challenge in the domain of NNs, which is non-application specific. It has led to many theoretical and application research studies, all with varying degrees of success, and may still be considered a totally unsolved problem. Nevertheless, the results attained to date and the complexity of problems which may be addressed using NNs will certainly lead to further investigations into their capabilities and applications in the future. In the domain of 12-lead ECG classification, results have shown that decomposing the problem into a number of smaller problems has had the overall result in improvement in the performance of the classification process. Nevertheless, the challenge lies in which part of the classification process the NN is to be applied. It is clear that their non-linear representation abilities can address highly complex problems, and it is this attribute which should be further exploited through usage of NNs to address a single element in the overall automated classification process.

The data driven nature of NNs also suits the 12-lead ECG problem well, given the lack of a well defined clinical rule set. Nevertheless, design and development of NNs are highly dependent on the quality of the dataset used for training. Although datasets exist, it is often difficult to attain a highly reliable and well validated dataset for developmental purposes. Development of NNs without a highly reliable validated dataset may inevitably introduce a negative bias into the classification process and even hamper the generalization abilities of the network.

The final challenge for NNs in 12-lead ECG classification will be their integration into commercial recording machines. For this to become a reality, certain CE Kite Mark and FDA regulations will need to be adhered to and, as such, a rigorous evaluation of their performance will need to be undertaken. This is an area which has recently been addressed, and guidelines for formal assessment are now becoming available (Smith et al., 2003).

As mentioned throughout, although the 12-lead ECG is the most widely used method of non-invasive cardiac assessment, BSPM offers significant improvements in diagnostic powers. The process of computerized BSPM is complicated by notions of *which* data to represent and *how* to visually represent the data. Nevertheless, advances in computing powers and clinical understanding have made the concept of computerized BSPM a reality. This area offers a number of challenges, the first of which can be considered clinical acceptance. Once this goal has been achieved, computational processing efforts can then be addressed. The lessons learned from the computerized classification of the 12-lead ECG should be considered and applied to the area of BSPM. This will allow efforts to be focused on the computational challenges within BSPM, for example, lead selection and classification of isointegrals and isopotentials with techniques such as NNs. Successfully solving these problems will offer the potential of further improvements in the process of CVD detection.

References

Andresen, A., Gasperina, M. D., Myers, R., Wagner, G. S., Warner, R. A., & Selvester, R. H. (2002). An improved automated ECG algorithm for detecting acute and prior myocardial infarction. *Journal of Electrocardiology, 35*(Suppl.), 105-110.

Barr, R. C., Spach, M. S., & Herman-Giddens, G. S. (1971). Selection of the number and position of measuring locations for electrocardiography. *IEEE Transactions on Biomedical Engineering, 18*, 125-138.

Baxt, W. G., Shofer, F. S., Sites, F. D., & Hollander, J. E. (2002). A neural computational aid to the diagnosis of acute myocardial infarction. *Annals of Emergency Medicine, 39*(4), 366-373.

Bortolan, G., Brohet, C., & Fusaro, S. (1996). Possibilities of using neural networks for ECG classification. *Journal of Electrocardiology, 29*, 10-16.

Bortolan, G., & Willems, J. L. (1993). Diagnostic ECG classification based on neural networks. *Journal of Electrocardiology, 26*, 75-79.

Guyton, A. C., & Hall, J. E. (2000). *Textbook of medical physiology*. London: W. B. Saunders Company.

Hole, J. W. (1998). *Human anatomy and physiology*. Europe: McGraw-Hill Education.

Horwitz, L. I. (1995). Current clinical utility of body surface mapping. *Journal of Invasive Cardiology, 7*(9), 265-274.

Hubbard, J., & Mechan, D. (1997). *The physiology of health and illness: With related anatomy*. Cheltenham: Stanley Thornes Ltd.

Kornreich, F., Rautaharju, P. M., Warren, J., Montague, T. J., & Horacek, B. M. (1985). Identification of the best electrocardiographic leads for diagnosing myocardial infarction by statistical analysis of body surface potential maps. *American Journal of Cardiology, 56*(13), 852-856.

Kors, J. A., & van Bemmel, J. H. (1990). Classification methods for computerized interpretation of the electrocardiogram. *Methods of Information in Medicine, 29*, 330-336.

Kowey, P. R., & Kocovic, D. Z. (2003). Ambulatory electrocardiographic recording. *Circulation, 108*, 31-33.

Kuncheva, L. I., & Whitaker, C. J. (2003). Measures of diversity in classifier ensembles and their relationship with classifier accuracy. *Machine Learning, 51*, 181-207.

Lopez, J. A. (2003). *Computational neural models for body surface cardiac data analysis*. Unpublished doctoral dissertation, University of Ulster, Northern Ireland, UK.

Lux, R. L. (1993). Electrocardiographic mapping: Noninvasive electrophysiological cardiac imaging. *Circulation, 87*(3), 1040-1042.

Lux, R. L. (2000). Uncertainty of the electrocardiogram: Old and new ideas for assessment and interpretation. *Journal of Electrocardiology, 33*(Suppl.), 203-208.

Lux, R. L. (2000a). Electrocardiographic potential correlations: Rationale and basis for lead selection and ECG estimation. *Journal of Electrocardiology, 35*(4), 1-5.

Lux, R. L. (2000b). Leads: How many and where? *Journal of Electrocardiology, 35,* 213-214.

Lux, R. L. (2003). Principal component analysis: An old but powerful tool for ECG analysis. *International Journal of Bioelectromagnetism, 5*(1), 342-345.

Lux, R. L., Burgess, M. J., Wyatt, R. F., Evans, A. K., Vincent, G. M., & Abilskov, J. A. (1979). Clinically practical lead systems for improved electrocardiography: Comparison with precordial grids and conventional lead systems. *Circulation, 50,* 356-363.

Lux, R. L., Smith, C. R., Wyatt, R. F., & Abilskov, J. A. (1978). Limited lead selection for estimation of body surface potential maps in electrocardiography. *IEEE Transactions in Biomedical Engineering, 25,* 270-276.

Menown, I. B. A., Mackenzie, G., & Adgey, A. A. J. (2000). Optimizing the initial 12-lead electrocardiographic diagnosis of acute myocardial infarction. *European Heart Journal, 21*(4), 275-283.

Maynard, S. J., Menown, I. B. A., Manoharan, G., Allen, J., McAnderson, J., & Adgey, A. A. J. (2003). Body surface mapping improves early diagnosis of acute myocardial infarction in patients with chest pain and left bundle branch block. *Heart, 89*(9), 998-1002.

Nugent, C. D., Webb, J. A. C., & Black, N. D. (2000). Feature and classifier fusion for 12-lead ECG classification. *Medical Informatics and the Internet in Medicine, 25*(3), 225-235.

Nugent, C. D., Webb, J. A. C., Black, N. D., & Wright, G. T. H. (1999). Electrocardiogram 2: Classification. *Automedica, 17,* 281-306.

Rowlandson, I. (1990). Computerized electrocardiography: A historical perspective. *Annals of the New York Academy of Sciences, 601*(Electrocardiography), 343-352.

Silipo, R., & Bortolan, G. (1997). Neural and traditional techniques in diagnostic ECG classification. *Proceedings of IEEE Conference on Acoustics, Speech and Signal Processing* (vol. 1, pp. 123-126).

Smith, A. E., Nugent, C. D., & McClean, S. I. (2003). Neural networks as decision support systems: Formal evaluation of inherent performance. *Artificial Intelligence in Medicine, 27*(1), 1-27.

Sun, S., Thomas, C. W., Liebman, J., Rudy, Y., Reich, Y., Stilli, D., & Macchi, E. (1988). Classification of normal and ischemia from BSPM by neural network approach. *Proceedings of the 10th Annual International Conference of the IEEE, Engineering in Medicine and Biology Society* (vol. 3, pp. 1504-1505).

Taccardi, B., Punske, B. B., Lux, R. L., MacLeod, R. S., Ershler, P. R., Dustman, T. J., & Vyhmeister, Y. (1998). Useful lessons from body surface mapping. *Journal of Cardiovascular Electrophysiology, 9,* 773-786.

Willems, J. L., Arnaud, P., van Bemmel, J. H., Degani, R., MacFarlane, P. W., & Zywietz, C. (1992). Comparison of diagnostic results of ECG computer programs and cardiologists. *Proceedings of Computers in Cardiology,* (pp. 93-96).

World Health Organization. (2004). *The atlas of heart disease and stroke.* Retrieved September 25, 2005, from http://www.who.int/cardiovascular_diseases/resources/atlas/en/

Yang, T. F., Devine, B., & MacFarlane, P. W. (1993). Deterministic logic versus software-based artificial neural networks in the diagnosis of atrial fibrillation. *Journal of Electrocardiology, 26,* 90-94.

Chapter IV

Neural Networks in ECG Classification:
What is Next for Adaptive Systems?

G. Camps-Valls, Universitat de València, Spain

J. F. Guerrero-Martínez, Universitat de València, Spain

Abstract

In this chapter, we review the vast field of application of artificial neural networks in cardiac pathology discrimination based on electrocardiographic signals. We discuss advantages and drawbacks of neural and adaptive systems in cardiovascular medicine and catch a glimpse of forthcoming developments in machine learning models for the real clinical environment. Some problems are identified in the learning tasks of beat detection, feature selection/extraction, and classification, and some proposals and suggestions are given to alleviate the problems of interpretability, overfitting, and adaptation. These have become important problems in recent years and will surely constitute the basis of some investigations in the immediate future.

Introduction

An electrocardiogram (ECG) is the graphical representation of the electrical activity of the heart as it is recorded from the body surface (Kilpatrick & Johnston, 1994). Non-invasive electrocardiography has proven to be a very interesting method of obtaining information about the state of a patient's heart and detecting cardiac pathologies. The goal of ECG discrimination is to classify the recorded signal into one of a possible number of diagnostic classes and, consequently, administer the most suitable treatment. The clinical staff can perform this process through visual inspection of the continuous ECG, but this process is time-consuming and requires intensive expertise and dedication. In addition, the ECG commonly presents high inter- and intra-patient variability, both in morphology and timing (Waltrous & Towell, 1995); thus, even experienced surgeons or cardiologists can misinterpret the data (Janet, 1997).

In this context, the use of *artificial neural networks* (ANN) in ECG processing has yielded promising results in cardiac pathology detection. In this chapter, we focus on *ECG classification*, which is concerned with discrimination of relevant pathologies such as arrhythmia, myocardial ischemia and infarction, ventricular tachycardia or fibrillation, or some other chronic alterations. The relevance of this topic has led to the appearance of computer-based classification approaches and their implementation in the daily clinical routine to produce more consistent and faster detection (Finlay et al., 2004; Mahalingam & Kumar, 1997; Nugent et al., 1999a; Willems et al., 1988).

The use of ANNs is commonly encouraged by their theoretical and practical advantages. In a neural approach, it is not strictly necessary to assume a specific relationship between variables; they provide non-linear flexible mappings, and they have proven to be effective techniques in a wide range of applications. In the literature, there are excellent reviews of applications of machine learning algorithms in medicine in general, and cardiology in particular (Abboud et al., 2002; Abreu-Lima & de Sa, 1998; Dybowski, 2000; Itchhaporia et al., 1996; Kumaravel et al., 1997; Lisboa, 2002; Miller et al., 1992; Molnar et al., 1998; Waltrous et al., 1996).

In this chapter, our aim is not only to provide a general overview of ANNs in ECG classification, but also to discuss the advantages and drawbacks of considering neural systems in cardiovascular medicine and to catch a glimpse of upcoming developments in neural models for ECG classification. The chapter is organized as follows. The *Background: Classification of ECG Signals with ANNs* section gives comprehensive background on the application of ANN in ECG classification. In the *Controversies and Problems* section, we discuss the relevant problems, advantages, and drawbacks in this arena. Finally, the *Solutions and Future Trends* section gives our particular viewpoint about future developments in the context of adaptive systems for ECG beat classification, its limitations, and needs.

Background: Classification of ECG Signals with ANNs

Although cardiac monitoring has made remarkable progress since the early work of Einthoven (1901), cardiovascular diseases are still a major cause of mortality. It has been demonstrated that rapid treatment leads not only to a decrease in the mortality rate, but also to a reduction in the infarct size (Ryan et al., 1999). As a consequence, intelligent systems capable of assisting doctors and staff in coronary intensive care units, and pharmacy services in hospitals are needed. Such systems should be easily implementable, scalable, accurate, robust, and stable. In addition, adaptability to uncommon situations is also desirable (Abboud et al., 2002).

Learning Scheme

Intelligent supervision systems (Passariello et al., 1993) appeared in the 1990s to overcome the drawbacks of first generation monitors (LeBlanc, 1986). Their aim was to integrate several sources of observation and several types of medical knowledge and to build interactive and helpful supervision systems. Their main objectives are: (1) to detect abnormal situations by analyzing the signals, (2) to predict the occurrence of abnormal events, (3) to give therapeutic advice, and (4) to explain the underlying mechanism generating the disorder.

In these approaches, three main tasks are clearly necessary: (1) the *acquisition step*, in which acquired ECGs and data from patients' follow-up is gathered; (2) the *signal processing step*, which processes the acquired signals and data to produce a relevant description of the signals; and (3) the *diagnosis step,* which has to detect potential pathologies as early as possible and characterize the situation on the basis of the previous processing steps. Figure 1 illustrates this general learning scheme for ECG classification.

In the following, we review the second and third steps in this diagram, since the first acquisition step is out of the scope of this chapter. The interested reader can find a more detailed analysis on the acquisition process in Nugent et al. (Ch. 3).

Figure 1. Schematic representation of a usual learning scheme *for ECG classification*

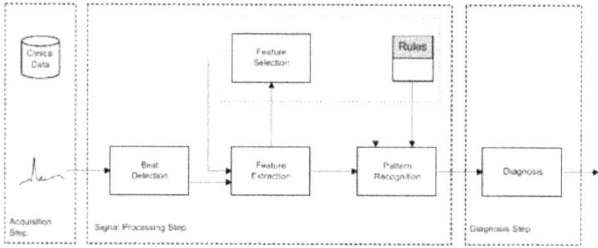

Signal Processing Step

The signal processing step has been previously formalized by some authors (Carrault et al., 2003; Nugent et al., 1999a). Various methodologies of automated ECG classification for simultaneous (or *posterior*) diagnosis are found in the literature. However, the entire process can be generally subdivided into a number of processing modules: (a) beat detection, (b) feature extraction/ selection, and (c) classification (see Figure 1).

a. *Detection.* The first preprocessing block of *beat detection* aims to locate each cardiac cycle QRS in each of the recording leads and insert reference markers indicating the beginning and end of each interwave component (see Chapter 3 in Nugent et al., 1999a for full details on the form of the cardiac cycle of an ECG). The accuracy of detection of each cardiac cycle is of great importance since it contributes significantly to the overall classification result. The markers are subsequently processed by the feature extraction step, where measurements are produced for wave amplitudes, frequencies, and durations.

b. *Feature selection/extraction.* In the majority of cases, detection of abnormal waves requires a preliminary feature extraction step, in which characteristics from the signal in time (duration, slope, amplitude of waves), frequency (energy in bands), or time-frequency domains (time and energy simultaneous feature scales) are extracted. An optional feature selection can be included in this process, by which the feature vector is reduced in dimension, including only the most relevant features necessary for discrimination and sometimes assisted by *a priori* knowledge or rules.

c.   *Pattern recognition.* The pattern recognition step involves development of intelligent systems dealing with the extracted and selected information in the previous step. A great many machine learning approaches have been used to identify different types of cardiac pathology. Chronologically, signal processing techniques were investigated first. Some of these approaches rely on model interpretation such as multistate Kalman filters (Gustafson et al., 1978) or Hidden Markov Models (Coast et al., 1990). Deterministic tests, ANNs, Bayesian networks, and decision trees have also been used for recognition (LeBlanc, 1986). More recently, artificial intelligence techniques have been proposed such as knowledge-based approaches using expert rules (Long, 1996), which are sometimes combined with fuzzy logic (Kundu et al., 1998). In this context, the majority of applications include the classical multilayer perceptron trained with the backpropagation learning algorithm, as identified in Lisboa (2002). Therefore, we will focus on the application of neural networks in relevant problems of cardiac anomaly detection in the Controversies and Problems section.

Diagnosis Step

The diagnosis step consists of detecting potential disorders and characterizing (or describing) the situation by means of abnormal features discovered during the pattern recognition step. Although apparently the same, there are conceptual differences between pattern recognition and diagnosis steps. In fact, it should be stressed that the diagnosis step can either directly exploit the classification provided by the signal-processing step (relevant features and classifier) or translate the information provided by the signal-processing step into the most accurate diagnosis according to a predetermined protocol of class label translation. In the first case, the classifier is trained to provide an explicitly defined diagnosis class. In the second, the clinical diagnosis is provided by means of a determined inductive principle from the signal-processing step. Abductive reasoning is generally associated with model-based diagnosis. However, these techniques are computationally demanding and useless for real-time monitoring. As a consequence, models closer to pure classification/recognition are usually preferred for diagnosis (Carrault et al., 2003).

Discrimination of Cardiac Disorders Using ANNs

In this section, we review the vast field of ECG signal classification in a categorized taxonomy based on the most relevant fields of application. The section does not intend to provide an exhaustive comparison among methods but presents the possible approaches followed in the literature.

Beat Classification

As we have seen in the previous section, an important step for ECG classification is beat detection. There are some interesting studies dealing with this specific issue by means of ANN. For example, in Edenbrandt et al. (1992), ANNs for classification of ECG ST-T segments were presented. Two thousand ST-T segments from the 12-lead ECG were visually classified into seven different groups. The material was divided into a training set and a test set. Computer-measured ST-T data were input to various ANNs, which correctly classified 90-95% of the individual ST-T segments in the test set.

A relevant example of a QRS detector can be found in the work of Xue et al. (1992), where an adaptive matched filtering algorithm based upon an ANNs for QRS detection was presented. The ANN adaptively modeled the lower frequencies of the ECG, which are inherently non-linear and non-stationary. The residual signal, which contains mostly higher frequency QRS complex energy, served a linear filter to detect the location of the QRS complex. In this case, the ANN acting as a filter was shown to be very effective in removing the time-varying, nonlinear noise characteristic of ECG signals.

In Hu et al. (1997), the authors presented a "mixture-of-experts" approach to develop a customized ECG beat classifier in an effort to further improve the performance of ECG processing and to offer individualized healthcare. A small, customized classifier was developed based on short time, patient-specific ECG data. It was combined with a global classifier, which was tuned to a large ECG patient database.

Finally, it is worth mentioning the work by Dokur and Olmez (2001), where a novel hybrid ANN structure for the classification of the ECG beats was presented. Two feature extraction methods for ECG beat classification, Fourier and wavelet analyses, were comparatively investigated in eight-dimensional feature space. ECG features were determined by dynamic programming according to the divergence value. In order to increase the classification performance and to decrease the number of nodes, the novel hybrid structure was trained by genetic algorithms (GAs). Ten types of ECG beats obtained from the Massachusetts Institute of Technology-Beth Israel Hospital (MIT-BIH) database and from a real-time ECG measurement system were correctly classified with a success rate of 96%.

Myocardial Infarction

Many studies have used ANNs for characterization of myocardial infarction (MI), which is one of the leading causes of death in Europe and the United States. Detection of MI has been extensively treated with ANNs by means of retrospective studies in which some clinical variables are used to train the models. Early diagnosis of acute myocardial infarction (AMI) in patients with severe chest pain presenting at emergency units has attracted considerable interest. In the early attempts, Baxt used an ANN to identify MI in patients presenting at an emergency department with anterior chest pain (Baxt, 1991; Baxt & White, 1995). Diagnosis of inferior MI with ANNs was also studied. Heden et al. (1994) obtained sensitivity of 84% and specificity of 97%, which was similar to results produced by Pahlm et al. (1990).

In another study, Kostis et al. (1993) used ANNs to estimate the prognosis of AMI. The purpose of the investigation was to use an ANN to estimate the future mortality of patients with AMI. The authors used a large database of long-term follow-ups and proposed a two-hidden-layer perceptron optimized by the ALOPEX algorithm, which yielded an overall accuracy of 74% with well-balanced sensitivity and specificity scores. Bortolan and Willems (1993) illustrated the use of ANNs in the problem of diagnostic classification of seven diagnostic classes (normal, left, right, and biventricular hypertrophy, and anterior, inferior, and combined MI) on the basis of ECG signals. More than 3,000 ECG signals were used, and results confirmed the potential of ANNs compared with classical methodologies. The authors further investigated and validated some characteristics of the approach for the same problems by considering three aspects: the normalization process, pruning techniques, and fuzzy preprocessing by use of radial basis functions (Bortolan et al., 1996).

Some other studies merit attention. For example, Heden et al. (1994) used 1,107 ECGs from patients who had undergone cardiac catheterization to train ANNs for the diagnosis of myocardial infarction. Different combinations of QRS and ST-T measurements were used as input to the ANNs. The networks correctly diagnosed anterior or inferior wall MI from the ECG, with higher sensitivity for anterior MI (80% vs. 68%) and similar specificity (about 95%) in both cases. The same authors performed a large-scale study for automated detection of AMI (Heden et al., 1997). A 20s trace was represented by six automatically generated ST-T measurements from each of the 12 leads and were inputs to a multilayer perceptron (MLP) trained with early stopping and the eight-fold cross-validation method. In Xue et al. (1998), the authors developed a pattern recognition model designed for ECG signal classification in general cases and for specific AMI recognition. The model combined a fuzzy logic inference system together with neural network adaptive learning, and promising results were obtained. Finally, in Ohlsson et al. (2001), the authors improved detection of AMI by incorporating previous ECGs, in addition to the current ECG, into the ANNs training. A total of 4,691 ECGs were recorded from patients admitted to an emergency department due to suspected AMI. ANNs were trained to detect AMI based on either the current ECG only or on the combination of the previous and the current ECG, which improved results.

Myocardial Ischemia

Myocardial ischemia is caused by a lack of oxygen and nutrients to the contractile cells of cardiac muscle and may lead to myocardial infarction with severe consequences of arrhythmia and heart failure. Bezerianos et al. (2000) originally proposed the network self-organizing map (NetSOM) model and applied it to the problem of myocardial ischemia detection. This network used radial basis functions in the neurons as local experts and improved the results of the basic self-organizing map (SOM), obtaining an average ischemic beat sensitivity of 77.7% and an average ischemic beat predictability of 74.1%. A different approach is found in Silipo and Marchesi (1998), where the authors successfully used static and recurrent neural networks (RNNs) for the classification of arrhythmia, myocardial ischemia, and chronic alterations. Finally, in Maglaveras et al. (1998a), a technique based on the Bidirectional Associative Memory (BAM) neural network was used to distinguish normal from ischemic beats. In this technique, the ECG beat is treated as a digitized image, which is then transformed into a *bipolar* vector suitable for input in the BAM. The results show that this method, when correctly tuned, can result in a fast and reliable ischemic beat detection algorithm.

In Maglaveras et al. (1998b), a supervised ANN was used for automated detection of ischemic episodes resulting from ST segment elevation or depression. The performance of the method was measured using the European ST-T database. In particular, the performance was measured in terms of both beat-by-beat ischemia detection and detection of ischemic episodes. An adaptive backpropagation (ABP) was used, which substantially reduced the training time and permitted real-time detection of ischemic episodes. Furthermore, the resulting model was capable of yielding average detection and duration sensitivities of 88% and 72%, respectively.

Arrhythmias

Among the high number of arrhythmias, the discrimination of wide QRS tachycardias in ventricular (VT) and supraventricular tachycardia (SVT) has become a complex area in electrocardiography. In fact, detection of ventricular fibrillation (VF) at an early stage is crucial in order to reduce the risk of sudden death and allow the specialist to have greater reaction time to give the patient appropriate therapy. Consequently, some relevant attempts have been made to develop classifiers and establish criteria for this differentiation (Brugada et al., 1991). More advanced developments have considered wavelet-based feature extraction and ANNs to obtain automatic detection and classification of arrhythmias (al-Fahoum & Howitt, 1999). In this work, nine different continuous and discrete wavelet transforms were considered in order to obtain the feature vector and train a radial basis function neural network (RBFNN) to detect arrhythmias. Utilizing the combination of Daubechies wavelet transform and RBFNN, an overall correct classification of 97.5% was obtained, with 100% correct classification for both ventricular fibrillation and ventricular tachycardia. In Rosado-Muñoz et al. (2002), the authors enhanced the discrimination accuracy of VF vs. VT obtained in a preliminary work (Rosado et al., 1999) by including more sophisticated feature selection techniques such as self-organizing maps (SOM) and decision trees in the scheme. The authors illustrated that with proper feature selection, higher recognition rates and simpler decision trees were obtained.

An important research area focuses on detection of paroxysmal atrial fibrillation (PAF). In Cubanski et al. (1994), a neural network system for detection of atrial fibrillation in ambulatory electrocardiograms was developed. The classification algorithm uses a rhythm analysis that considers the ECG to be a time series of RR interval durations. This is combined with an analysis of baseline morphology that considers the morphological characteristics of the non-QRS portions of the waveform. A backpropagation-based ANN was used as part of the classifier implementation. When applied to a database consisting exclusively of 42,970 examples of atrial fibrillation (AF) and other supraventricular rhythm disturbances validated by an experienced cardiologist, the algorithm demonstrated sensitivity of 82.4% for 10-beat runs of PAF and a specificity of 96.6%. An excellent review of methods for PAF detection was recently presented in the *Computers in Cardiology 2001 Challenge* (http://www.physionet.org/challenge/2001), where some neural approaches were developed with good competitive results.

The detection of premature ventricular contraction (PVC) has also captured the interest of many researchers. In Ham and Han (1996), for instance, the authors used fuzzy adaptive resonance theory mapping (ARTMAP) to classify cardiac arrhythmias. Two different conditions were analyzed: normal and abnormal PVC. The test results showed that the fuzzy ARTMAP ANN can classify cardiac arrhythmias with greater than 97% sensitivity and 99% specificity. Later, Maglaveras et al. (1998a) proposed a nonlinear ECG mapping preprocessing step and a classification which used a shrinking algorithm based on ANNs.

The technique was applied to the PVC detection problem with good results. Recently, a novel method for detecting PVC from Holter records has been proposed by Shyu et al. (2004). The method takes advantage of the information used during the QRS detection by first using wavelet transform feature extraction and then using a fuzzy neural network (FNN) classifier. The QRS duration in scale three and the area under the QRS complex in scale four were selected as the input features. It was found that the R-wave amplitude had a marked influence on the computation of proposed characteristic features, and, consequently, normalization of these features became necessary in order to reduce the effect of alternating R-wave amplitude and achieve reliable PVC detection. The observed accuracy for PVC classification was excellent (about 99.8%).

Additional interesting studies are found in the literature. In Usher et al. (1997), the authors used an adaptive fuzzy classifier to discriminate between intracardiac arrhythmias, showing the potential of such a system for use in implantable defibrillators. A non-linear predictor using the adaptive neuro-fuzzy inference system (ANFIS) was used to classify the arrhythmias and hence distinguish if defibrillation was required. A training structure utilizing desired input-output data pairs of target ECG waveforms (i.e., the intra-cardiac arrhythmia) was based on a hybrid learning procedure. The system resulted in correct arrhythmia detection and classification based on the lowest prediction. Lagerholm et al. (2000) employed SOMs in conjunction with Hermite basis functions for the purpose of beat clustering to identify and classify ECG complexes in arrhythmia. SOMs topological structure was beneficial in interpretation of the data. The experimental results were claimed to outperform other supervised learning methods using the same data. Recently, Osowski et al. (2004) proposed a committee of experts formed by several support vector machines (SVM). Two different preprocessing methods for generation of features were applied: higher order statistics and Hermite characterization of QRS complexes. The good results for the recognition of 13 heart rhythm types confirmed the reliability of the proposed approach. Finally, in Acharya et al. (2004), the authors developed an ANN with fuzzy relationships for the classification of cardiac rhythms. The feature extraction step was based on heart rate variation measurement (instantaneous heart rate against time), which has become a popular, non-invasive tool for assessing the autonomic nervous system. The results indicated a high level of efficacy, with an accuracy level of 80-85%.

Other Applications

In this section, we review some relevant additional applications of ANN in the context of ECG classification. This is the case in detection of ventricular late potentials (VLP), in which intelligent analysis of ECG data has been used for beat-to-beat detection (Shuicai et al., 2001). The system extracts features from the VLP time-frequency distribution of the filtered ECG using a wavelet transform. The wavelet coefficients are presented to an ANN for VLP recognition. Results showed that the method could detect beat-to-beat VLP with a sensitivity of 80% and a specificity of 77%, and overall accuracy of 78%. In Strauss et al. (2001), the authors used an adapted wavelet-packet decomposition to extract discriminating features in endocardial electrograms representing antegrade and retrograde activation patterns. The goal was to study the discrimination of ventricular tachycardias with 1:1 retrograde conduction from sinus tachycardia.

Another interesting research field is fetal monitoring. Multilayer recurrent ANN has been compared with conventional algorithms for recognizing fetal heart rate abnormality (Lee et al., 1999). This study revealed that the performance of ANNs is excellent compared to conventional systems, even with adjusted thresholds. More recently, Camps-Valls et al. (2004) have introduced dynamic ANNs, such as FIR and Gamma ANNs, in the problem of fetal ECG extraction. In this problem, the goal of the ANN is to reduce the maternal contribution to the acquired signal; thus, the network is introduced in the well-known adaptive noise cancellation (ANC) scheme. Results showed that the maternal contribution was greatly attenuated in synthetic (with several noise sources) and real registers and served as a good preprocessor of the acquired abdominal ECG signal for fetal monitoring.

Finally, left ventricular mass (LVM) and hypertrophy (LVH), using both clinical information and the ECG, have been predicted using ANNs (Hopkins et al., 2000). A backpropagation ANN was constructed. It was trained on 217 patients and tested on a further 100. Left ventricular mass and hypertrophy were successfully predicted with 79% and 82% accuracies, respectively. The ANN integrated clinical and ECG data efficiently, obtaining better accuracies than those obtained using conventional ECG diagnostic criteria.

Controversies and Problems

As presented in the previous sections, ANNs have been shown to be powerful tools in the enhancement of cardiac diagnosis systems in the last few decades. In Partridge et al. (1996), several advantages of ANNs over conventional models and manual analysis in medical applications were identified: (1) system implementation was possible using data instead of (possibly) ill-defined rules; (2) ANNs can deal with noise and novel situations automatically via data generalization, (3) ANNs can be automated for fast, reliable real-time analysis and diagnosis; and (4) they eliminate error associated with human fatigue and habituation. In the work of Passold et al. (1996), some additional benefits of ANNs were identified. ANNs can (1) process massive input data, (2) simulate diffuse medical reasoning, (3) obtain higher performances than statistical approaches, (4) self-organize to extrapolate data, and (5) easily update the encoded knowledge.

However, an evident gap exists between the theoretical properties of ANNs and their real implementation in clinical practice, mainly due to the special characteristics and requirements for an acceptable method in this field of application. Although ANNs have shown excellent results in many clinical applications, there are some shortcomings seen by the medical community such as the issue of interpretability of the decisions or complexity of the formulation that can restrict their acceptance in this domain. In Dassen et al. (1993), the authors identified the need for developing convincing, well-performed studies when working with ANNs. This is because, despite great acceptance in other application domains, the use of ANNs in medicine requires additional efforts in terms of assessment of the model's stability and robustness, which, in most cases, is not carried out. These are important concerns that must be addressed in the near future, as the machine learning and medical communities enclose each other in concepts and standardization of their common practice.

In the following, we review the main problems encountered in the literature when developing ANNs for the ECG classification problem. Following the learning scheme in Figure 1, it is easy to find problems in all steps of model development.

Quality and Representativity of the Available Data

When a problem is addressed following a *learning from samples* scheme, a critical issue is the quality and representativity of the available data, which is particularly relevant in diagnosis of cardiac pathologies. In this context, the majority of databases contain few, missing or erratic annotations, contradictory instances, all types of noise, and so forth. These issues make it difficult to train any statistical classifier or ANN. A good example in the literature is the work by Kostis et al. (1993), in which no unique output value for identical input cases were observed in the database. Consequently, the authors developed a specific ANN-based method for this case study. In Edenbrandt et al. (1992), the importance of the size and representativity of the training set was clearly demonstrated, and Selker et al. (1995) concluded that an important limitation of the predictive performance was the unavailability of reliable data, rather than the need for more algorithmic development.

Detection Algorithms

Problems in detection of the QRS complex have already been studied (LeBlanc, 1986). The main problem is due to the presence of various types of noise (slow baseline drift, high frequency noise, impulsive noise) and the great variability of patterns, which depend on the patient and change over time. New solutions based on multiband filters and multicadence theory (Afonso et al., 1999) are still emerging today. The detection of atrial activities (P-wave detection) has been investigated, but no satisfactory response has been found in Holter and intensive care units applications. The industrial systems focus on QRS detection and generally neglect P-wave detection, which is acceptable as far as sinusal rhythm is concerned, but is unsatisfactory for atrial disorders such as atrio-ventricular block or atrial bigeminy. Clearly, a gap still exists between the academic results and those observed daily in clinical practice, where high rates of false alarms are found (Coiera, 1994).

Feature Selection/Extraction

A very important aspect of the feature extraction/selection is that the extracted features should not only make sense, but also be meaningful for diagnosis. Nadal and deBossan (1993) used PCA and the RR intervals of QRS complexes to evaluate arrhythmias, which are one of the risks of sudden cardiac arrest in coronary care units. In this study, the authors used the first and second principal component coefficients to reduce the data dimension of each QRS complex and fed them to an ANN for detecting several pathologies. When four principal component coefficients were used, the classification results were improved. Despite the authors trying different numbers of coefficients, in the end, the selection was based on trial-and-error. Certainly, the problem of estimating the correct number of input features (or eliminating redundant clinical data) is still an unsolved problem in the machine learning community and, by extension, in ECG classification problems.

Other feature extraction methods can be used. Recently, time-frequency methods and wavelet decomposition methods have been used in the context of ECG signal classification. In Rosado et al. (1999), the authors extracted features from time-frequency distributions and then fed a mixture of ANNs. On some occasions, the feature extraction step involves a clustering process of the input data in order to simplify the task of the classifier by splitting the input space into similar feature regions. In Silipo et al. (1993), the authors extracted beat features from both morphologic and prematurity information and used an ANN which obtained good classification results for ventricular ectopic beats.

Classification Step

In the classification/diagnosis steps, four main problems exist: (1) how to define the diagnosis classes, (2) how to select the most suitable classifier, (3) how to train the selected classifier, and (4) how to measure the quality of the classifier. In the following, we review these issues.

Standardizing the Diagnosis Class

The most pertinent problem with computerized classification is that few works have faced the problems of standardization, the classification rules, and definition of what information should be considered during diagnosis (Kors & van Bemmel, 1990; van Bemmel et al., 1990). This mainly affects rule-based classifiers, as they are dependent on the knowledge provided by the human expert, which, in some cases, may be based on trial-and-error procedures. These problem may explain the recent popularity of ANNs, where no rules are initially required and the human input merely annotates and selects the cross-validation sets. The former process could be correctly based upon a set (or subset) of class categories described in the Common Standards for Quantitative Electrocardiography Committee (Willems et al., 1990).

Selection of the Most Suitable Classifier

In the task of ECG classification, the classical feedforward ANN trained with the backpropagation learning algorithm is usually employed. However, further improvement can be obtained when using more elaborate neural or kernel methods. After a thorough revision of the literature, the conclusion is that researchers and medical staff often use sophisticated approaches in *easy* problems and vice versa. In Selker et al. (1995), the authors noticed poor performance and lack of interpretability of the MLP compared to simpler models. They concluded from this study that the selection of the classification technique should be made on the basis of specific application needs, rather than assuming that any of the methods tried are intrinsically more powerful than the others.

Model Development

The problem of selecting the most suitable classifier and methodology for model development in a given ECG classification problem is related to several aspects.

For instance, practitioners should think (before selecting a model family) about their suitability for the problem, that is, the capability of dealing with noise and changing dynamics, of working efficiently with high input space dimension problems, of working with low numbers of training samples, or of being included in efficient multiclassification schemes. In addition, the risk of falling into local minima, the specific learning algorithm, or the need for techniques to avoid overfitting (regularization, early stopping, pruning, feature selection wrappers) should be discussed in the specific context of application.

An important problem is overfitting when working with low numbers of (representative) training samples compared to the number of input dimensions. Some comprehensive discussions about overfitting problems in ECG classification are found in Jorgensen et al. (1996), Pedersen et al. (1996), and Polak et al. (1997). Almost all of the papers invariably use the multilayer perceptron with early stopping to prevent overfitting. The problem of overfitting is dramatic in itself, but it can lead to misleading conclusions when a sensitivity (saliency) analysis is carried out using the trained network. In Baxt and White (1995), for instance, a network was trained to recognize high risk of AMI, and the sensitivity analysis required bootstrap techniques to correct sample bias. Other authors propose Bayesian-based ANNs to alleviate the problem of skewed distributions in pathology discrimination (Lisboa et al., 2000).

The real implementation and the induced concepts of scalability, real-time performance, and adaptation should also be considered. These issues are not commonly discussed in the literature before adopting a determined classifier. In the excellent review by Lisboa (2002), some crucial themes in model design and calibration, such as regularization, variable selection, validation, benchmarking, robustness, and stability, were highlighted. These are certainly major topics that should be addressed in the future.

Accuracy Assessment

Some suggestions for performing exhaustive evaluation of intelligent medical decision support systems based on ANNs are provided in Smith et al. (2003). The authors reviewed some necessary concepts to perform a thorough model accuracy evaluation. As they indicated, many of the well-known concepts drawn from mathematics are not familiar to the medical community and vice versa. Therefore, sometimes an ANN is evaluated in terms of meaningful criteria for the machine learning community but with few benefits for the medical community. This implies that ANNs should be compared to standard, accepted statistical techniques in the field. Furthermore, model comparison should be carried out to demonstrate accuracy and bias performance through the use of widely recognized sets of performance measurements, and additional statistical tests should be performed to identify significant differences among models.

Solutions and Future Trends

Some of the problems previously described can be alleviated following a correct methodology for model development. In any case, the quality and representativity of the available data will give an upper bound for the model's performance. When few samples are available, some methodologies can be useful. For example, the usual cross-validation methodologies for selecting the optimal free parameters will surely give a suboptimal and potentially biased solution. Bootstrap resampling, V-fold cross-validation, or leaving-one-out could deal efficiently with the problem and yield less biased results (see Efron & Tibshirani, 1998; Lisboa, 2002 for details on cross-validation methods). Also, replication of training samples by adding small noise perturbation has demonstrated good results in terms of accuracy and model robustness.

With regard to the feature extraction/selection step, the present methodologies (PCA, wavelets, time-frequency domains) can provide rich enough representations to the classifiers. The relevance of this step also appears when the given features are used to explain the achieved results. Being able to explain the obtained solution (in terms of the selected input features) becomes as relevant as obtaining the best possible answer (accuracy of the subsequent classifier). In ECG signal classification, the feature selection is also relevant because data are usually scarce compared to the number of features (even order of magnitudes); therefore, overfitting is likely to occur, significantly reducing the performance of the system. Some promising alternatives to this problem include: (1) combination of feature extractors, (2) Walsh expansions and genetic algorithms, (3) the use of kernel-based methods, (4) wrappers and embedded methods, and (5) nested subset methods. A recent review of feature and variable selection can be found in Guyon and Elisseeff (2003).

SVM is a well-known regularized kernel-based method which can handle large input spaces efficiently and can effectively work with reduced datasets, alleviate overfitting by controlling the margin, and automatically identify the most critical informative examples in the training set, namely *support vectors*. In fact, an important issue in model development, previously highlighted in Lisboa (2002), is model *regularization*, which allows us to obtain smooth and robust solutions, combating, in a certain way, the overfitting problem. There are some works aimed at obtaining fast and regularized neural-network solutions, using heuristic methods (Mahalingam & Kumar, 1997). However, kernel methods provide more elegant formulations to the regularization task, which is drawn naturally from the minimizing function that follows the principle of Structural Risk Minimization.

An additional critical issue is the extensive use of the MLP, which is justified because of its good results and flexibility. However, this network performs a *static* mapping; there are no internal dynamics. In order to introduce dynamic capabilities in a static neural network, we can either substitute the static synaptic weights by dynamic connections or introduce recurrent loops in the hidden layer. These types of networks are especially appropriate for time-series processing. Recently, Camps-Valls et al. (2004) introduced dynamic networks in the context of fetal ECG monitoring with good performances.

Finally, an important issue that merits comment is the feasibility of implementation of a neural classifier of ECG pathologies in a clinical environment, whether in a local software, hardware monitor, or Web-based system (Bosnjak et al., 1995; Carrault et al., 2003; Hernandez et al., 2001; Passariello et al., 1993). Recently, integration of ANNs in the real clinical environment has received great attention, and systems are not only required to be accurate, but also fast, adaptive, easily scalable, and robust to noise and changing dynamics. The final user demands accurate and real-time diagnosis; thus, systems and standards of implementation and data transmission are challenging in the design of simple but powerful classifiers.

Concluding Remarks

In this chapter, we have reviewed the field of application of ANNs in cardiac pathology discrimination based on ECG signals. We have reviewed the learning scheme for the application of ANNs in ECG signal classification, in which three standard consecutive steps constitute the scheme: (1) acquisition, (2) processing, and (3) diagnosis. We have looked more closely at the second step, in which the ECG signal is processed to extract relevant and meaningful features that feed a neural classifier trained to discriminate cardiac pathologies. Development and application of network-based classifiers in a given environment is full of pitfalls and problems which are even more difficult in ECG processing, given the dimensionality problem, the wide inter- and intra-subject variability, and the need for combined and individualized strategies for both developing feature extraction/selection and multiclassification schemes.

In this context, we have reviewed some of the most crucial applications of ANNs in ECG signal classification and additionally discussed advantages and drawbacks of neural and adaptive systems in cardiovascular medicine. Some proposals and suggestions have been given to alleviate the problems of interpretability, overfitting, and adaptation. These have all arisen as important problems in the recent years and will surely constitute the basis of some studies in the future.

References

Abboud, M. F., Linkens, D. A., Mahfouf, M., & Dounias, G. (2002). Survey on the use of smart and adaptive engineering systems in medicine. *Artificial Intelligence in Medicine, 26*(3), 179-209.

Abreu-Lima, C., & de Sa, J. P. (1998). Automatic classifiers for the interpretation of electrocardiograms. *Revista Portuguesa de Cardiologia, 17*(5), 415-428.

Acharya, R., Kumar, A., Bhat, P. S., Lim, C. M., Iyengar, S. S., Kannathal, N., & Krishnan, S. M. (2004). Classification of cardiac abnormalities using heart rate signals. *Medical & Biological Engineering and Computing, 42*(3), 288-293.

Afonso, V. X., Tompkins, W. J., Nguyen, T. Q., & Luo, S. (1999). ECG beat detection using filter banks. *IEEE Transactions on Biomedical Engineering, 46*(2), 192-202.

al-Fahoum, A. S., & Howitt, I. (1999). Combined wavelet transformation and radial basis neural networks for classifying life-threatening cardiac arrhythmias. *Medical & Biological Engineering and Computing, 37*(5), 566-573.

Baxt, W. G. (1991). Use of an artificial neural network for the diagnosis of myocardial infarction. *Annals of Internal Medicine, 115*(11), 843-848.

Baxt, W. G., & White, H. (1995). Bootstrapping confidence intervals for clinical input variable effects in a network trained to identify the presence of acute myocardial infarction. *Neural Computation, 7*(3), 624-638.

Bezerianos, A., Vladutu, L., & Papadimitriou, S. (2000). Hierarchical state space partitioning with a network self-organising maps for the recognition of ST-T segment changes. *Medical & Biological Engineering and Computing, 38*(4), 406-415.

Bortolan, G., Brohet, C., & Fusaro, S. (1996). Possibilities of using neural networks for ECG classification. *Journal of Electrocardiology, 29*(Suppl.), 10-16.

Bortolan, G., & Willems, J. L. (1993). Diagnostic ECG classification based on neural networks. *Journal of Electrocardiology, 26*(Suppl.), 75-79.

Bosnjak, A., Bevilacqua, G., Passariello, G., Mora, F., Sanso, B., & Carrault, G. (1995). An approach to intelligent ischaemia monitoring. *Medical & Biological Engineering and Computing, 33*(6), 749-56.

Brugada, P., Brugada, J., Mont, L., Smeets, J., & Andries, E. W. (1991). A new approach to the differential diagnosis of a regular tachycardia with a wide QRS complex. *Circulation, 83*(5), 1649-1659.

Camps-Valls, G., Martinez-Sober, M., Soria-Olivas, E., Magdalena-Benedito, R., Calpe-Maravilla, J., & Guerrero-Martinez, J. (2004). Foetal ECG recovery using dynamic neural networks. *Artificial Intelligence in Medicine, 31*(3), 197-209.

Carrault, G., Cordier, M. O., Quiniou, R., & Wang, F. (2003). Temporal abstraction and inductive logic programming for arrhythmia recognition from electrocardiograms. *Artificial Intelligence in Medicine, 28*(3), 231-263.

Coast, D. A., Stern, R. M., Cano, G. G., & Briller, S. A. (1990). An approach to cardiac arrhythmia analysis using hidden Markov models. *IEEE Transactions on Biomedical Engineering, 37*(9), 826-836.

Coiera, E. (1994, May 5-7). Designing for decision support in a clinical monitoring environment. In C. Schizas & G. Chistodoulides (Eds.), *Proceedings of the International Conference on Medical Physics and Biomedical Engineering,* University of Cyprus, Nicosia (pp.130-142).

Cubanski, D., Cyganski, D., Antman, E. M., & Feldman, C. L. (1994). A neural network system for detection of atrial fibrillation in ambulatory electrocardiograms. *Journal of Cardiovascular Electrophysiology, 5*(7), 602-608.

Dassen, W. R., Mulleneers, R. G., den Dulk, K., & Talmon, J. L. (1993). Artificial neural networks and ECG interpretation. Use and abuse. *Journal of Electrocardiology, 26*(Suppl.), 61-65.

Dokur, Z., & Olmez, T. (2001). ECG beat classification by a novel hybrid neural network. *Computer Methods and Programs in Biomedicine, 66*(2-3), 167-181.

Dybowski, R. (2000). Neural computation in medicine: Perspective and prospects. *Proceedings of the ANNIMAB-1 Conference (Artificial Neural Networks in Medicine and Biology).* Heidelberg, Germany: Springer-Verlag.

Edenbrandt, L., Devine, B., & Macfarlane, P. W. (1992). Neural networks for classification of ECG ST-T segments. *Journal of Electrocardiology, 25*(3), 167-173.

Efron, B., & Tibshirani, R.J. (1998). *An introduction to the bootstrap.* London: Chapman & Hall.

Einthoven, W. (1901). Un nouveau galvanometre. *Arch Neerland Sci Exact Nat, 6*, 625-633.

Finlay, D., Nugent, C., McCullagh, P., Lopez, J., & Black, N. (2004). The use of prediction models in the development of ECG classifiers based on ANNs. *Medinfo, 2004*(CD), 1593.

Gustafson, D. E., Willsky, A. S., Wang, J. Y., Lancaster, M. C., & Triebwasser, J. H. (1978). ECG/VCG rhythm diagnosis using statistical signal analysis—I. Identification of transient rhythms. *IEEE Transactions on Biomedical Engineering, 25*(4), 353-361.

Guyon, I., & Elisseeff, A. (2003). An introduction to variable and feature selection. *Journal of Machine Learning Research, 3*, 1157-1182.

Ham, F. M., & Han, S. (1996). Classification of cardiac arrhythmias using fuzzy ARTMAP. *IEEE Transactions on Biomedical Engineering, 43*(4), 425-430.

Heden, B., Edenbrandt, L., Haisty, W. K., Jr., & Pahlm, O. (1994). Artificial neural networks for the electrocardiographic diagnosis of healed myocardial infarction. *American Journal of Cardiology, 74*(1), 5-8.

Heden, B., Ohlin, H., Rittner, R., & Edenbrandt, L. (1997). Acute myocardial infarction detected in the 12-lead ECG by artificial neural networks. *Circulation, 96*(6), 1798-1802.

Hernandez, A. I., Mora, F., Villegas, G., Passariello, G., & Carrault, G. (2001). Real-time ECG transmission via Internet for nonclinical applications. *IEEE Transactions on Biomedical Engineering, 5*(3), 253-257.

Hopkins, C. B., Suleman, J., & Cook, C. (2000). An artificial neural network for the electrocardiographic diagnosis of left ventricular hypertrophy. *Critical Reviews in Biomedical Engineering, 28*(3-4), 435-438.

Hu, Y. H., Palreddy, S., & Tompkins, W. J. (1997). A patient-adaptable ECG beat classifier using a mixture of experts approach. *IEEE Transactions on Biomedical Engineering, 44*(9), 891-900.

Itchhaporia, D., Snow, P. B., Almassy, R. J., & Oetgen, W. J. (1996). Artificial neural networks: Current status in cardiovascular medicine. *Journal of the American College of Cardiology, 28*(2), 515-521.

Janet, F. (1997). Artificial neural networks improve diagnosis of acute myocardial infarction. *Lancet, 350*(9082), 935.

Jorgensen, J. S., Pedersen, J. B., & Pedersen, S. M. (1996). Use of neural networks to diagnose acute myocardial infarction. I. Methodology. *Clinical Chemistry, 42*(4), 604-612.

Kilpatrick, D., & Johnston, P. R. (1994). Origin of the electrocardiogram. *IEEE Transactions on Biomedical Engineering*, 479-486.

Kors, J., & van Bemmel, J. H. (1990). Classification methods for computerised interpretation of the electrocardiogram. *Methhods of Information in Medicine, 29*, 33-36.

Kostis, W., Yi, C., & Micheli-Tzanakou, E. (1993). Estimation of long-term mortality of myocardial infarction using a neural network based on the ALOPEX algorithm. In M. Cohen & D. Hudson (Eds.), *Comparative approaches in medical reasoning.*

Kumaravel, N., Rajesh, J., & Nithiyanandam, N. (1997). Equivalent tree representation of electrocardiogram using genetic algorithm. *Biomedical Science Instrumentation, 33*, 573-578.

Kundu, M., Nasipuri, M., & Basu, D. (1998). A knowledge-based approach to ECG interpretation using fuzzy logic. *IEEE Transactions on Systems, Man and Cybernetics, 28*(2), 237-243.

Lagerholm, M., Peterson, C., Braccini, G., Edenbrandt, L., & Sornmo, L. (2000). Clustering ECG complexes using Hermite functions and self-organizing maps. *IEEE Transactions on Biomedical Engineering, 47*(7), 838-848.

LeBlanc, A. R. (1986). Quantitative analysis of cardiac arrhythmias. *Critical Reviews in Biomedical Engineering, 14*(1), 1-43.

Lee, C., Ulbricht, G., & Dorffner A. (1999). Application of artificial neural networks for detection of abnormal fetal heart rate pattern: A comparison with conventional algorithms. *Journal of Obstetrics and Gynaecology, 19*(5), 482-485.

Lisboa, P. J. (2002). A review of evidence of health benefit from artificial neural networks in medical intervention. *Neural Networks, 15*(1), 11-39.

Lisboa, P. J., Vellido, A., & Wong, H. (2000). Bias reduction in skewed binary classification with Bayesian neural networks. *Neural Networks, 13*(4-5), 407-410.

Long, W. (1996). Temporal reasoning for diagnosis in a causal probabilistic knowledge base. *Artificial Intelligence in Medicine, 8*(3), 193-215.

Maglaveras, N., Stamkopoulos, T., Pappas, C., & Strintzis, M. (1998a). ECG processing techniques based on neural networks and bidirectional associative memories. *Journal of Med Eng Technol, 22*(3), 106-111.

Maglaveras, N., Stamkopoulos, T., Pappas, C., & Strintzis, M. G. (1998b). An adaptive backpropagation neural network for real-time ischemia episodes detection: Development and performance analysis using the European ST-T database. *IEEE Transactions on Biomedical Engineering, 45*(7), 805-813.

Mahalingam, N., & Kumar, D. (1997). Neural networks for signal processing applications: ECG classification. *Australas Phys Eng Sci Med, 20*(3), 147-151.

Miller, A. S., Blott, B. H., & Hames, T. K. (1992). Review of neural network applications in medical imaging and signal processing. *Medical & Biological Engineering and Computing, 30*(5), 449-464.

Molnar, B., Papik, K., Schaefer, R., Dombovari, Z., Feher, J., & Tulassay, Z. (1998). Medical use of artificial neural networks. *Orv Hetil, 139*(1), 3-9.

Nadal, J., & deBossan, M. C. (1993). Classification of cardiac arrhythmias based on principal components analysis and feedforward neural networks. *Proceedings of the Computers in Cardiology Conference* (pp. 341-344)

Nugent, C. D., Webb, J. A., Black, N. D., Wright, G. T., & McIntyre, M. (1999a). An intelligent framework for the classification of the 12-lead ECG. *Artificial Intelligence in Medicine, 16*(3), 205-222.

Ohlsson, M., Ohlin, H., Wallerstedt, S. M., & Edenbrandt, L. (2001). Usefulness of serial electrocardiograms for diagnosis of acute myocardial infarction. *Amercan Journal of Cardiology, 88*(5), 478-481.

Osowski, S., Hoai, L. T., & Markiewicz, T. (2004). Support vector machine-based expert system for reliable heartbeat recognition. *IEEE Transactions on Biomedical Engineering, 51*(4), 582-589.

Pahlm, O., Case, D., Howard, G., Pope, J., & Haisty, W. K. (1990). Decision rules for the ECG diagnosis of inferior myocardial infarction. *Comput Biomed Res, 23*(4), 332-345.

Partridge, D., Abidi, S. S. R., & Goh, A. (1996). Neural network applications in medicine. *Proceedings of National Conference on Research and Development in Computer Science and Its Applications (REDECS'96),* Universiti Pertanian Malaysia, Kuala Lampur (pp. 20-23).

Passariello, G., Mora, F., Carrault, G., & Le Pichon, J. -P. (1993). Intelligent patient monitoring and management systems: A review. *IEEE Engineering in Medicine and Biology Magazine, 12*(4), 23-33.

Passold, F., Ojeda, R. G., & Mur, J. (1996). Hybrid expert system in anesthesiology for critical patients. *Proceedings of the 8th IEEE Mediterranean Electrotechnical Conference, MELECON'96 (ITALIA)* (vol. 3, pp. 1486-1489).

Pedersen, S. M., Jorgensen, J. S., & Pedersen, J. B. (1996). Use of neural networks to diagnose acute myocardial infarction. II. A clinical application. *Clin Chem, 42*(4), 613-617.

Polak, M. J., Zhou, S. H., Rautaharju, P. M., Armstrong, W. W., & Chaitman, B. R. (1997). Using automated analysis of the resting twelve-lead ECG to identify patients at risk of developing transient myocardial ischaemia—an application of an adaptive logic network. *Physiol Meas, 18*(4), 317-325.

Rosado, A., Guerrero, J., Serrano, A. J., Soria, E., Martínez, M., & Camps, G. (1999). Ventricular fibrillation detection method using pseudo Wigner-Ville time-frequency representation. *Proceedings of the Fifth Conference of the European Society for Engineering & Medicine,* Barcelona, Junio (pp. 379-380).

Rosado-Muñoz, A., Camps-Valls, A., Guerrero-Martínez, J., Francés-Villora, J. V., MuDoz-Marí, J., & Serrano-López, A. (2002, September 22-25). Enhancing feature extraction for VF detection using data mining techniques. *Proceedings of the Computers in Cardiology Conference* (vol. 29, pp. 209-212).

Ryan, T. J., Antman, E. M., Brooks, N. H., Califf, R. M., Hillis, L. D., Hiratzka, L. F., Rapaport, E., Riegel, B., Russell, R. O., Smith, E. E., III, Weaver, W. D., Gibbons, R. J., Alpert, J. S., Eagle, K. A., Gardner, T. J., Garson, A., Jr., Gregoratos, G., & Smith, S. C., Jr. (1999). 1999 update: ACC/AHA guidelines for the management of patients with acute myocardial infarction: Executive summary and recommendations: A report of the American College of Cardiology/American Heart Association Task Force on Practice Guidelines (Committee on Management of Acute Myocardial Infarction). *Circulation, 100*(9), 1016-1030.

Selker, H. P., Griffith, J. L., Patil, S., Long, W. J., & D'Agostino, R. B. (1995). A comparison of performance of mathematical predictive methods for medical diagnosis: Identifying acute cardiac ischemia among emergency department patients. *J Investig Med, 43*(5), 468-476.

Shuicai, W., Yongxian, Q., Zhiyong, G., & Jiarui, L. (2001). A novel method for beat-to-beat detection of ventricular late potentials. *IEEE Transactions on Biomedical Engineering, 48*(8), 931-935.

Shyu, L. Y., Wu, Y. H., & Hu, W. (2004). Using wavelet transform and fuzzy neural network for PVC detection from the Holter ECG. *IEEE Transactions on Biomedical Engineering, 51*(7), 1269-1273.

Silipo, R., Gori, M., & Marchesi, C. (1993, September 5-8). Autoassociator structured neural network for rhythm classification of long-term electrocardiogram. *Proceedings of the Computers in Cardiology Conference* (vol. 20, pp. 349-352).

Silipo, R., & Marchesi, C. (1998). Artificial neural networks for automatic ECG analysis. *IEEE Transactions on Signal Processing, 46*(5), 1417-1425.

Smith, A. E., Nugent, C. D., & McClean, S. I. (2003). Evaluation of inherent performance of intelligent medical decision support systems: Utilising neural networks as an example. *Artificial Intelligence in Medicine, 27,* 1-27.

Strauss, D., Jung, J., Rieder, A., & Manoli, Y. (2001). Classification of endocardial electrograms using adapted wavelet packets and neural networks. *Ann Biomed Eng, 29*(6), 483-492.

Usher, J., Campbell, D., Vohra, J., & Cameron, J. (1997). Fuzzy classification of intra-cardiac arrhythmias. *Proceedings of the 18th Annual International Conference of the IEEE Engineering in Medicine and Biology Society,* Amsterdam, The Netherlands (vol. 3, pp. 997-998).

van Bemmel, J., Zywietz, C., & Kors, J. A. (1990). Signal analysis for ECG interpretation. *Meth Inf Med, 29,* 317-329.

Waltrous, R., & Towell, G. (1995). A patient-adaptive neural network ECG patient monitoring algorithm. *Proceedings of the Computer in Cardiology Conference* (vol. 22, pp. 229-232).

Waltrous, R. L., Towell, G., & Glassman, M. S. (1996). Synthesize, optimize, analyze, repeat (SOAR): Application of neural network tools to ECG patient monitoring. *Procceedings of the Third International Conference on Neural Networks and Expert Systems in Medicine and Healthcare* (pp. 560-570).

Willems, J. L., Abreu-Lima, C., Arnaud, P., van Bemmel, J. H., Brohet, C., Degani, R., Denis, B., Graham, I., van Herpen, G., Macfarlane, P. W., et al. (1988). Effect of combining electrocardiographic interpretation results on diagnostic accuracy. *Eur Heart J, 9*(12), 1348-1355.

Willems, J. L., Arnaud, P., van Bemmel, J. H., Degani, R., MacFarlane, P., & Zywietz, C. (1990). Common standards for quantitative electrocardiography: Goals and main results. *Methods of Information in Medicine, 29,* 263-271.

Xue, Q., Hu, Y. H., & Tompkins, W.J. (1992). Neural-network-based adaptive matched filtering for QRS detection. *IEEE Transactions on Biomedical Engineering, 39*(4), 317-329.

Xue, Q., Taha, B., Reddy, S., & Aufderheide, T. (1998). An adaptive fuzzy model for ECG interpretation. *Proceedings of the 20th Annual International Conference of the IEEE Engineering in Medicine and Biology Society,* Piscataway, NJ.

Chapter V

A Concept Learning-Based Patient-Adaptable Abnormal ECG Beat Detector for Long-Term Monitoring of Heart Patients

Peng Li, Nanyang Technological University, Singapore

Kap Luk Chan, Nanyang Technological University, Singapore

Sheng Fu, Nanyang Technological University, Singapore

Shankar M. Krishnan, Nanyang Technological University, Singapore

Abstract

In this chapter, a new concept learning-based approach is presented for abnormal ECG beat detection to facilitate long-term monitoring of heart patients. The novelty in our approach is the use of complementary concept— "normal" for the learning task. The concept "normal" can be learned by a v-support vector classifier (v-SVC) using only normal ECG beats from a specific patient to relieve the doctors from annotating the training data beat by beat to train a classifier. The learned model can then be used to detect abnormal beats in the long-term ECG recording of the same patient. We have compared with other methods, including multilayer feedforward neural networks, binary support vector machines, and so forth. Experimental results on MIT/BIH arrhythmia ECG database demonstrate that such a patient-adaptable concept learning model outperforms these classifiers even though they are trained using tens of thousands of ECG beats from a large group of patients.

Introduction

Electrocardiogram (ECG) is a recording of the electric potential variation due to the cardiac activities, which is often used by doctors to obtain reliable information about the performance of the heart function. The analysis of heart beat cycles in ECG signal is very important for long-term monitoring of heart patients. However, it is very costly for the medical expert to analyze the ECG recording beat by beat since the ECG records may last for hours. Therefore, it is justified to develop a computer-assisted technique to examine and annotate the ECG recording to facilitate review by medical experts. This computer annotation will assist doctors to select only the abnormal beats for further analysis.

Annotation of ECG recording requires the detection of various types of heart beats. This is a pattern recognition task. Very often, a classifier is to be trained to recognize different types of beats. The training set of the classifier, such as a multilayer neural network, is usually a large database which consists of the ECG beats from a large pool of patients. However, these classifiers suffer from the problem of poor generalization because there are usually some variations in the "normal" range among human beings. Even doctors may experience difficulty in assessing abnormal ECG beats if only considering the reference values based on the general patient population. There is a need to incorporate local information of a specific patient to improve the recognition of abnormal ECG beats and thus help to improve the generalization.

In this chapter, we proposed to approach this problem based on kernel concept learning. The benefit of concept learning is that only the information from one class is needed for training a classifier (a class density estimator to be precise). A concept learning model, called one-class support vector machine (SVM), is investigated to learn the concept "normal" and then used to detect the normal beats in ECG recording; hence, the abnormal beats are revealed as the complementary of the normal beats. Such model can relieve the doctors from annotating the ECG beats one by one for training a binary classifier such as neural networks and binary support vector machines. The proposed method is compared to the generally used methods such as multilayer perceptron, using MIT/BIH arrhythmia ECG database (Massachusetts Institute of Technology, 1997).

Background

Electrocardiogram (ECG) is a recording of the heart's electrical currents obtained with the electrocardiograph, an instrument designed for recording the electrical currents that traverse the heart and initiate its contraction (Yanowitz, 2003). A typical ECG signal is illustrated in Figure 1 where different segments of the ECG signal characterize different cardiac activities. For example, P wave indicates the sequential activation (depolarization) of the left and right atria, ST-T wave signifies ventricular repolarization, QRS complex reveals the left and right ventricular depolarization, and so forth (Yanowitz, 2003). The main objectives of ECG monitoring include:

1.   Detecting arrhythmias that occur intermittently or during certain physical activities.

2.   Evaluating symptoms (such as chest pain, dizziness, or fainting) of possible heart disease.

Figure 1. A typical ECG beat

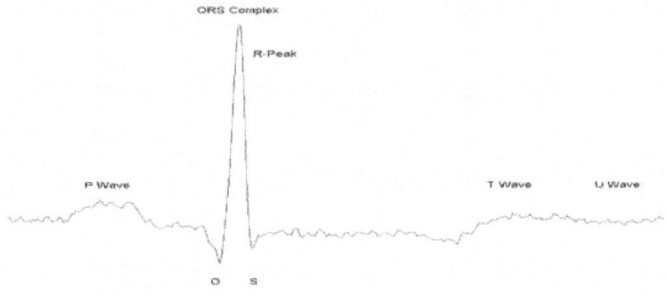

3.   Detecting poor blood flow to heart muscle (ischemia), which may indicate coronary artery disease.

4.   Monitoring the effectiveness of treatment (such as medication or a pacemaker or automatic defibrillator) for irregular heart rhythms.

Since ECG signal provides reliable information about the performance of the heart, the analysis of heart beat cycles in ECG signal is very important for long-term monitoring and diagnosis of patients' heart conditions in an intensive care unit or at patients' homes through a telemedicine network. However, it is very costly for the doctor to analyze the ECG records beat by beat since the ECG records may last for hours. Therefore, it is meaningful to develop some computer-assisted techniques to examine the ECG records and select only the abnormal beats for further analysis.

The problem at hand can be considered as a machine learning or data mining problem. Many algorithms have been applied to ECG beat cycle analysis, among which, neural networks are the most generally used model. Kohonen self-organizing maps were investigated in ECG beat recognition (Baig et al., 2001; Hu et al., 1997). Learning vector quantization was employed in Hu et al. (1997) and Baig et al. (2001). Stamkopoulos et al. (1998) proposed to detect ischemia using non-linear PCA neural networks. Guler and Ubeyh (2005) developed a combined multilayer perceptron neural network model for ECG beat classification. A survey of ECG pattern recognition based on nonlinear transformations and neural networks can be found in Maglaveras et al. (1998). There were also some attempts to incorporate fuzzy logic into the neural networks for ECG analysis (Engin, 2004; Osowski & Linh, 2001; Shyu et al., 2004). Recently, support vector machines, a new method emerging from the neural network research community, were introduced for ECG signal recognition (Millet-Roig et al., 2000; Osowski et al., 2004; Strauss et al., 2001).

One of the challenges faced by these ECG beat recognition algorithms is the large variation in the morphologies of ECG signals from different patients. The range of "normal beats" is different among the patients, which causes a so-called poor generalization problem; that is, a finely tuned ECG detector to the training data from a group of people may perform badly to the ECG beats of a new patient. Hu et al. (1997) attempted to solve this problem using a mixture of expert approaches. Such a mixture of expert structures was formed by combining the knowledge of a global expert trained using ECG data from a large database and a local expert trained using 3 to 5 minutes of ECG signals from a specific patient. When the mixture of expert systems was used to classify the ECG beats from the specific patient, the classification performance was improved compared to that based on the global expert. However, the major drawback of such an approach is that a local expert has to be constructed for each patient, and the

ECG records of each patient have to be annotated by a doctor in order to train the local expert, even with only 5 minutes of a patient's ECG recording. Such an annotation process is very costly and discourages the practical application of this approach. Another problem lies in the unbalanced data problem. In the scenario of long-term monitoring of heart patients, normal ECG beats usually dominate the ECG records. It takes a long time to collect sufficient and balanced normal and abnormal ECG data to construct a good local expert; otherwise, the local expert may suffer from the unbalanced data problem (Japkowicz & Stephen, 2002).

In this chapter, a kernel concept learning-based approach is proposed to solve such a generalization problem. One-class support vector classifier (v-SVC) (Scholkopf et al., 2001) is a concept learning model whose goal is to find a decision boundary to include patterns from one class (called targets) and exclude the patterns from the other classes (called outliers). A particular benefit of v-SVC is that it can be trained using only the data from one class. In the scenario of long-term monitoring of heart patients, the normal ECG beats usually dominate the ECG records; that is, the number of abnormal ECG beats is far less than that of the normal ones. Furthermore, there are many kinds of abnormal ECG beats corresponding to different cardiac diseases, such as atrial premature beats, ventricular escape beats, fusion of ventricular and normal beats, left bundle branch block beats, right bundle branch block beats, supraventricular premature or ectopic beats, premature ventricular contraction beats, and so on. Some of the typical abnormal beats and a normal ECG beat are illustrated in Figure 2. On one hand, these abnormal ECG beats appear differently in morphology. On the other hand, the normal ECG beats usually appear similar to each other and show less variation, which implies that the concept "normal" is more compact compared to that of the concept "abnormal" and thus easier to learn using few samples. Since normal ECG beats can be easily obtained from the patients, a v-SVC can be trained using only the normal ECG beats from each specific patient to learn the concept "normal." The trained v-SVC can then be used to detect from ECG records of the same patient and find "normal" ECG beats and thus detect the complementary abnormal beats. Such a kernel concept learning model can relieve the doctors from annotating the ECG beats from each patient beat by beat. Our experimental results using MIT/BIH arrhythmia ECG database (Massachusetts Institute of Technology, 1997) show that the patient-adaptable v-SVC, constructed using only hundreds of normal ECG beats from a specific patient, outperforms all the other classifiers trained using tens of thousands of data from a group of patients in detecting the abnormal ECG beats of the specific patient. This suggests that our approach has good potential for practical clinical application.

Figure 2. Eight samples of normal and abnormal ECG beats using data from MIT/BIH arrhythmia database (Massachusetts Institute of Technology, 1997)

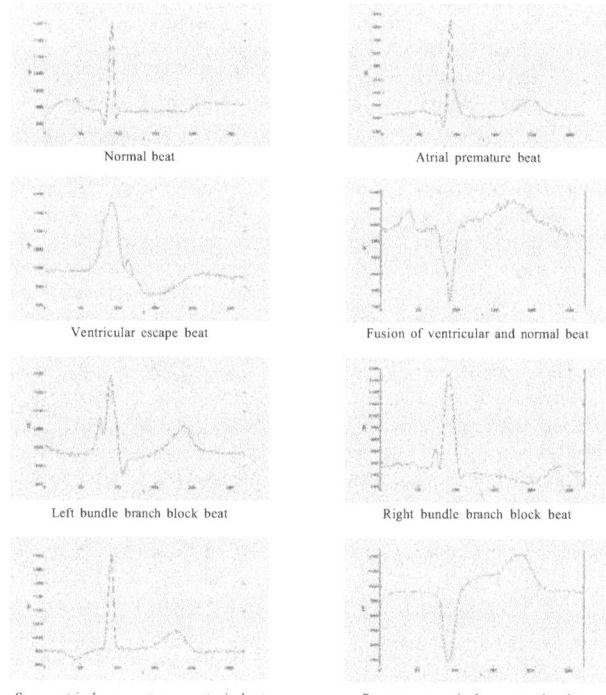

Normal beat

Atrial premature beat

Ventricular escape beat

Fusion of ventricular and normal beat

Left bundle branch block beat

Right bundle branch block beat

Supraventricular premature or ectopic beat

Premature ventricular contraction beat

Generalization Problem in ECG Beat Detection

A fundamental assumption in the field of pattern recognition is that the distribution of the training samples is the same as that of the test samples (Duda et al., 2001). However, such an assumption may not hold in practical applications. The abnormal ECG beat detection problem is one of such examples. Figure 3 illustrates the distribution of the first two principal components of the original 39 dimensional feature vectors of ECG beats obtained by using Karhunen-Loeve transform (principal component analysis—PCA) from 4 records of MIT/BIH arrhythmia ECG database, where the red asterisks indicate normal ECG beats, and the blue crosses are abnormal ones. Although some discriminative information may be lost using PCA, it can be observed that the distribution of "normal" ECG beats are different in each patient. We may even plot such data distribution of the whole database, but the difference of the ECG beats among patients still exists. This is the difference between the population and a specific patient. Although an ECG detector can be finely trained using the ECG beats from a large database which consists of the records of different patients, it may perform badly in detecting ECG beats of other patients not in the database. This is the so-called generalization problem.

Figure 3. Scatterplot of ECG data of six patients in MIT/BIH arrhythmia database showing the first two principal components of PCA projection

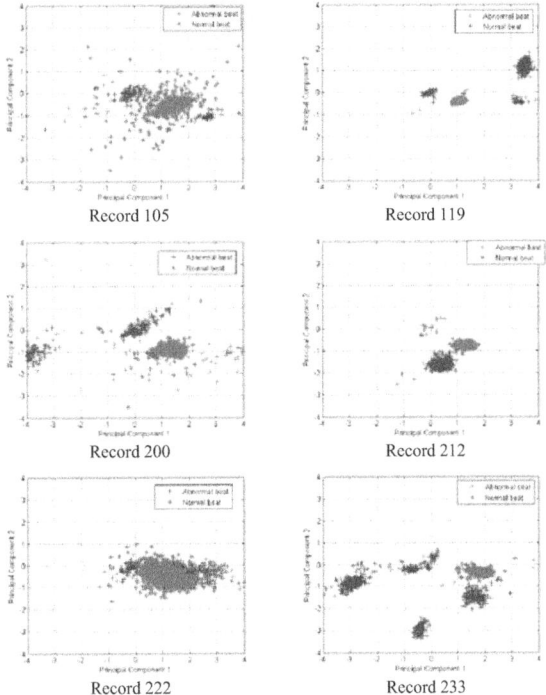

The solution of such generalization problem lies in the incorporation of local information of a specific patient to the ECG detector. Since the distribution of the training samples is not the same as that of the test samples, some information about the test samples has to be added to train the ECG detector properly. It is infeasible to ask the doctors to annotate the ECG beats directly from the specific patient to be used for training the classifier due to the high cost of the process (de Chazal et al., 2004; Hu et al., 1997), and also the unbalanced data problem usually exists in the training data. Therefore, a concept learning-based approach is proposed to construct a patient-adaptable abnormal ECG detector.

Concept Learning

Concept learning is also called one-class classification or novelty detection (Tax, 2001). The goal of concept learning is to find a descriptive model for a set of data. Different from classical binary classification, in concept learning, only data from one class (called the target) are used in the training stage, while no information is used about the other class (called the outliers). The philosophy behind concept learning is in agreement with the way human beings learn a concept. Suppose we expect to teach a child the concept of "tiger." We need to give him or her some examples of tigers and do not need to give the examples of non-"tiger," such as horse, elephant, or chicken. That is to say, people can learn a concept using only the examples of the target. Of course, the information about non-target or outliers is helpful to improve the discrimination between the target and non-target classes. However, using the examples from only the target class is sufficient to learn the concept of the target and recognize whether a new example belongs to the target or not.

One-Class Support Vector Classifier

One-class support vector classifier (v-SVC) is a kind of support vector machine (Scholkopf et al., 2001) which can be used as a concept learning tool. Given a set of target data $X = \{x_i \quad R^d \mid i = 1,2, \quad , \quad \}$, the goal of v-SVC is to find a decision function $f(x)$ such that most of the target data will have $f(x) \quad 0$ while most of the outliers will have $f(x) < 0$. It might be difficult to find such a decision function directly in the original space; therefore, the target data are mapped into a higher dimensional space called feature space $\phi(x)$ (illustrated in Figure 4) in which the dot product can be computed using some kernel function

Figure 4. Illustration of the kernel mapping of v-SVC

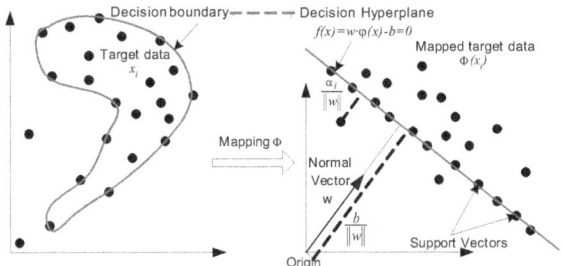

$$k(x_i, x_j) = \phi(x_i) \cdot \phi(x_j) \tag{1}$$

such as a Gaussian radial basis function (RBF) kernel

$$k(x_i, x_j) = e^{-\frac{\|x_i - x_j\|^2}{\sigma}} \tag{2}$$

where σ>0 is the width parameter of the Gaussian.

The mapped target data are separated from the origin with maximum margin using a hyperplane where the origin corresponds to the outliers. The hyperplane can be found by solving the following problem

$$\min_{w, \alpha_i, b} \frac{\|w\|^2}{2} + \frac{1}{vN} \sum_{i=1}^{N} \alpha_i - b \tag{3}$$

subject to

$$w \cdot \phi(x_i) - b + \alpha_i \geq 0, \; \alpha_i \geq 0, \; i = 1, 2, \cdots, N \tag{4}$$

where α_i is a slack variable, and $v \in (0,1]$ is a regularization parameter to control the effect of outliers and allows for target samples falling outside of the decision boundary (see Figure 4). The decision function corresponding to the hyperplane is

$$f(x) = w \cdot \phi(x) \cdot b \tag{5}$$

where w is a weight vector and b is a bias item, similar to those of the neural networks.

The function in (3) is called the objective function and in (4) are called inequality constraints. (3) and (4) form a constrained optimization problem, which is usually dealt with by introducing Lagrange multipliers $\alpha_i \geq 0$, $\beta_i \geq 0$, and a Lagrangian (Amari, 1998) for this can be written as

$$L(w, \alpha_i, b, \xi_i, \beta_i) = \frac{\|w\|^2}{2} + \frac{1}{N} \sum_{i=1}^{N} \alpha_i b - \sum_{i=1}^{N} \beta_i \xi_i - \sum_{i=1}^{N} \alpha_i (w \cdot \phi(x_i) \cdot b + \xi_i) \tag{6}$$

Setting the partial derivatives of Lagrangian with respect to w, ξ_i, and b to zero, the new constraints are

$$\sum_{i=1}^{N} \alpha_i = 1 \tag{7}$$

$$\frac{1}{N} - \alpha_i - \beta_i = 0 \tag{8}$$

$$w = \sum_{i=1}^{N} \alpha_i \phi(x_i) \tag{9}$$

Substituting (7-9) to the Lagrangian (6) and using kernel function (1), the dual problem is

$$\max \frac{1}{2} \sum_{i,j=1}^{N} \alpha_i \alpha_j k(x_i, x_j) \tag{10}$$

subject to

$$\sum_{i=1}^{N} \alpha_i = 1 \tag{11}$$

$$0 \leq \alpha_i = \frac{1}{N} \quad \alpha_i \quad \frac{1}{N} \tag{12}$$

This is a quadratic programming problem which can be solved using some standard algorithms such as sequential minimization optimization (Scholkopf et al., 2001).

The decision function in (5) can be reformulated as follows using (9) and kernel function (1)

$$f(x) = \sum_{i=1}^{N} \alpha_i (\langle \phi(x_i) \cdot \phi(x) \rangle) \quad b = \sum_{i=1}^{N} \alpha_i k(x_i, x) \quad b \tag{13}$$

At the optimal point, a set of conditions have to be satisfied, known as the Karush-Kuhn-Tucker (KKT) optimal conditions (Kuhn & Tucker, 1951). Exploiting the KKT conditions, the following three cases of α_is can be the result:

1. $\alpha_i = \frac{1}{N}$: $f(x_i) < 0$, the target data x_i is outside the decision hyperplane (incorrectly classified). Such a x_i is called bounded support vector (BSV).

2. $0 < \alpha_i < \frac{1}{N}$: $f(x_i) = 0$, the target data x_i is on the decision hyperplane. Such a x_i is called unbounded support vector (USV).

3. $\alpha_i = 0$: $f(x_i) > 0$, the target data x_i is inside the decision hyperplane (correctly classified).

All of the target data whose $\alpha_i > 0$ are called support vectors (SVs), including both BSVs and USVs. It can be observed from (13) that only support vectors contribute to the decision function. The number of support vectors is usually far less than that of the target samples. These support vectors can be regarded as a sparse representation or compact template of the whole target dataset. Given a new pattern, it is compared with the support vectors in the decision function (13). If the new pattern is from the targets, the decision function has a large positive value. If the new pattern is from the outlier class, it is different from the support vectors, and the decision function has a large negative value. The larger the value of the decision function, the more confident the decision. From these, we can see the great similarity between the support vector machines and neural networks.

At the optimal point, the constraints in (4) become equalities. Both $_i$ and $_i$ are in $(0, \frac{1}{N})$. The bias b can be recovered using one of such a USV $_k$ corresponding to the target sample x_k

$$b = w \quad (x_k) = \sum_{i=1}^{N} {}_i k(x_i, x_k) \tag{14}$$

Another kernel concept learning model is support vector data description (SVDD) (Tax & Duin, 1999). It is proved that when a RBF kernel (2) is used, SVDD is equivalent to v-SVC (Scholkopf et al., 2001; Tax, 2001). Therefore, only v-SVC is investigated in the current study.

Model Selection

Model selection for concept learning with v-SVC is still an open problem because only the data from one class is used in the training stage and no outlier is available. Some attempts have been made to select the model parameters of concept learning with v-SVC using only the information from the target data. For example, Tax proposed the use of consistency of the classifiers to select model parameters based on the error on the target class only (Tax & Muller, 2004). But this may be biased since no information of the outliers is used. Another solution is generating artificial outliers, uniformly distributed in a hypersphere or hypercube, which are used to estimate the outlier error (Tax & Duin, 2002). The latter is investigated in the current problem.

There are two hyperparameters to be tuned in v-SVC using RBF kernel, the width parameter in (2) and the regularization parameter v in (3). Let N_{SV} be the number of support vectors. Since the constraint in (11) is $\sum_{i=1}^{N} {}_i = 1$, and the upper bound of $_i$ in (12) is $\frac{1}{N}$, the following equation can be written

$$N_{SV} \frac{1}{N} \quad 1 \tag{15}$$

thus

$$\frac{N_{SV}}{N} \tag{16}$$

Obviously, v is the upper bound of the fraction of support vectors among all the target data. This observation can help to select the value of v. The larger the value of v, the more target samples will be excluded from the decision boundary, and this leads to larger error of the target class. Therefore, the value of v cannot be very large. Here it is fixed as 0.01, which means the training error of the target class cannot be larger than 1%.

The value of   can be selected using an artificial validation set (Tax & Duin, 2002). Given a set of target samples, some outlier samples are generated randomly with the assumption that the outliers are uniformly distributed around the target class. The union of targets and generated outliers is used as a validation

Figure 5. Flowchart of the proposed framework for abnormal ECG beat detection

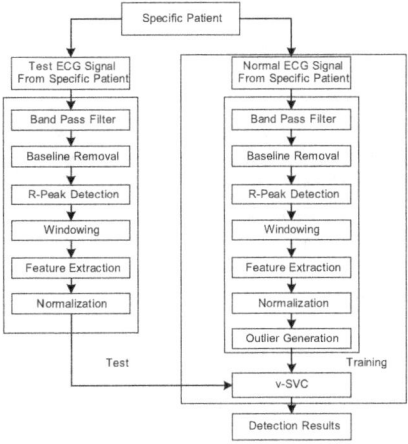

set. The value of   is chosen so that the error of both target class and outlier class on the validation set is minimized.

The selection of   depends on the distribution of the generated outliers. From Figure 3, it is observed that the normal ECG data are usually in the center of the feature space, and the abnormal ones are distributed around the normal data. Therefore, the assumption of uniformly distributed outliers approximately holds, which is demonstrated in the experimental results.

Proposed Framework

Figure 5 illustrates the flowchart of the proposed framework for ECG beat detection. The details are as follows.

ECG Signal Preprocessing

The ECG signal is usually coupled with noise and baseline shift due to power line interference, respiration and muscle tremors, and so forth, which have to be removed in favor of further analysis. The ECG signal is first processed using two averaging filters (Christov, 2004):

1. *Electromyogram noise suppression:* averages samples in an interval of 28 ms.
2. *Power line interference suppression:* averages samples in a period of the interference frequency of the power line.

The baseline of the ECG signal can be obtained using two consecutive median filters to the ECG signal after noise suppression whose widths are 200ms and 600ms, respectively (de Chazal et al., 2004). The baseline is subtracted from the original signal, and the resulted signal is then baseline-corrected.

After noise suppression and baseline correction, the R-peak of the ECG signal can be detected using the first derivative of the ECG signal (Christov, 2004), which is used in the following process.

Feature Extraction

Many features have been proposed for ECG beat recognition, such as time domain representation (Hu et al., 1997), heartbeat interval features (de Chazal et al., 2004), Hermite functions (Gopalakrishnan et al., 2004), autoregressive modeling-based representation (Zhang et al., 2004), and wavelet transform-based representation (Engin, 2004; Millet-Roig et al., 2000; Shyu et al., 2004). Here we investigate the use of raw amplitude of the time domain ECG signals after noise suppression and baseline shift removal as feature vectors to represent the ECG beats. After the R-peak is found, the ECG signal in a window of 550 ms is taken as an ECG beat. The lengths of the signal before and after the R-peak in each beat are 140 ms and 410 ms, respectively, such that the window covers most of the characterization of the ECG beat. The signal in each window is then down-sampled uniformly to form a feature vector of 38-dimensions. It has been shown that R-R interval (the interval between two consecutive R-peaks) (de Chazal et al., 2004; Hu et al., 1997) is useful in recognition of some abnormal ECG beats. Therefore, it is also used in this study by appending it to the 38-dimensional feature vector. The length of the feature vector to represent the ECG beat is then 39.

There are some variations in the amplitude ranges of ECG signals among human beings, which imply that a normalization procedure is necessary to the ECG feature vectors. The feature vectors are then divided by the mean value of R peaks in the training data of each patient, such that the maximum amplitude in each ECG beat window is around 1. The normalized ECG feature vectors are then used.

Learning the Concept Normal for Abnormal ECG Beat Detection

In order to detect abnormal beats from the long-term ECG records of a patient, an abnormal ECG beat detector can be constructed using v-SVC based on a short period of the normal ECG beats from the same patient such that the model can learn the concept of "normal" beat of the patient. A new ECG beat can be classified to the "normal" class or non-"normal" class by the trained v-SVC. The abnormal ECG beats are thus annotated automatically for the doctors for further review.

Experimental Results and Discussions

An experiment is conducted using MIT/BIH arrhythmia ECG database to demonstrate the feasibility of the proposed patient-adaptable concept learning approach. The details of the experiment are as follows.

Data Preparation

MIT/BIH arrhythmia ECG database consists of 48 annotated records from 47 patients, and each record is about 30 minutes in length. The labels in the annotation file made by cardiologists are used as the ground truth in training and evaluating the classifiers. The ECG beats labeled as "normal" (NOR) are taken as the target class whose number in the database is more than 70,000. All of the other beats are regarded as outlier class or "abnormal" class, including atrial premature beats, nodal premature beats, ventricular escape beats, fusion of ventricular and normal beats, and so forth, which totals around 30,000.

Table 1. Classification performance of the classifiers in each recording of the test set

Record #	Number of Beats			v-SVC				LSVC			
	Abnormal	Normal	Total	TP	FN	FP	TN	TP	FN	FP	TN
100	30	1862	1892	24	6	75	1787	28	2	440	1422
103	8	1731	1739	8	0	484	1247	6	2	17	1714
105	141	2098	2239	141	0	261	1837	130	11	1362	736
113	5	1488	1493	5	0	20	1468	5	0	47	1441
117	4	1275	1279	4	0	442	833	3	1	267	1008
119	448	1294	1742	448	0	52	1242	333	115	37	1257
121	12	1548	1560	11	1	202	1346	12	0	824	724
123	3	1259	1262	3	0	60	1199	3	0	2	1257
200	891	1432	2323	854	37	25	1407	828	63	69	1363
202	78	1707	1785	78	0	1399	308	75	3	807	900
210	223	2011	2234	218	5	127	1884	206	17	355	1656
212	1507	792	2299	1506	1	47	745	1396	111	64	728
213	530	2212	2742	430	100	144	2068	237	293	3	2209
215	161	2669	2830	160	1	4	2665	95	66	6	2663
219	212	1711	1923	205	7	129	1582	186	26	79	1632
221	348	1700	2048	348	0	70	1630	345	3	176	1524
222	539	1629	2168	429	110	752	877	207	332	649	980
228	362	1419	1781	314	48	0	1419	329	33	83	1336
230	177	1875	2052	177	0	18	1857	174	3	21	1854
231	1370	302	1672	1370	0	24	278	770	600	0	302
233	758	1865	2623	752	6	39	1826	683	75	115	1750
234	63	2237	2300	62	1	42	2195	39	24	9	2228
Total	7870	36116	43986	7547	323	4416	31700	6090	1780	5432	30684

Four records (102, 104, 107, and 217), including paced beats, are excluded from the study in compliance with the standards recommended for reporting performance results of cardiac rhythms by the Association for the Advancement of Medical Instrumentation (AAMI) (Mark & Wallen, 1987). Among the remaining 44 records, 22 records are used to train classical binary classifiers, including SVMs and other neural networks for comparison with the concept learning method. They are records 101, 106, 108, 109, 111, 112, 114, 115, 116, 118, 122, 124, 201, 203, 205, 207, 208, 209, 214, 220, 223, and 230. This dataset is called DB1. The other 22 records are split into two parts. The normal ECG beats in the first one sixth of each of the 22 records (Table 1) (each about 300 beats) are used as the training set to construct the v-SVCs. These data form DB2. The remaining five sixth of each of the 22 records is used as a test set to evaluate the performance of the v-SVCs and the binary classifiers trained on the other 22 ECG records. Such a dataset is called DB3. The 22 records in Table 1 are selected so that most of the ECG beats are normal, which is appropriate to simulate the real ECG records captured in a long-term monitoring scenario.

The original signals in the MIT/BIH arrhythmia database are two-leads, sampled at 360 Hz. The ECG signal of Lead 1 is used in this study. The ECG signals are processed following the procedure described in the previous section. Each ECG beat is represented by a 39-D feature vector.

Evaluating Criteria

Table 2 illustrates the full classification matrix for calculating the evaluating criteria, including true positives (TP), true negatives (TN), false positives (FP), and false negatives (FN). The criteria used to evaluate the performance of ECG beat classification include sensitivity, specificity, and balanced classification rate. Sensitivity (SEN) is the fraction of abnormal ECG beats that are correctly detected among all the abnormal ECG beats.

$$SEN = \frac{TP}{TP+FN} \tag{17}$$

Table 2. Full classification matrix for calculating the evaluation measure

Ground Truth	Classification Results	
	Abnormal	Normal
Abnormal	True Positive (TP)	False Negative (FN)
Normal	False Positive (FP)	Truth Negative (TN)

Specificity (SPE) is the fraction of normal ECG beats that are correctly classified among all the normal ECG beats.

$$SPE = \frac{TN}{TN+FP} \tag{18}$$

The generally used average classification rate (ACR) is the fraction of all correctly classified ECG beats, regardless of normal or abnormal among all the ECG beats.

$$ACR = \frac{TP+TN}{TP+TN+FP+FN} \tag{19}$$

As mentioned in the previous section, the "normal" class dominates the test set. Commonly used average classification rate is not valid in such an imbalanced dataset. For example, if a classifier is trained to classify all the test data as normal beats, it has SPE = 100% and SEN = 0%, but the ACR is still high because the number of abnormal beats is too small. Therefore, another evaluation measure is used in this study, balanced classification rate (BCR). BCR is the average value of SEN and SPE.

$$BCR = \frac{SEN+SPE}{2} \tag{20}$$

Only when both SEN and SPE have large values can BCR have a large value. Therefore, the use of BCR can have a balanced performance in the evaluation of the classifiers which favor both lower false positives and false negatives. This measure is more suitable for the current study than ACR.

Training Global Binary Classifiers for Comparison

A set of commonly used binary classifiers are trained using 22 ECG records outside the test records to compare with the proposed concept learning method. The training set DB1 consists of 31,069 "normal" beats and 19,661 "abnormal" beats. There are some classifiers that have problems with training using such a large database; therefore, a smaller subset of these training sets is formed by randomly selecting 4,000 "normal" beats and 4,000 "abnormal" beats, called DB11. A Matlab toolbox called PRTOOLS (Duin et al., 2004) is used in our experiment to construct most of these classifiers otherwise mentioned. The classifiers include:

1. *Linear Bayes normal classifier (LDC):* The linear classifier between the two classes by assuming normal densities with equal covariance matrices.

2. *Quadratic Bayes normal classifier (QDC):* The quadratic classifier between the two classes by assuming normal densities.

3. *Nearest mean classifier (NMC):* The nearest mean classifier between the two classes. The test pattern is classified so the class whose mean value is closer to the test pattern in the feature space.

4. *Backpropagation feedforward neural network classifier (BNN):* A feedforward neural network classifier with m units in a hidden layer, the training is stopped after l epochs. The hyperparameters m and l are optimized using 5-fold cross validation on the training set. The optimal values in DB1 are $m = 44$ and $l = 2000$, respectively.

5. *Binary support vector machines:* Including a linear SVM (LSVC) and a SVM with RBF kernel (RSVC). LIBSVM is used in this study (Chang & Lin, 2001). The hyperparameters are similar to v-SVC, which are optimized using 5-fold cross validation on the training set. SVMs have problem to deal with large training dataset (Cristianini & Shawe-Taylor, 2000). So the compact subset DB11 (8,000 ECG beats) is used for training SVMs. The hyperparameters are optimized using 5-fold cross validation on the training set DB11. The optimal values are regularization parameter $C = 4096$ for LSVC and $C = 16$, $= 0.7$ for RSVC.

The classification results of using these binary classifiers trained on the large dataset and the v-SVC trained using only "normal" ECG beats from the specific patient are illustrated in Table 3. The results are averaged over 22 test ECG records. In accordance with AAMI recommendations to present the results

Table 3. Comparison of abnormal ECG beat detection using v-SVC trained with only normal data from the specific patient and the binary classifiers trained with large database excluding the specific patient

Classifier	v-SVC	LSVC	RSVC	LDC	QDC	NMC	BNN
BCR	0.917	0.840	0.814	0.833	0.773	0.730	0.838
SPE	0.958	0.823	0.819	0.822	0.696	0.494	0.766
SEN	0.876	0.856	0.808	0.844	0.850	0.965	0.909
ACR	0.883	0.831	0.803	0.828	0.845	0.883	0.851

tape-by-tape, the classification results of *v*-SVC and the best binary classifier LSVC of each record are shown in Table 1.

Discussions

From Table 3, it can be observed that the patient-adaptable concept learning model, *v*-SVC trained on DB2, outperforms all the binary classifiers trained using large database DB1 excluding the specific patient to be tested. The best binary classifier is LSVC and BNN whose BCRs are about 84%. The BCR of *v*-SVC is about 92%, which is much greater than all of the binary classifiers. It indicates that the local information is very important in the classification of the ECG beats from a specific patient. The incorporation of such local information can help deal with the gap between the distribution of training dataset and test dataset, which helps to improve the generalization.

Another observation is that it seems that the linear classifier shows better performance than those of the non-linear classifier. RBF SVM is usually superior to Linear SVM in the classification. However, in Table 3, the linear SVM outperforms RBF SVM. This is caused by the difference of training dataset and test dataset. RBF SVM can produce a more flexible decision boundary than linear SVM. Since it is tuned to fit to the training set, it cannot generalize well in the test set due to the difference between the two datasets. On the other hand, the linear SVM shows more robustness although it produces larger error in the training set. Therefore, the proposed concept learning method is suitable to solve the problem at hand.

The performance of *v*-SVC varies among the 22 test sets. The *v*-SVC model performs well in most of these test sets. Only in some of them, it does not perform well. For example, the BCR in record 222 is only about 67%. Figure 3 illustrates the data distribution of this record. It shows that the "normal" ECG beats and "abnormal" beats overlap greatly in these two records. In this case, even the optimal Bayesian classifier may produce a large error rate. More efficient features are needed to further improve the classification between the two classes, which is our future work.

The classification results in Table 2 and Table 3 show that the features used are quite efficient in discriminating abnormal ECG beats from those of the normal ones. Compared to other features, such as heartbeat interval features (de Chazal et al., 2004), Hermite functions (Gopalakrishnan et al., 2004), autoregressive modeling-based representation (Zhang et al., 2004), and wavelet transform-based representation (Engin, 2004; Millet-Roig et al., 2000; Shyu et al., 2004), the currently used features are simpler to implement because only R-peak of each

ECG beat needs to be detected to extract these features and no further detection such as QRS detection or other transform is necessary anymore. Therefore, its computation complexity is far less than those of the other features.

Hu et al. (1997) concentrated on the classification of normal beats and ventricular ectopic beats using a mixture of two classifiers. The sensitivity and specificity achieved are 82.6% and 97.1%, which means its BCR is about 90%. De Chazal et al. (2004) have claimed that they achieved comparable performance to the method of Hu's using a linear discriminant classifier. Our concept learning-based method achieved a balanced classification rate of 92% although only some "normal" ECG beats from each patient are used to train the v-SVC model. Furthermore, the data records including the test data and the training data of v-SVC are seriously unbalanced. Hu et al. (1997) and de Chazal et al. (2004)'s methods have problems in training a good classifier in such cases. Therefore, our proposed method shows better or at least comparable performance compared to Hu et al. (1997) and de Chazal et al. (2004). Another advantage of our method is that it can relieve the doctors from annotating the ECG beats one by one as needed in Hu et al. (1997), and it is easier to be constructed to adapt to the specific patient.

Conclusion

In this chapter, a new concept learning-based approach is proposed to detect abnormal ECG beats for long-term monitoring of heart patients. A kernel concept learning model, v-SVC, can be trained to extract the concept "normal" using only some "normal" ECG beats from a patient, which can then be used to detect "abnormal" ECG beats in long-term ECG records of the same patient. Such an approach can relieve doctors from annotating the training ECG data beat by beat and also addresses the generalization problem in ECG signal classification among patients. Experiments were conducted using 44 ECG records of MIT/BIH arrhythmia database. The experimental results demonstrate the good performance of our proposed concept learning method and suggest its potential for practical clinical application.

Acknowledgment

The authors wish to acknowledge the support by Distributed Diagnosis and Home Healthcare project (D2H2) under Singapore-University of Washington

Alliance (SUWA) Program and Biomedical Engineering Research Center at Nanyang Technological University in Singapore. Also, the first author would like to express gratitude for the research scholarship from the School of Electrical and Electronic Engineering, Nanyang Technological University, Singapore.

References

Amari, S. I. (1998). Natural gradient works efficiently in learning. *Neural Computation, 10*(2), 251-276.

Baig, M. H., Rasool, A., & Bhatti, M. I. (2001, October). Classification of electrocardiogram using SOM, LVQ and beat detection methods in localization of cardiac arrhythmias. *Proceedings of the 23rd Annual International Conference of the IEEE Engineering in Medicine and Biology Society, 2*, 1684-1687.

Chang, C. C., & Lin, C. J. (2001). *LIBSVM: A library for support vector machines.* Retrieved October 7, 2005, from http://www.csie.ntu.edu.tw/~cjlin/libsvm

Christov, I. (2004). Real time electrocardiogram QRS detection using combined adaptive threshold. *BioMedical Engineering Online, 3.* Retrieved October 7, 2005, from http://www.biomedical-engineering-online.com/content/3/1/28

Cristianini, N., & Shawe-Taylor, J. (2000). *An introduction to support vector machines.* New York: Cambridge University Press.

de Chazal, P., O'Dwyer, M., & Reilly, R. B. (2004). Automatic classification of heartbeats using ECG morphology and heartbeat interval features. *IEEE Transactions on Biomedical Engineering, 51*, 1196-1206.

Duda, R. O., Hart, P. E., & Stork, D. G. (2001). *Pattern classification* (2nd ed.). New York: John Wiley & Sons.

Duin, R. P. W., Juszczak, P., Paclik, P., Pekalska E., de Ridder, D., & Tax, D. M. J. (2004). *PRTools4, A Matlab Toolbox for pattern recognition.* Delft University of Technology. Retrieved October 7, 2005, from http://www.prtools.org/

Engin, M. (2004). ECG beat classification using neuro-fuzzy network. *Pattern Recognition Letters, 25*, 1715-1722.

Gopalakrishnan, R., Acharya, S., & Mugler, D. H. (2004, April). Automated diagnosis of ischemic heart disease using dilated discrete Hermite functions. *Proceedings of the IEEE 30th Annual Northeast Bioengineering Conference* (pp. 97-98).

Guler, I., & Ubeyh, E. D. (2005). ECG beat classifier designed by combined neural network model. *Pattern Recognition, 38*, 199-208.

Hu, Y. H., Palreddy, S., & Tompkins, W.J. (1997). A patient-adaptable ECG beat classifier using a mixture of experts approach. *IEEE Transactions on Biomedical Engineering, 44*, 891-900.

Japkowicz, N., & Stephen, S. (2002). The class imbalance problem: A systematic study. *Intelligent Data Analysis, 6*, 429-450.

Kuhn, H. W., & Tucker A. W. (1951). Nonlinear programming. *Proceedings of the 2nd Berkeley Symposium on Mathematical Statistics and Probabilistics, 481-492*

Maglaveras, N., Stamkopoulos, T., Diamantaras, K., Pappas, C., & Strintzis. M. (1998). ECG pattern recognition and classification using non-linear transformations and neural networks: A review. *International Journal of Medical Informatics, 52*, 191-208.

Mark, R., & Wallen, R. (1987). *AAMI-recommended practice: Testing and reporting performance results of ventricular arrhythmia detection algorithms.* Association for the Advancement of Medical Instrumentation, Arrhythmia Monitoring Subcommittee. AAMI ECAR-1987.

Massachusetts Institute of Technology. (1997). *MIT-BIH Arrhythmia database.* Retrieved October 7, 2005, from http://ecg.mit.edu/

Millet-Roig, J., Ventura-Galiano, R., Chorro-Gasco, F.J., & Cebrian, A. (2000). Support vector machine for arrhythmia discrimination with wavelet-transform-based feature selection. *Computers in Cardiology, 28*, 407-410.

Osowski, S., Hoai, L. T., & Markiewicz, T. (2004). Support vector machine-based expert system for reliable heartbeat recognition. *IEEE Transactions on Biomedical Engineering, 51*, 582-589.

Osowski, S., & Linh, T. H. (2001). ECG beat recognition using fuzzy hybrid neural network. *IEEE Transactions on Biomedical Engineering, 48*, 1265-1271.

Scholkopf, B., Platt, J. C., Shawe-Taylor J., Smola, A. J., & Williamson, R. C. (2001). Estimating the support of a high-dimensional distribution. *Neural Computation, 13*, 1443-1471.

Shyu, L. Y., Wu, Y. H., & Hu, W. (2004). Using wavelet transform and fuzzy neural network for VPC detection from the holter ECG. *IEEE Transactions on Biomedical Engineering, 51*, 1269-1273.

Stamkopoulos, T., Diamantaras, K., Maglaveras, N., & Strintzis, M. (1998). ECG analysis using nonlinear PCA neural networks for ischemia detection. *IEEE Transactions on Signal Processing, 46*, 3058-3067.

Strauss, D., Steidl, G., & Jung, J. (2001). Arrhythmia detection using signal-adapted wavelet preprocessing for support vector machines. *Computers in Cardiology, 28,* 497-501.

Tax, D. M. J. (2001). *One-class classification: Concept-learning in the absence of counter-examples.* ASCI Dissertation Series, Delft University of Technology. Retrieved October 7, 2005, from http://www.ph.tn.tudelft.nl/~davidt/thesis.pdf

Tax, D. M. J., & Duin, R. P. W. (1999). Support vector data description. *Pattern Recognition Letters, 20*(11-13), 1191-1199.

Tax, D. M. J., & Duin, R. P. W. (2002). Uniform object generation for optimizing one-class classifiers. *Journal of Machine Learning Research, 2,* 155-173. Retrieved October 7, 2005, from http://www.ingentaselect.com/rpsv/cgi-bin/cgi?body=linker&reqidx=1532-4435(2002)2:2L.155

Tax, D. M. J., & Muller, K. R. (2004, August). A consistency-based model selection for one-class classification. *Proceedings of the 17th International Conference on Pattern Recognition (ICPR),* Cambridge, UK.

Yanowitz, F. G. (2003). *The Alan E. Lindsay ECG Learning Center.* Retrieved October 7, 2005, from http://medlib.med.utah.edu/kw/ecg/

Zhang, Z. G., Jiang, H. Z., Ge, D. F., & Xiang, X. J. (2004, June). Pattern recognition of cardiac arrhythmias using scalar autoregressive modeling. *Proceedings of the Fifth World Congress on Intelligent Control and Automation (WCICA 2004), 6,* 5545-5548.

Section III

Electromyography

Chapter VI

A Recurrent Probabilistic Neural Network for EMG Pattern Recognition

Toshio Tsuji, Hiroshima University, Japan

Nan Bu, Hiroshima University, Japan

Osamu Fukuda, National Institute of Advanced Industrial
Science and Technology, Japan

Abstract

In the field of pattern recognition, probabilistic neural networks (PNNs) have been proven as an important classifier. For pattern recognition of EMG signals, the characteristics usually used are: (1) amplitude, (2) frequency, and (3) space. However, significant temporal characteristic exists in the transient and non-stationary EMG signals, which cannot be considered by traditional PNNs. In this article, a recurrent PNN, called recurrent log-linearized Gaussian mixture network (R-LLGMN), is introduced for EMG pattern recognition, with the emphasis on utilizing temporal characteristics. The structure of R-LLGMN is based on the algorithm of a hidden Markov model (HMM), which is a routinely used technique for modeling stochastic time series. Since R-LLGMN inherits advantages from both HMM and neural computation, it is expected to have higher representation ability and show better performance when dealing with time series like EMG signals. Experimental results show that R-LLGMN can achieve high discriminant accuracy in EMG pattern recognition.

Introduction

Electromyographic (EMG) signals provide information about neuromuscular activities and have been recognized as efficient and promising resources for human-machine interface (HMI) used for the rehabilitation of people with mobility limitations and those with severe neuromuscular impairment. Typically, a pattern recognition process is applied to *translate* EMG signals into control commands for the HMIs, such as powered prostheses and functional electrical stimulation devices (Englehart et al., 2001; Fukuda et al., 2003; Hudgins et al., 1993; Lusted & Knapp, 1996). Generally speaking, a successful EMG pattern recognition technique relies on two principle elements: a pattern classifier with reliable discrimination accuracy and efficient representation of EMG feature characteristics.

Probabilistic neural networks (PNNs) developed in the field of pattern recognition make a decision according to the probability density distribution of patterns in the feature space (Specht, 1990; Tsuji et al., 1999). Since PNNs integrate statistical models into the neural networks' architecture as prior knowledge, outstanding performance has been reported. Recently, PNNs have become widely accepted as important classifiers and have been proven to be efficient, especially for complicated problems such as pattern recognition of bioelectric signals.

For EMG pattern recognition using PNNs, the feature characteristics usually used include: (1) amplitude, (2) frequency, and (3) spatial information from multiple channels of EMG signals. However, significant temporal characteristics exist in the transient and non-stationary EMG signals, which cannot be considered by the traditional PNNs based on static stochastic models, and, in some cases, temporal characteristics could be the only clues for reliable recognition.

This chapter introduces a recurrent PNN called recurrent log-linearized Gaussian mixture network (R-LLGMN) (Tsuji et al., 2003) into EMG pattern recognition, with emphasis on utilizing temporal characteristics. The structure of R-LLGMN is based on the hidden Markov model (HMM) algorithm, which is a routinely used technique for modeling stochastic time series. Since R-LLGMN inherits the advantages from both HMM and neural computation, it is expected to have higher representation ability and exhibit better classification performance when dealing with time series like EMG signals.

After a review of the literature, the structure and algorithm of R-LLGMN are explained. The proposed EMG pattern recognition method using R-LLGMN is then described, and experiments on filtered EMG and raw EMG signals are presented. Based on the experimental results, the possibility of applying the proposed method to practical human interface control is discussed. The final section offers some concluding remarks.

Background

Up to now, many techniques have been developed for EMG pattern recognition using statistical methods and neural networks (NNs). Kang et al. (1995) proposed a maximum likelihood method (MLM) based on Mahalanobis distances between input pattern and the prototypes, and the Bayes decision rule is applied in this method. A traditional linear discriminant analysis (LDA) classifier is used in an EMG classification scheme for multifunction myoelectric control (Englehart et al., 2001).

Due to NNs' learning capability of finding near-optimum functional relationships between the class memberships and the EMG patterns, several NN-based EMG pattern recognition methods have been presented. For example, Hiraiwa et al. (1989) used a multilayer perceptron (MLP) NN to perform pattern discrimination of five finger motions. Kelly et al. (1990) applied an MLP to classify four arm functions. Hudgins et al. (1993) devised a control system for powered upper-limb prostheses using a set of time-domain features extracted from EMG signals and a simple MLP as a classifier. Also, similar studies have been developed using MLPs to classify EMG features, such as autoregressive (AR) parameters (Lamounier et al., 2002) and features of filtered EMG signals (Tsuji et al., 1993). However, several factors have hindered the extension of MLP classifiers for other applications, such as the choice of network structure, slow learning convergence, the need for a large amount of training data, and local minima.

To tackle these problems, numerous attempts have been made by the pattern recognition community to integrate statistical models, as prior knowledge, into the classifier's architecture, to take advantage of both statistical classification methods and neural computation. Consequently, probabilistic neural networks

(PNNs) have been developed for pattern recognition (Specht, 1990; Zhang, 2000). In particular, Tsuji et al. (1999) proposed a feedforward PNN, a log-linearized Gaussian mixture network (LLGMN), which is based on the Gaussian mixture model (GMM) and a log-linear model. Although weights of the LLGMN correspond to a non-linear combination of the GMM parameters, such as mixture coefficients, mean vectors, and covariance matrices, constraints on the parameters in the statistical model are relieved in the LLGMN. Therefore, a simple backpropagation-like learning algorithm can be derived, and the parameters of LLGMN are trained according to a criterion of maximum likelihood (ML). The LLGMN has been successfully applied to EMG pattern recognition, where eight motions of the forearm have been classified using EMG signals measured by several pairs of electrodes (Fukuda et al., 2003). Also, the LLGMN has been further used to develop interface applications like prosthetic devices and EMG-based pointing devices (Fukuda et al., 1997, 1999; Fukuda et al., 2003).

However, since the GMM is a *static* stochastic model, it cannot make efficient use of temporal (time-varying) characteristics in EMG signals. Generally, pattern recognition using LLGMN is made under the assumption that feature patterns are stationary or change very slowly. EMG signals, in fact, are non-stationary and vary significantly in amplitude and frequency, even in the space domain. Due to the complicated nature of EMG signals, it is widely accepted that the temporal characteristic contains information important for pattern recognition (Englehart et al., 1999).

In order to cope with the time-varying characteristics of EMG signals, a pattern recognition method using an MLP classifier and a neural filter (NF) was applied (Tsuji et al., 2000). Continuous motions by the operators can be discriminated with sufficient accuracy even using the non-stationary time series of EMG signals. In addition to improving the classifiers, time-frequency representations of EMG signals have been adopted to gain a high level of discrimination accuracy (Englehart et al., 1999, 2001; Hussein & Granat, 2002). Although these methods can generate sufficient discrimination accuracy, there may be some criticism due to more complicated signal processing required or more intricate structure of classifiers. Also more parameters in the algorithm(s) of the signal processing and/or the classifier need to be determined by the user. Optimization of the whole pattern recognition method is almost impossible, and it is hard to gain a high performance of discrimination, especially in practical applications.

The present study focuses on the classifier aspect of EMG pattern recognition and introduces a recurrent PNN to improve discrimination accuracy when dealing with non-stationary EMG signals.

A Recurrent Probabilistic
Neural Network

The recurrent PNN, R-LLGMN (Tsuji et al., 2003), is based on the algorithm of continuous density hidden Markov model (CDHMM), which is a combination of the GMM and the HMM (Rabiner, 1989). The probability density function (pdf) of input patterns is estimated using GMM; HMM is used simultaneously to model the time-varying characteristics in stochastic time series. In the R-LLGMN, recurrent connections are incorporated into the network structure to make efficient use of the time-varying characteristics of EMG signals. With the weight coefficients well trained using a learning scheme of the backpropagation through time (BPTT) algorithm, R-LLGMN can calculate posterior probabilities of the discriminating classes.

HMM-Based Dynamic Probabilistic Model

First, let us consider a dynamic probabilistic model, as shown in Figure 1. There are C classes in this model, and each class c ($c \in \{1, \cdots, C\}$) is composed of K_c states. Suppose that, for the given time series $\tilde{\mathbf{x}} = \mathbf{x}(1), \mathbf{x}(2), \cdots, \mathbf{x}(T)$ ($\mathbf{x}(t) \in \Re^d$), at any time $\mathbf{x}(t)$ must occur from one state k of class c in the model. With this model, the posterior probability for class c, $P(c \mid \tilde{\mathbf{x}})$, is calculated as

$$P(c \mid \tilde{\mathbf{x}}) = \sum_{k=1}^{K_c} P(c, k \mid \tilde{\mathbf{x}}) = \sum_{k=1}^{K_c} \frac{\alpha_k^c(T)}{\sum_{c'=1}^{C} \sum_{k'=1}^{K_{c'}} \alpha_{k'}^{c'}(T)}. \tag{1}$$

Here, $\alpha_k^c(T)$ is the forward variable, which is defined as the probability for time series $(\mathbf{x}(1), \mathbf{x}(2), \cdots, \mathbf{x}(T))$ to be generated from class c, and vector $\mathbf{x}(T)$ occurs from state k in class c. According to the forward algorithm (Rabiner, 1989), it can be derived as

$$\alpha_k^c(1) = \pi_k^c b_k^c(\mathbf{x}(1)), \tag{2}$$

$$\alpha_k^c(t) = \sum_{k'=1}^{K_c} \alpha_{k'}^c(t-1) \gamma_{k',k}^c b_k^c(\mathbf{x}(t)) \quad (1 < t \le T), \tag{3}$$

Figure 1. HMM-based dynamic probabilistic model with C classes and K_c states in class c

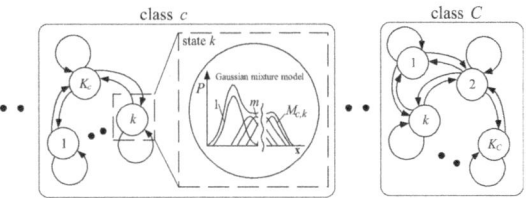

where $\gamma_{k',k}^{c}$ is the probability of the state changing from k' to k in class c, and $b_k^c(\mathbf{x}(t))$ is defined as the posterior probability for state k in class c corresponding to $\mathbf{x}(t)$. Also, the prior probability π_k^c is equal to $P(c,k)|_{t=0}$.

In this model, the posterior probability $b_k^c(\mathbf{x}(t))$ is approximated by summing up $M_{c,k}$ components of a Gaussian mixture distribution, and $\gamma_{k',k}^c b_k^c(\mathbf{x}(t))$ on the right side of (3) is derived in the form

$$
\begin{aligned}
\gamma_{k',k}^{c} b_k^c(\mathbf{x}(t)) &= \sum_{m=1}^{M_{c,k}} \gamma_{k',k}^{c} r_{c,k,m} g(\mathbf{x}(t); \boldsymbol{\mu}^{(c,k,m)}, \Sigma^{(c,k,m)}) \\
&= \sum_{m=1}^{M_{c,k}} \gamma_{k',k}^{c} r_{c,k,m} (2\pi)^{-\frac{d}{2}} \left| \Sigma^{(c,k,m)} \right|^{-\frac{1}{2}} \exp\Bigg[-\frac{1}{2} \sum_{j=1}^{d} \sum_{l=1}^{j} (2-\delta_{jl}) s_{jl}^{(c,k,m)} x_j(t) x_l(t) \\
&\quad + \sum_{j=1}^{d} \sum_{l=1}^{d} s_{jl}^{(c,k,m)} \mu_j^{(c,k,m)} x_l(t) - \frac{1}{2} \sum_{j=1}^{d} \sum_{l=1}^{d} s_{jl}^{(c,k,m)} \mu_j^{(c,k,m)} \mu_l^{(c,k,m)} \Bigg],
\end{aligned}
\tag{4}
$$

where $r^{(c,k,m)}$, $\boldsymbol{\mu}^{(c,k,m)} = (\mu_1^{(c,k,m)}, \cdots, \mu_d^{(c,k,m)})^{\mathrm{T}}$, $\Sigma^{(c,k,m)} \in \Re^{d \times d}$, $s_{jl}^{(c,k,m)}$ and $x_j(t)$ stands for the mixing proportion, the mean vector, the covariance matrix of each component $\{c,k,m\}$, the element of the inverse of covariance matrix $\Sigma^{(c,m,k)-1}$, and the element of $\mathbf{x}(t)$.

The R-LLGMN is developed from the model defined above. For an input time series $\tilde{\mathbf{x}}$, the posterior probability for each class can be estimated with a well-trained R-LLGMN. The R-LLGMN network structure and learning algorithm are explained in the following.

Figure 2. The structure of R-LLGMN

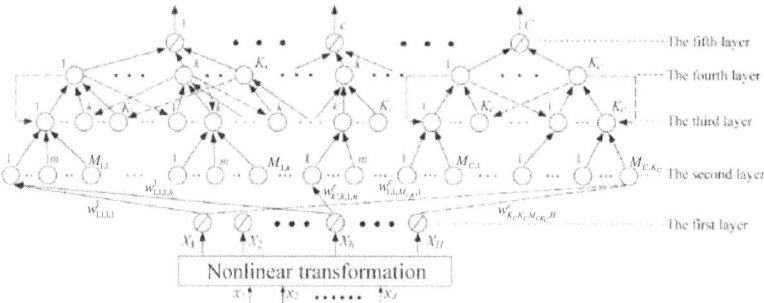

Network Architecture

R-LLGMN is a five-layer recurrent NN with feedback connections between the fourth and the third layers, the structure of which is shown in Figure 2. First, the input vector series $\mathbf{x}(t) \in \Re^d$ $(t=1,\cdots,T)$ is preprocessed into the modified input series $\mathbf{X}(t) \in \Re^H$ as follows:

$$\mathbf{X}(t) = (1, \mathbf{x}(t)^\mathsf{T}, x_1(t)^2, x_1(t)x_2(t), \cdots, x_1(t)x_d(t),$$
$$x_2(t)^2, x_2(t)x_3(t), \cdots, x_2(t)x_d(t), \cdots x_d(t)^2)^\mathsf{T}, \tag{5}$$

where the dimension H is determined as $H = 1 + d(d+3)/2$. The vector $\mathbf{X}(t)$ acts as the input of the first layer, and the identity function is used to activate each unit. The output of the hth $(h = 1,\cdots,\mathrm{H})$ unit in the first layer is defined as $^{(1)}O_h(t)$. Unit $\{c,k,k',m\}$ $(c = 1,\cdots,C;\ k',k = 1,\cdots,K_c;\ m = 1,\cdots,M_{c,k})$ in the second layer receives the output of the first layer, weighted by the coefficient $w_{k',k,m,h}^c$. The input $^{(2)}I_{k',k,m}^c(t)$ and the output $^{(2)}O_{k',k,m}^c(t)$ are defined as

$$^{(2)}I_{k',k,m}^c(t) = \sum_{h=1}^{H} {}^{(1)}O_h(t)w_{k',k,m,h}^c , \tag{6}$$

$$^{(2)}O_{k',k,m}^c(t) = \exp(^{(2)}I_{k',k,m}^c(t)), \tag{7}$$

where C is the number of discriminating classes, K_c is the number of states in class c, and $M_{c,k}$ denotes the number of GMM components in the state k of class c. In (7), the exponential function is used in order to calculate the probability of the input pattern.

The outputs of units $\{c,k,k',m\}$ in the second layer are summed and input into a unit $\{c,k,k'\}$ in the third layer. Also, the output of the fourth layer is fed back to the third layer. These are expressed as follows:

$$^{(3)}I^c_{k',k}(t) = \sum_{m=1}^{M_{c,k}} {}^{(2)}O^c_{k',k,m}(t), \tag{8}$$

$$^{(3)}O^c_{k',k}(t) = {}^{(4)}O^c_{k'}(t-1)^{(3)}I^c_{k',k}(t), \tag{9}$$

where $^{(4)}O^c_{k'}(0) = 1.0$ is for the initial phase. The recurrent connections between the fourth and the third layers play an important role in the process, which corresponds to the forward computation; see Equation (3).

The activation function in the fourth layer is described as

$$^{(4)}I^c_k(t) = \sum_{k'=1}^{K_c} {}^{(3)}O^c_{k',k}(t), \tag{10}$$

$$^{(4)}O^c_k(t) = \frac{^{(4)}I^c_k(t)}{\sum_{c'=1}^{C} \sum_{k'=1}^{K_{c'}} {}^{(4)}I^{c'}_{k'}(t)}. \tag{11}$$

In the fifth layer, the unit c integrates the outputs of K_c units $\{c,k\}$ $(k = 1, \cdots, K_c)$ in the fourth layer. The relationship in the fifth layer is defined as:

$$^{(5)}I^c(t) = \sum_{k=1}^{K_c} {}^{(4)}O^c_k(t), \tag{12}$$

$$^{(5)}O^c(t) = {}^{(5)}I^c(t). \tag{13}$$

In R-LLGMN, the posterior probability of each class is defined as the output of the last layer. After optimizing the weight coefficients $w_{k',k,m,h}^c$ between the first layer and the second layer, the NN can estimate the posterior probability of each class. Obviously, the R-LLGMN's structure corresponds well with the HMM algorithm. R-LLGMN, however, is not just a copy of HMM. The essential point of R-LLGMN is that the parameters in HMM are replaced by the weight coefficients $w_{k',k,m,h}^c$, and this replacement removes restrictions of the statistical parameter in HMM (e.g., $0 \le$ the transition probability ≤ 1, and standard deviations > 0). Therefore, the learning algorithm of R-LLGMN is simplified and can be expected to have higher generalization ability than that of HMMs. That is one of the major advantages of R-LLGMN.

A Maximum Likelihood Training Algorithm

A set of input vector streams $\tilde{\mathbf{x}}^{(n)} = (\mathbf{x}(1)^{(n)}, \mathbf{x}(2)^{(n)}, \cdots, \mathbf{x}(T_n)^{(n)})$ $(n = 1, \cdots, N)$ and the teacher vector $\mathbf{T}^{(n)} = (T_1^{(n)}, \cdots, T_c^{(n)}, \cdots, T_C^{(n)})^{\mathrm{T}}$ are given for the learning of R-LLGMN. We assume that the network acquires the characteristics of the data through learning if, for all the streams, the last output of stream $\tilde{\mathbf{x}}^{(n)}$, namely $^{(5)}O^c(T_n)$ $(c = 1, \cdots, C)$, is close enough to the teacher signal $\mathbf{T}^{(n)}$. The objective function for the network is defined as

$$J = \sum_{n=1}^{N} J_n = -\sum_{n=1}^{N} \sum_{c=1}^{C} T_c^{(n)} \log {}^{(5)}O^c(T_n). \tag{14}$$

The learning process attempts to minimize J, that is, to maximize the likelihood that each teacher vector $\mathbf{T}^{(n)}$ is obtained for the input stream $\tilde{\mathbf{x}}^{(n)}$.

The weight modification $\Delta w_{k',k,m,h}^c$ for $w_{k',k,m,h}^c$ is defined as

$$\Delta w_{k',k,m,h}^c = \eta \sum_{n=1}^{N} \frac{\partial J_n}{\partial w_{k',k,m,h}^c}, \tag{15}$$

in a collective learning scheme, where $\eta > 0$ is the learning rate. Due to the recurrent connections in R-LLGMN, a learning algorithm based on the BPTT algorithm has been applied. It is supposed that the error gradient within a stream is accumulated, and weight modifications are only computed at the end of each stream; the error is then propagated backward to the beginning of the stream.

The term $\frac{\partial J_n}{\partial w^c_{k',k,m,h}}$ in (15) can be defined as

$$
\begin{aligned}
\frac{\partial J_n}{\partial w^c_{k',k,m,h}} &= \sum_{t=0}^{T_n-1}\sum_{c'=1}^{C}\sum_{k''=1}^{K_{c'}} {}^{(n)}\Delta^{c'}_{k''}(t)\frac{\partial^{(4)}O^{c'}_{k''}(T_n-t)}{\partial^{(4)}I^c_k(T_n-t)}\frac{\partial^{(4)}I^c_k(T_n-t)}{\partial^{(3)}O^c_{k',k}(T_n-t)}\\
&\quad \times \frac{\partial^{(3)}O^c_{k',k}(T_n-t)}{\partial^{(3)}I^c_{k',k}(T_n-t)}\frac{\partial^{(3)}I^c_{k',k}(T_n-t)}{\partial^{(2)}O^c_{k',k,m}(T_n-t)}\\
&\quad \times \frac{\partial^{(2)}O^c_{k',k,m}(T_n-t)}{\partial^{(2)}I^c_{k',k,m}(T_n-t)}\frac{\partial^{(2)}I^c_{k',k,m}(T_n-t)}{\partial w^c_{k',k,m,h}}\\
&= \sum_{t=0}^{T_n-1}\sum_{c'=1}^{C}\sum_{k''=1}^{K_{c'}} {}^{(n)}\Delta^{c'}_{k''}(t)(\Gamma_{(c',k''),(c,k)} - {}^{(4)}O^{c'}_{k''}(T_n-t))\\
&\quad \times \frac{{}^{(4)}O^{c'}_{k''}(T_n-t)}{{}^{(4)}I^{c'}_{k''}(T_n-t)}\,{}^{(4)}O^c_{k'}(T_n-t-1)^{(2)}O^c_{k',k,m}(T_n-t)X_h(T_n-t),
\end{aligned}
$$

$$(16)$$

where $\Gamma_{(c',k''),\,(c,k)}$ is defined as

$$
\Gamma_{(c',k''),(c,k)} = \begin{cases} 1 & (c'=c; k''=k)\\ 0 & (\text{otherwise}) \end{cases},
$$

$$(17)$$

and ${}^{(n)}\Delta^{c'}_{k''}(t)$ is the partial differentiation of J_n to ${}^{(4)}O^{c'}_{k''}(T_n-t)$,

$$
{}^{(n)}\Delta^{c'}_{k''}(0) = \frac{T^{(n)}_{c'}}{{}^{(5)}O^c(T_n)},
$$

$$(18)$$

$$
\begin{aligned}
{}^{(n)}\Delta^{c'}_{k''}(t+1) &= \sum_{c''=1}^{C}\sum_{k'''=1}^{K_{c''}} {}^{(n)}\Delta^{c''}_{k'''}(t)\sum_{k'''=1}^{K_{c'}}(\Gamma_{(c'',k'''),(c',k''')} - {}^{(4)}O^{c''}_{k'''}(T_n-t))\\
&\quad \times \frac{{}^{(4)}O^{c''}_{k'''}(T_n-t)}{{}^{(4)}I^{c''}_{k'''}(T_n-t)}\,{}^{(3)}I^{c'}_{k'',k'''}(T_n-t).
\end{aligned}
$$

$$(19)$$

Figure 3. Structure of the proposed EMG pattern recognition system

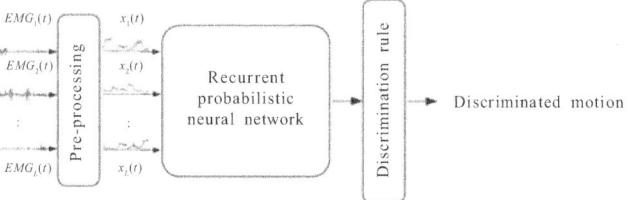

It should be mentioned that all intermediate values of the R-LLGMN's feedforward computation are used in the calculation of Equations (16)-(19).

EMG Pattern Recognition Using R-LLGMN

The structure of the proposed EMG pattern recognition system is shown in Figure 3. This system consists of three parts in sequence: (1) EMG signal processing, (2) recurrent probabilistic neural network, and (3) discrimination rule.

1. *EMG signal processing*

    The EMG signals are processed to extract the feature patterns. In this study, feature patterns extracted from filtered EMG signals and raw EMG signals are used for motion discrimination. Also, the force information is extracted for motion onset detection and to determine the speed of the motion classified.

2. *Recurrent probabilistic neural network*

    The R-LLGMN described in the previous section is employed for motion discrimination. Using samples labeled with the corresponding motions, R-LLGMN learns the non-linear mapping between the EMG patterns and the forearm motions. Given an EMG feature stream with length T, the output $^{(5)}O^c(T)$ ($c = 1, \cdots, C$) presents the posterior probability of each discriminating motion.

3. *Discrimination rule*

    In order to recognize whether the motion has really occurred or not, the force information $\sigma(t)$ is compared with a prefixed motion appearance

Figure 4. Six motions used in the experiments

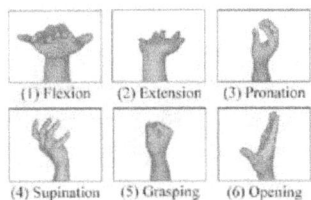

(1) Flexion   (2) Extension   (3) Pronation

(4) Supination   (5) Grasping   (6) Opening

threshold M_d. The motion is considered to have occurred if $\sigma(t)$ exceeds M_d. The entropy of R-LLGMN's outputs is also calculated to prevent the risk of misdiscrimination. The entropy is defined as

$$H(t) = -\sum_{c=1}^{C} {}^{(5)}O^c(t)\log_2 {}^{(5)}O^c(t).$$ (20)

If the entropy $H(t)$ is less than the discrimination threshold H_d, the specific motion with the largest probability is determined according to the Bayes decision rule. If not, the determination is suspended.

The discriminated motion can be used as *control commands* for HMIs, for example, powered prosthetic limbs.

Experimental Conditions

Five subjects (amputee subjects A and B, and normal subjects C, D, and E) participated in this study. Six pairs of Ag/AgCl electrodes (NT-511G: NIHON KOHDEN Corp.) with conductive paste were attached to the forearm and upper arm (Flexor Carpi Radialis (FCR), Extensor Carpi Ulnaris (ECU), Flexor Carpi Ulnaris (FCU), Biceps Brachii (BB), Triceps Brachii (TB): two pairs on FCR and one pair on the others). The subjects were asked to continuously perform six motions ($C = 6$) : flexion, extension, supination, pronation, hand grasping, and hand opening. The motions are shown in Figure 4.

The differential EMG signals were amplified (70 [dB]) and filtered out with a low-pass filter (cut-off frequency: 100 [Hz]) by a multi-telemeter (Web5000:

Figure 5. The multi-telemeter (Web5000) and electrodes (NT-511G) used in the experiments

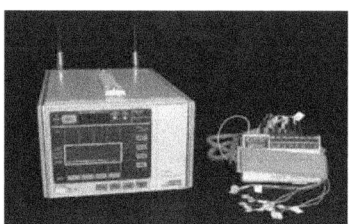

NIHON KOHDEN Corp.), as shown in Figure 5, then digitized by an A/D converter (sampling frequency: 200 [Hz]; quantization: 12 [bits]).

In the experiments, the network structure of R-LLGMN is set as ($C = 6$), $K_c = 1$ ($c = 1, \cdots C$), and the component for each unit in the third layer is one. The parameters used are chosen to make conditions of comparison experiments as equal as possible. The lengths of training sample streams, T_n ($n = 1, \cdots, N$), are set as T, which was determined with respect to the EMG features. In accordance with previous researches on EMG pattern classification (Tsuji et al., 1993; Fukuda et al., 2003), the determination threshold H_d was set to 0.5, and the motion appearance threshold M_d to 0.2. All pattern recognition experiments were conducted off-line.

Pattern Recognition of Filtered EMG Signals

First, motion discrimination experiments using filtered EMG signals were conducted to examine the performance of the proposed method. In the experiments, the training sample consists of 20 EMG patterns extracted from the filtered EMG signals for each motion.

Six channels of EMG signals ($L = 6$) are rectified and filtered by a second-order Butterworth filter (cut-off frequency: 1 [Hz]). The filtered EMG signals are defined as $FEMG_l(t)$ ($l = 1, \cdots, L$) and are normalized to make the sum of L channels equal to 1:

$$x_l(t) = \frac{FEMG_l(t) - FEMG_l^{st}}{\sum_{l'=1}^{L} FEMG_{l'}(t) - FEMG_{l'}^{st}} \quad (l = 1, \cdots L),$$
(21)

where $FEMG_l^{st}$ is the mean value of $FEMG_l(t)$ measured while the arm is relaxed. The feature vector $\mathbf{x}(t) = [x_1(t), x_2(t), \cdots x_L(t)]$ is used for the input of the neural classifier, R-LLGMN, where the dimension of R-LLGMN's input, d, is set as $d = L$. In this study, it is assumed that the amplitude level of EMG signals varies in proportion to muscle force. Force information $\sigma_F(t)$ for the input vector $\mathbf{x}(t)$ is defined as follows:

Figure 6. Example of the discrimination results for filtered EMG signals (subject A)

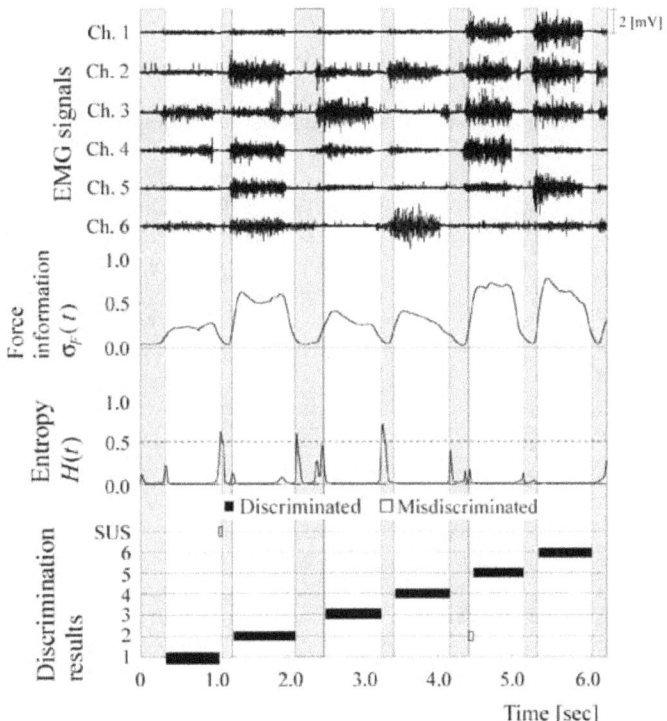

Table 1. Discrimination results of five subjects with filtered EMG signals

Type of the method s		MLP	LLGMN	R-LLGMN
Subject A	DR	73.4	94.0	99.1
(Amputee)	SD	7.9	5.5	0.0
Subject B	DR	46.5	82.8	89.3
(Amputee)	SD	12.3	0.0	0.4
Subject C	DR	44.2	88.5	93.0
(Normal)	SD	10.4	0.0	0.1
Subject D	DR	69.8	88.7	93.5
(Normal)	SD	10.0	0.2	0.0
Subject E	DR	69.2	89.3	92.8
(Normal)	SD	7.0	0.1	0.0

DR : Discrimination rate [%],   *SD* : Standard deviation [%]

$$\sigma_F(t) = \frac{1}{L} \sum_{l=1}^{L} \frac{FEMG_l(t) - FEMG_l^{st}}{FEMG_l^{max} - FEMG_l^{st}},$$ (22)

where $FEMG_l^{max}$ is the mean value of $FEMG_l(t)$ measured while maintaining the maximum arm voluntary contraction.

An example of the discrimination results of subject A is shown in Figure 6. The subject was an amputee (51-year-old male), whose forearm, three cm from the left wrist joint, was amputated when he was 18 years old as the result of an accident. He has never used EMG controlled prosthetic limbs and usually uses a cosmetic hand. In the experiments, he was asked to perform six motions in the order continuously for six seconds. Figure 6 plots six channels of the input EMG signals, the force information $\sigma_F(t)$, the entropy $H(t)$, and the discrimination results. The labels of the vertical axis in the discrimination results correspond to the motions shown in Figure 4, and SUS means that the determination was suspended. The gray areas indicate that no motion was determined because the force information was less than M_d. Incorrect determination was eliminated using the entropy. Figure 6 demonstrates that the proposed method achieves high discrimination accuracy with filtered EMG signals during continuous motion.

The discrimination accuracy for five subjects was then investigated, and LLGMN and an MLP classifier were used for comparison. The same preprocessing method and discrimination rule were applied to the experiments using LLGMN and MLP. The number of units in the input layer of LLGMN was equal to the dimension of input signal (L). Units in the hidden layer corresponded to the Gaussian components in GMM, the number of which was set in the same manner as for the R-LLGMN. The output layer included C units, and each unit gave the posterior probability for the input pattern. In contrast, MLP had four layers (two

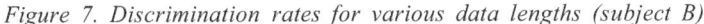

Figure 7. Discrimination rates for various data lengths (subject B)

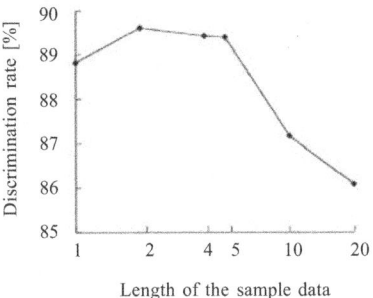

hidden layers), and the units of the layers were set at 6, 10, 10, and 6. Each output of MLP corresponded to a motion, and all six outputs were normalized to make the sum of all outputs equal 1.0 for comparison with R-LLGMN and LLGMN. The learning procedure of MLP continued until the sum of the square error was less than 0.01, where the learning rate was 0.01. However, if the sum of the square error after 50,000 iterations was still not less than 0.01, the learning procedure was stopped. In all three methods, ten different sets of initial weights (all randomized between [0, 1]) were used.

Discrimination rate, which is defined as the ratio of correctly classified data to the total test set, is used to evaluate discrimination accuracy of three methods. The mean values and the standard deviations of the discrimination rates are shown in Table 1. It can be seen that R-LLGMN achieved the best discrimination rate among all three methods and had the smallest standard deviation.

Also, the classification results were examined by altering the experiment conditions, such as the length of sample data. Experiments were performed using various lengths of sample data. For each sample data, R-LLGMN was trained with ten different sets of initial weights, which were randomly chosen in the range [0, 1]. The mean values of the discrimination rates for each length are shown in Figure 7, where the standard deviations are all very small, close to 0. It can be seen from Figure 7 that the discrimination rate maintains a high level when the sample data is of an appropriate length (T). However, if $T > 5$, it is too long to train R-LLGMN using filtered EMG signals. The discrimination rate tends to deteriorate because R-LLGMN, which was trained using the long-length sample data, failed to discriminate the switching of motions.

Pattern Recognition of Raw EMG Signals

This subsection presents pattern recognition experiments of time series of raw EMG signals. In the previously proposed methods for classifying the intended motion of an operator, the filtered or smoothed EMG signals (Fukuda et al., 1997, 2003; Kelly et al., 1990; Tsuji et al., 1993, 2000) or the extracted characteristics in a fixed time window (Hiraiwa et al., 1989; Hudgins et al., 1993) have been used as the input vector to the NN classifier. However, these signal-processing steps result in considerable phase delay and time delay caused by the low-pass filtering and the time window operation. To avoid such delay, raw EMG signals without any preprocessing are used as the input to R-LLGMN. The experiments were performed with the subjects (A, B, C, D, and E) who had experience in manipulating the EMG signals.

As raw EMG signals, six channels of EMG signals ($L = 6$) sampled from the input of multi-telemeter are denoted by $REMG_l(t)$ ($l = 1, \ldots, L$). For the case of raw EMG signals, force information $_R(t)$ is obtained calculating moving average within the length T:

$$_R(t) = \frac{1}{L} \sum_{l=1}^{L} \frac{\overline{REMG_l}(t)}{\overline{REMG_l}^{max}}, \tag{23}$$

$$\overline{REMG_l}(t) = \frac{1}{T} \sum_{j=0}^{T-1} \left| REMG_l(t-j) \right|, \tag{24}$$

where $\overline{REMG_l}^{max}$ is the premeasured integral EMG of each channel under the maximum voluntary contraction. Also, it should be noted that $REMG_l(t-j) = 0$ when $t - j < 0$.

The input vector $\mathbf{x}(t)$ ($t = 1, \ldots, T$) of R-LLGMN is normalized $REMG_l(t)$ with $_R(t)$ as

$$x_l(t) = _R^{-1}(T)REMG_l(t). \tag{25}$$

Here, the normalization enables R-LLGMN to discriminate motions from a pattern of all channels as well as from the amplitude of the raw EMG signals.

In pattern recognition experiments of raw EMG signals, the length of training sample stream T is set as 20. Eight sample streams are used for each motion. The threshold for motion onset detection M_d is 0.155.

Figure 8 provides an example of the classification results of subject A. The figure shows six channels of the raw EMG signals, the force information $_R(t)$, the entropy $H(t)$ calculated from the output probability of R-LLGMN, and the classification results of the R-LLGMN. The discrimination rate was about 95.5% in this experiment. It can be seen that R-LLGMN generates acceptable classification results during continuous motion, and the entropy is low during motions except for the motion one (Flexion). It indicates that R-LLGMN can discriminate the hand and forearm motions from the raw EMG signals, even for control purposes.

Comparisons were conducted with discrimination results of MLP, LLGMN, and R-LLGMN using filtered EMG signals. It should be noted that due to the stochastic nature of raw EMG signals, MLP and LLGMN could not learn motion patterns of raw EMG signals. The network structures of MLP and LLGMN were set to the same as those in pattern recognition experiments of filtered EMG, and the beginning and ending of motions were recognized according to the force information $_R(t)$. The discrimination threshold H_d was not used in the comparison, so that all classification results were used for comparison. Each experiment was repeated ten times with different randomly chosen initial weights. Table 2 depicts the mean values and the standard deviations of the discrimination rates for five subjects. Due to the filtering processes, onsets of the filtered EMG signals are delayed, and the EMG patterns vary significantly in time domain during the transient phase. Since MLP cannot deal well with time-varying patterns, MLP's discrimination result is the worst among these methods. Although LLGMN shows better discrimination accuracy than MLP due to the statistical model incorporated in its structure, it still provides poor discrimination accuracy since the model is static. Consequently, it is can be concluded that phase delay due to the filtering processes is one of the major causes of degradation in the discrimination results in cases of MLP and LLGMN. In contrast, R-LLGMN provides superior discrimination results for both the filtered EMG signals and the raw EMG. Also, we found that patterns of raw EMG signals are much more complicated than that of filtered EMG signals, and training and estimation of R-LLGMN using raw EMG signals are more difficult. Therefore, the classification performance of R-LLGMN with filtered EMG signals is a little higher than that using raw EMG signals. However, since no signal processing is used, the latter has a faster response. There is thus a trade-off between discrimination accuracy and response speed.

The response time of raw EMG-based motion discrimination was further investigated, and the proposed method and traditional classifiers (MLP and LLGMN) were compared. Figure 9 illustrates the signals magnified from 6.3 s to 9.9 s in Figure 8 during the wrist extension motion. This figure depicts the EMG signal of the channel 3, the filtered EMG signal that is rectified and filtered out by the second-order Butterworth low-pass filter (cut-off frequency: 1.0 [Hz]),

Figure 8. Example of the discrimination result for raw EMG signals (subject A)

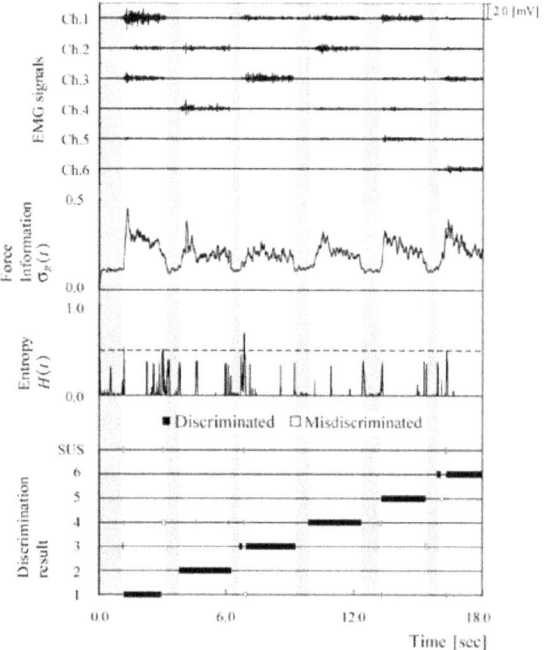

Table 2. Motion discrimination results for raw EMG signals, comparing with methods using filtered EMG signals

Type of the methods		MLP (Filtered EMG)	LLGMN (Filtered EMG)	R-LLGMN (Filtered EMG)	R-LLGMN (Raw EMG)
Subject A (Amputee)	DR	66.1	89.8	96.1	93.8
	SD	14.0	0.0	0.0	0.0
Subject B (Amputee)	DR	70.1	89.3	92.5	91.2
	SD	10.8	0.0	0.0	1.3
Subject C (Normal)	DR	80.5	82.9	94.2	94.1
	SD	8.1	0.0	0.0	0.4
Subject D (Normal)	DR	78.9	88.3	97.4	90.4
	SD	4.1	0.0	0.0	0.9
Subject E (Normal)	DR	75.8	85.9	90.7	91.0
	SD	4.5	0.0	0.0	1.8

DR : Discrimination rate [%],   *SD* : Standard deviation[%]

Figure 9. Changes of the discrimination results by three types of neural networks (subject A)

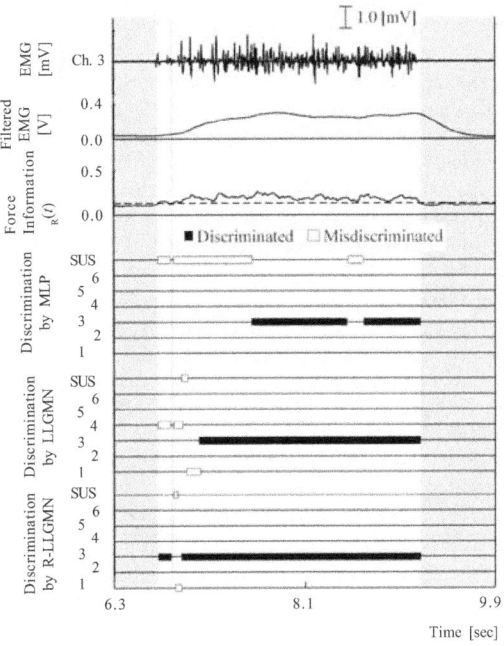

Table 3. Discrimination results for five subjects

Type of the method s		BPNN	LLGMN	R-LLGMN
Subject A (Amputee)	DR	30.4	58.3	89.6
	SD	13.6	4.1	0.3
Subject B (Amputee)	DR	67.2	63.7	75.0
	SD	11.0	0.2	0.0
Subject C (Normal)	DR	49.4	50.0	91.7
	SD	11.5	0.0	0.0
Subject D (Normal)	DR	52.8	58.3	73.8
	SD	3.8	0.0	0.0
Subject E (Normal)	DR	64.4	63.3	66.7
	SD	3.0	0.0	0.0

DR : Discrimination rate [%],   *SD* : Standard deviation [%]

the force information $_{R}(t)$, and the discrimination results of three comparison methods. The MLP and LLGMN used the features extracted from filtered EMG signals as the input, while the R-LLGMN achieved motion discrimination based on the raw EMG signals. It can be seen from the figure that there is a considerable phase delay between the raw EMG and the filtered EMG signals, which causes the misdiscrimination in the results of MLP and LLGMN. In contrast, using the raw EMG signals, R-LLGMN achieves higher discrimination accuracy than the others, and a correct classification is made just after the beginning of motion. It was also found that the discrimination rates of both MLP and LLGMN decreased considerably when the cut-off frequency of the low-pass filter increased. The increase of the cut-off frequency results in filtered EMG signals containing high frequency components, so that the learning of the NNs becomes very difficult.

Then, discrimination accuracy during the beginning and ending of motions was investigated. In these experiments, EMG signals during 100 msec from onset and 100 msec before ending of each motion were used. Similarly, MLP and LLGMN using filtered EMG signals were used for comparison. Table 3 presents the discrimination results for five subjects using three different methods. The mean values and the standard deviations of the discrimination rates are computed for ten randomly chosen initial weights. From this table, it can be seen that R-LLGMN attained the best discrimination rates during the beginning and ending of motions; therefore, the R-LLGMN provides superior response performance.

Discussions

A new EMG pattern recognition method using R-LLGMN is proposed to improve discrimination accuracy when dealing with non-stationary EMG signals. R-LLGMN performs both the filtering process and pattern classification within the same network architecture, so the proposed method outperforms the previous methods with filtered EMG and raw EMG patterns. What is even more encouraging is that the response time of discrimination results can also be shortened by using raw EMG signals.

In the studies on human-machine interfaces (HMIs), it is widely believed that the response time is an important aspect, especially for practical application systems. For HMIs used in daily activities, it has been mentioned that techniques for real-time classification are needed in order to decrease global time delay of response, which would reduce the operator's mental burden and increase the range of applications and number of potential users (Chang et al., 1996; Vuskovic & Du, 2002). A classification system based on digital signal processors (DSP) was used to realize the pattern classification algorithm for fast processing (Chang et al., 1996). Vuskovic and Du (2002) attempted to simplify a fuzzy ARTMAP network used for EMG classification, which resulted in overall smaller computational times. On the other hand, since the EMG signals include high-frequency components, adequate signal processes such as low-pass filtering are necessary in order to extract meaningful information for HMIs. Actually, this low-pass filtering process increases the time delay.

In contrast to these previous studies, which focus on reduction of the computational time (complexity) of classifiers, a pattern recognition technique that directly uses raw EMG signals is an interesting choice. Given the experimental results in the previous section, it is expected that improved response performance is possible by adopting the proposed raw EMG pattern recognition scheme into traditional HMIs, which use filtered EMG patterns (Fukuda et al., 1997, 2003; Kelly et al., 1990; Tsuji et al., 1993, 2000). Further studies should focus on this idea.

This chapter introduced R-LLGMN in order to make effective use of the non-stationary (time-varying) characteristics in EMG signals. In recent years, time-frequency analysis has attracted increasing attention for representing the non-stationary essence of frequency domain (Englehart et al., 1999, 2001; Hussein & Granat, 2002). Since the wavelet transform results in a good time-frequency resolution, it has become a very popular feature extraction method for time-frequency representation of EMG signals. Based on the idea of building prior information into neural network design, the algorithm of wavelet transform can be incorporated into the probabilistic neural network, so that the PNNs could process frequency information of EMG signals more effectively.

Summary

This chapter proposes a new EMG pattern recognition method based on a recurrent log-linearized Gaussian mixture network (R-LLGMN). Because of the recurrent connections in the R-LLGMN's structure, the temporal information of EMG signals can be used to improve discrimination accuracy.

To examine the discrimination capability and accuracy of the proposed method, EMG pattern recognition experiments were conducted with five subjects. In the experiments, the proposed method achieved high discrimination accuracy for varying EMG signals, and its discrimination results are superior to those of the LLGMN and MLP classifiers. We found that the discrimination results change when different lengths of sample stream T are used. The length T should be well modulated according to the input signals. For example, to discriminate filtered EMG signals, T should be less than five.

Even more encouraging is the outcome of EMG pattern recognition experiments using the non-stationary time series of raw EMG signals. Results of these experiments demonstrate that R-LLGMN performs both the filtering process and pattern recognition within the same network architecture and can realize a relatively high discrimination rate that is good enough for control purposes. It should be noted that there is a trade-off between discrimination accuracy and response speed when using R-LLGMN as a classifier. In practical applications, such as prosthetic control, the latter may be preferred.

References

Chang, G. C., Kang, W. J., Luh, J. J., Cheng, C. K., Lai, J. S., Chen, J. J., & Kuo, T. S. (1996). Real-time implementation of electromyogram pattern recognition as a control command of man-machine interface. *Medical Engineering & Physics, 18*, 529-537.

Englehart, E., Hudgins, B., & Parker, A. (2001). A wavelet-based continuous classification scheme for multifunction myoelectric control. *IEEE Transactions on Biomedical Engineering, 48*, 302-311.

Englehart, E., Hudgins, B., Parker, A., & Stevenson, M. (1999). Classification of the myoelectric signal using time-frequency based representations. *Medical Engineering & Physics, 21*, 431-438.

Fukuda, O., Tsuji, T., & Kaneko, M. (1997). An EMG controlled robotic manipulator using neural networks. *Proceedings of the IEEE International Workshop on Robot and Human Communication*, 442-447.

Fukuda, O., Tsuji, T., & Kaneko, M. (1999). An EMG-controlled pointing device using a neural network. *Proceedings of the 1999 IEEE International Conference on Systems, Man, and Cybernetics, 4*, 63-68.

Fukuda, O., Tsuji, T., Kaneko, M., & Ohtsuka, A. (2003). A human-assisting manipulator teleoperated by EMG signals and arm motions. *IEEE Transactions on Robotics and Automation, 19*, 210-222.

Hiraiwa, A., Shimohara, K., & Tokunaga, Y. (1989). EMG pattern analysis and classification by neural network. *Proceedings of the IEEE International Conference on Systems, Man, and Cybernetics, 3*, 1113-1115.

Hudgins, B., Parker, P., & Scott, R.N. (1993). A new strategy for multifunction myoelectric control. *IEEE Transactions on Biomedical Engineering, 40*, 82-94.

Hussein, S. E., & Granat, M. H. (2002). Intention detection using a neuro-fuzzy EMG classifier. *IEEE Engineering in Medicine and Biology Magazine, 21*(6), 123-129.

Kang, W. J., Shiu, J. R., Cheng, C. K., Lai, J. S., Tsao, H. W., & Kuo, T. S. (1995). The application of cepstral coefficients and maximum likelihood method in EMG pattern recognition. *IEEE Transactions on Biomedical Engineering, 42,* 777-785.

Kelly, M. F., Parker, P. A., & Scott, R. N. (1990). The application of neural networks to myoelectric signal analysis: A preliminary study. *IEEE Transactions on Biomedical Engineering, 37,* 221-230.

Lamounier, E., Soares, A., Andrade, A., & Carrijo, R. (2002). A virtual prosthesis control based on neural networks for EMG pattern classification. *Proceedings of the 6ᵗʰ IASTED International Conference on Artificial Intelligence and Soft Computing,* 456-461.

Lusted, H. S., & Knapp, R. B. (1996, October). Controlling computers with neural signals. *Scientific American,* 82-87.

Rabiner, L.R. (1989). A tutorial on hidden Markov model and selected applications in speech recognition. *Proceedings of the IEEE, 77,* 257-286.

Specht, D.F. (1990). Probabilistic neural networks. *Neural Networks, 3,* 109-118.

Tsuji, T., Bu, N., Fukuda, O., & Kaneko, M. (2003). A recurrent log-linearized Gaussian mixture network. *IEEE Transactions on Neural Networks, 14,* 304-316

Tsuji, T., Fukuda, O., Ichinobe, H., & Kaneko, M. (1999). A log-linearized Gaussian mixture network and its application to EEG pattern classification. *IEEE Transactions on Systems, Man, and Cybernetics, Part C: Applications and Reviews, 29,* 60-72.

Tsuji, T., Fukuda, O., Kaneko, M., & Ito, K. (2000). Pattern classification of time-series EMG signals using neural networks. *International Journal of Adaptive Control and Signal Processing, 14,* 829-848.

Tsuji, T., Ichinobe, H., Ito, K., & Nagamachi, M. (1993). Discrimination of forearm motions from EMG signals by error back propagation typed neural network using entropy (in Japanese). *Transactions of the Society of Instrument and Control Engineers, 29,* 1213-1220.

Vuskovic, M., & Du, S. (2002). Classification of prehensile EMG patterns with simplified fuzzy ARTMAP networks. *Proceedings of the 2002 International Joint Conference on Neural Networks,* 2539-2545.

Zhang, G.D. (2000). Neural network for classification: A survey. *IEEE Transactions on Systems, Man and Cybernetics, Part C: Applications and Reviews, 30,* 451-462.

Chapter VII

Myoelectric Teleoperation of a Dual-Arm Manipulator Using Neural Networks

Toshio Tsuji, Hiroshima University, Japan

Kouji Tsujimura, OMRON Corporation, Japan

Yoshiyuki Tanaka, Hiroshima University, Japan

Abstract

In this chapter, an advanced intelligent dual-arm manipulator system teleoperated by EMG signals and hand positions is described. This myoelectric teleoperation system employs a probabilistic neural network, so called log-linearized Gaussian mixture network (LLGMN), to gauge the operator's intended hand motion from EMG patterns measured during tasks. In addition, an event-driven task model using Petri net and a non-contact impedance control method are introduced to allow a human operator to maneuver a couple of robotic manipulators intuitively. A set of experimental results demonstrates the effectiveness of the developed prototype system.

Introduction

Many researchers have actively studied teleoperation technology as an effective human interface for supporting an operator in various tasks. However, current technology is still far from realizing an autonomous robotic system that has high intelligence for auto-recognition and judgment in human task situations. If the operator can control a tele-exist slave-robot as his own arm with natural feeling, task performance will increase.

In this chapter, an advanced intelligent dual-arm manipulator system teleoperated by EMG signals and hand positions is described. The presented myoelectric teleoperation system employs a probabilistic neural network, so called log-linearized Gaussian mixture network (LLGMN), to gauge the operator's intended hand motion from EMG patterns measured during tasks. In addition, an event-driven task model using Petri net and a non-contact impedance control method are introduced to allow a human operator to maneuver a couple of robotic manipulators intuitively. A set of experimental results demonstrates the effectiveness of the developed prototype system.

Background

In the late 1940s, Argonne National Laboratory developed the first teleoperation system that could handle radioactive materials in a nuclear reactor using a robotic manipulator from outside. The motion of the master-arm was transmitted to the slave-arm in the nuclear reactor via a mechanical link structure (Sheridan, 1992). Fundamental concept of current teleoperation systems using electric signals was proposed by Goertz (1954). Since then, many researchers have actively studied teleoperation technology as an effective human interface for supporting an operator in various tasks (Shimamoto, 1992; Yokokohji & Yoshikawa, 1994; Yoon et al., 2001; Mobasser et al., 2003; Ueda & Yoshikawa, 2004).

Some teleoperation tasks require dexterous manipulation of a robotic arm. If the operator can control a tele-exist slave-robot as his own arm with natural feeling, task performance will increase. However, controlling the robot manipulator by means of a conventional interface system, such as a joystick or a master-arm robot, is difficult because it requires highly skilled and experienced system operators. Experimental studies utilizing bioelectric signals, such as electroencephalogram (EEG) and electromyogram (EMG) as an input of the interface system have been undertaken (Farry et al., 1996; Kim et al., 2001; Englehart & Hudgins, 2003; Suryanarayanan & Reddy, 1997; Tsujiuchi et al., 2004; Wolpaw et al., 1998). However, since previous studies focused mainly on reproducing the specified operator's motions by a robotic device, it is almost impossible to apply those proposed systems to practical situations in an actual task environment in which human-like skillful and flexible movements, as well as the cooperative operation of a dual arm, will be required.

This chapter argues cybernetic control of a dual-arm manipulator system teleoperated by EMG signals and hand positions, in which the operator can control two manipulators intuitively by his arm movements with regulating muscle contraction levels. To realize skillful cooperative operations of the dual arm in general task environments, the developed system employs an event-driven task model and a non-contact impedance control method. Moreover, high recognition performance is achieved by using a posterior neural network that can adapt the variation of the EMG signals caused by individual differences, electrode locations, physical fatigue, and perspiration.

An Intelligent EMG-Based Dual-Arm Manipulator System

Figure 1 illustrates the control structure of the proposed teleoperation system using EMG signals, where the system consists of the forearm control part and the upper arm control part for each arm. The prosthetic hand (Imasen lab.) is attached as each end-effector of two robotic manipulators (Move Master RM-501: Mitsubishi Electric Corp.), and each arm has seven DOFs as illustrated in Figure 2. In this system, the section from the first to third link is defined as the upper arm part, while the rest, including the end-effector, as the forearm part. The positive joint rotational direction and the standard link posture of the forearm are presented in Figure 2.

Forearm Control Part

The forearm control part processes the measured EMG signals transmitted by the wireless equipment and extracts feature patterns corresponding to the operator's intended motion. This subsection explains one arm of the dual-arm system. Each motion of the forearm's joints (J_{4w}, J_{5w}, J_{6w}, J_{7w}) is controlled according to the operator's intended motion, estimated by the trained neural network. System parameters are then regulated automatically so that dynamic properties of the robotic arm are adapted for the task model of a given task. In addition, the forearm motion uses impedance control to realize human-like skillful

Figure 1. The dual-arm manipulator system using EMG signals

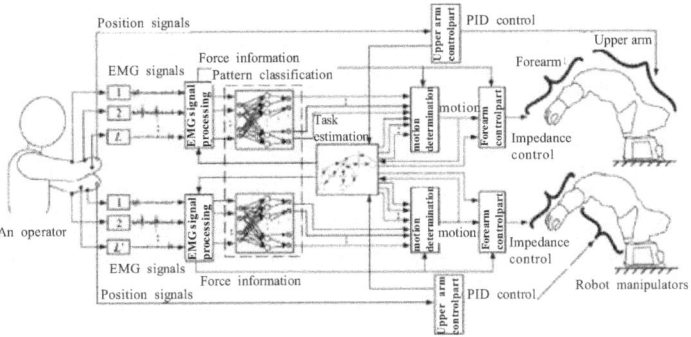

Figure 2. A link model of the robot manipulator

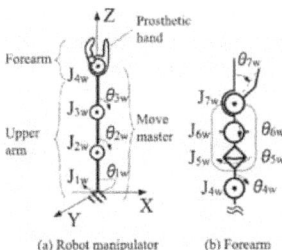

movements in the coordinated task by dual arms. Detailed explanations of each function in the control system are given below.

EMG Signal Processing

EMG signals measured from L pairs of electrodes attached at one arm of the operator are digitized by an analog-to-digital (A/D) converter (sampling frequency 1.0 [kHz]). Then, the digitized data are amplified, rectified, and filtered through a digital second-order Butterworth filter (cut-off frequency: 1.0 [Hz]). These sampled signals are defined as $EMG_l(n)$ ($l = 1, 2, \ldots, L$).

EMG patterns are extracted from a set of $EMG_l(n)$ and represented as a feature pattern vector $\mathbf{x}(n) = [x_1(n), x_2(n), \cdots, x_L(n)]^{\mathrm{T}} \in \mathfrak{R}^L$ by

$$x_l(n) = \frac{EMG_l(n) - \overline{EMG_l}^{st}}{EMG_l^{max} - \overline{EMG_l}^{st}} \sum_{l=1}^{L} \frac{EMG_l^{max} - \overline{EMG_l}^{st}}{EMG_l(n) - \overline{EMG_l}^{st}}, \tag{1}$$

where $\overline{EMG_l}^{st}$ denotes the mean value of $EMG_l(n)$ measured in relaxing the muscles, and EMG_l^{max} are the values of EMG signals measured in the maximum voluntary contraction. Notice that $\mathbf{x}(n)$ is normalized to make its norm equal 1.

Also, using EMG signals, the force information in arm movements is calculated by

$$F_{EMG}(n) = \frac{1}{L} \sum_{l=1}^{L} \frac{EMG_l(n) - \overline{EMG_l}^{st}}{EMG_l^{max} - \overline{EMG_l}^{st}}. \tag{2}$$

The value of $F_{EMG}(n)$ is utilized as a measurement to decide whether the operator takes an action for operating the robotic arm or not.

Pattern Classification Using Probabilistic Neural Networks

An extracted EMG pattern is regarded as a stochastic one since the EMG signal is the composition of spike potentials generated in the muscle fibers. In this study, a log-linearized Gaussian mixture network (LLGMN) (Tsuji et al., 1994, 1999; Fukuda et al., 2003) is utilized as a neural network to estimate the intended hand motion of an operator. This network approximates a probability density function of discriminating data by a Gaussian mixture model through learning with sample data and can calculate *a posteriori* probability of the operator's motion with high discrimination performance from EMG patterns. Accordingly, the proposed system can be manipulated by an operator who does not have knowledge of EMG signals.

The input of the LLGMN $\mathbf{X}(n) \in \mathfrak{R}^H$ is calculated with the vector $\mathbf{x}(n) \in \mathfrak{R}^L$ as follows:

$$\mathbf{X}(n) = [1, \mathbf{x}(n)^{\mathrm{T}}, x_1(n)^2, x_1(n)x_2(n), \cdots, x_1(n)x_L(n),$$
$$x_2(n)^2, x_2(n)x_3(n), \cdots, x_2(n)x_L(n), \cdots, x_L(n)^2]^{\mathrm{T}} \tag{3}$$

The first layer consists of $H(=1+L(L+3)/2)$ units corresponding to the dimension of $\mathbf{X}(n)$, and the identity function is used for an activation function of each unit. The output of the unit h, $^{(1)}O_h(n)$, is the same value of $^{(1)}I_h(n)$:

$$^{(1)}I_h(n) = \mathbf{X}_h(n), \tag{4}$$

$$^{(1)}O_h(n) = {}^{(1)}I_h(n). \tag{5}$$

The second layer consists of the same number of units as the total number of components of the Gaussian mixture network. Each unit of the second layer receives the output of the first layer $^{(1)}O_h(n)$ weighted by the coefficient $w_h^{(k,m)}$, and outputs *a posteriori* probability of each component. The relationship between the input $^{(2)}I_{k,m}(n)$ and the output $^{(2)}O_{k,m}(n)$ in the second layer is defined as

$$^{(2)}I_{k,m}(n) = \sum_{h=1}^{H} {}^{(1)}O_h(n)w_h^{(k,m)}, \tag{6}$$

$$^{(2)}O_{k,m}(n) = \frac{\exp[{}^{(2)}I_{k,m}(n)]}{\sum_{k'=1}^{K}\sum_{m'=1}^{M_{k'}}\exp[{}^{(2)}I_{k',m'}(n)]}, \tag{7}$$

where $w_h^{(K,M_K)} = 0$ $(h = 1,2,\cdots,H)$. Note that (7) can be considered a generalized sigmoid function (Tsuji et al., 1994).

The unit k in the third layer integrates the outputs of M_k units in the second layer, and the relationship between the input $^{(3)}I_k(n)$ and the output $^{(3)}O_k(n)$ is described as

$$^{(3)}I_k(n) = \sum_{m=1}^{M_k} {}^{(2)}O_{k,m}(n), \tag{8}$$

Table 1. Structure of the LLGMN (Fukuda et al., 2003)

The 1st layer	Number of units	H
	Input	$X_d(n)$
	Output	$^{(1)}O_d(n)$
	I/O function	Identity function
The 2nd layer	Number of units	$\sum_{d=1}^{3} M_d$
	Input	$^{(2)}I_{k,m}(n)=\sum_{h=1}^{H_{(2)}}{}^{(1)}O_d(n)w_h^{(k,m)}$
	Output	$^{(2)}O_{k,m}(n)$
	I/O function	Generalized sigmoid function
The 3rd layer	Number of units	K
	Input	$^{(3)}I_k(n)=\sum_{m=1}^{M_k(3)}{}^{(2)}O_{k,m}(n)$
	Output	$^{(3)}O_k(n)$
	I/O function	Identity function
Weight coefficients from 1st layer to 2nd layer		$w_h^{(k,m)}$
Weight coefficients from 2nd layer to 3rd layer		1

$$Y_k(n)={}^{(3)}I_k(n). \tag{9}$$

The output of the third layer $Y_k(n)$ corresponds to *a posteriori* probabilities of the class k for the inputted EMG pattern $\mathbf{x}(n)$. The detailed structure of the LLGMN is presented in Table 1.

Next, the network's learning method is explained. Consider a supervised learning with a teacher vector $\mathbf{T}^{(n)}=[T_1^{(n)},\cdots,T_k^{(n)},\cdots,T_K^{(n)}]^{\mathrm{T}}$ for the nth input vector $\mathbf{x}(n)$. If a teacher provides a perfect classification, $T_k^{(n)}=1$ for the particular class k and $T_k^{(n)}=0$ for all other classes. LLGMN is trained using a given set of N data $\mathbf{x}(n)$ $(n=1,2,\cdots,N)$ to maximize the likelihood function. The employed energy function J for the network training is defined as

$$J=\sum_{n=1}^{N}J_n=-\sum_{n=1}^{N}\sum_{k=1}^{K}T_k^{(n)}Y^k(n), \tag{10}$$

and the learning is performed to minimize this energy function (i.e., to maximize the likelihood function). The learning rule is designed with the concept of terminal attractor (TA) so that the convergence time of the function can be specified (Fukuda et al., 2003; Tsuji et al., 1994).

The proposed system uses off-line learning in the preliminary stage to perceive the EMG patterns corresponding to each of Kth target motions, while the online learning method adapts for the variation of EMG properties caused by muscle fatigue, sweat, and so on.

Task Estimation Using Petri Nets

In operating a dual-arm system, the operator has to skillfully coordinate the motions of right and left robotic arms. However, the classification results from the EMG pattern cannot be adopted directly because they are not considered to other arm conditions. This part estimates a task state of the coordinated tasks by the dual arms based on the time history of task states.

Let us imagine that an operator is pouring water into a cup held by the left arm from a bottle held by the right arm. In this task, a human should not drop a glass or bottle from their hand while pouring water. In this study, such a task flow is described with a task model using Petri nets (Reisig, 1988) that are proper for dealing with an event-driven task. Thus, the proposed system can estimate current task states and can regulate control parameters according to the estimated task states.

A task model $N = (P,T;F,M)$ can be expressed with the place set $P = \{p_0, p_1, \cdots, p_P\}$, the transition set $T = \{t_0, t_1, \cdots, t_T\}$, the arc set $F \, \hat{I} \, (P \times T) \cup (T \times \Pi)$, and the initial marking set $M : P \rightarrow N \cup \{\omega\}$. N indicates a set of positive integers, and ω is the infinity. T and P denote the numbers of transitions and places. The initial marking $m_0 \in M$ is settled on the place p_0 that corresponds to the standby state (Fukuda et al., 2002).

Figure 3 presents an example of the task model using Petri nets, where a token denotes the current state (the standby state), and the branch subnets connecting this place represent the details of each task. The tree structure of the task model is suitable for recomposing its structure according to the change of tasks.

The task model calculates a modifying vector γ_m according to the estimated task state by

$$\gamma_m = [\gamma_{m0}, \gamma_{m1}, \cdots, \gamma_{mK}, \gamma_{m(K+1)}]^T \tag{11}$$

where $m \in \{0,1,2,\cdots,P\}$ is the index of the place in the task model; $\gamma_{m1}, \cdots, \gamma_{mK}$ indicates the weights corresponding to the motions; γ_{m0} and $\gamma_{m(K+1)}$ the modifying weights of a do-nothing operation and a suspending motion, respectively.

The modifying vector is then sent to the motion determination part. Also, the estimated power $F_{EMG}(n)$ given in (2) is modified using the parameters f_m as

$$F_{EMG}(n) = \frac{1}{L} \sum_{i=1}^{L} \frac{EMG_i(n) - \overline{EMG_i}^{st}}{EMG_i^{max} - \overline{EMG_i}^{st}} f_m. \tag{12}$$

Motion Determination

Motion is determined by the estimated force $F_{EMG}(n)$ given in (12), and the probability of the do-nothing operation $Y_0(n)$ is calculated by the following membership function:

$$Y_0(n) = -\frac{1}{\pi}\tan^{-1}\{A_1(F_{EMG}(n) - B_1)\} + 0.5, \tag{13}$$

where A_1 and B_1 are positive constants. The value of $Y_0(n)$ approaches 1 as $F_{EMG}(n)$ approaches 0, while $Y_0(n)$ decreases as $F_{EMG}(n)$ increases as presented in Figure 4(a).

Next, to evaluate the accuracy of discrimination results by the neural network, the probabilities of suspending motion $Y_k(n)$ ($k = 1, 2, \cdots, K$: K is the number of target motions) is defined with the entropy $H(n)$:

$$H(n) = -\sum_{k=1}^{K} Y_k(n) \log Y_k(n). \tag{14}$$

The entropy is calculated by *a posteriori* probabilities of the operator's motions that are the output of the trained LLGMN, which may be interpreted as a risk of ill recognition. For example, the entropy is low when the energy function is thoroughly reduced, in which one of *a posteriori* probabilities takes a remarkably large value and the other ones are close to 0. In contrast, when the output of LLGMN is ambiguous, the entropy is high. This entropy tends to increase when EMG patterns are disturbed by an unexpected external event, such as the switching of the operator's motions and unexpected noise signals.

Figure 3. An example of the task model

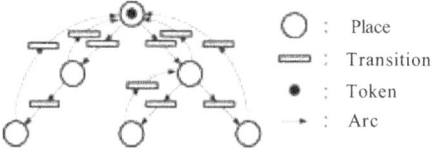

○ : Place

▭ : Transition

● : Token

→ : Arc

By means of the entropy given by (14), the probability of suspending motion $Y_{K+1}(n)$ is defined as

$$Y_{K+1}(n) = \frac{1}{\pi} \tan^{-1}\{A_2(H(n) - B_2)\} + 0.5, \tag{15}$$

where A_2 and B_2 are positive constants. If the entropy $H(n)$ is close to 0, $Y_{K+1}(n)$ becomes close to 0. However, if $H(n)$ increases, $Y_{K+1}(n)$ is close to 1 as indicated in Figure 4(b).

Finally, the motion k with the maximum value of the probability $O_k(n)$ is selected as the operator's intended motion:

$$O_k(n) = \frac{\gamma_{mk} Z_k(n)}{\sum_{j=1}^{K+1} \gamma_{mj} Z_j(n)}, \tag{16}$$

where $Z_k(n)$ $(k = 0,1,\cdots,K,K+1)$ is calculated using $Y_0(n)$, $Y_{K+1}(n)$, and $Y_k(n)$ $k = 0,1,\cdots,K)$ as

$$Z_k(n) = \begin{cases} Y_k(n) & (k = 0) \\ (1 - Y_0(n))(1 - Y_{K+1}(n))Y_k(n) & (k = 1,2,\cdots,K), \\ (1 - Y_0(n))Y_k(n) & (k = K+1) \end{cases} \tag{17}$$

Adaptive Learning Algorithm

When the operator controls the dual-arm manipulator for many hours, it is necessary to consider variations of EMG properties resulting from muscle fatigue, sweat, and the change of the characteristics and the electrode position. The muscles of a non-dominant arm fatigue more readily compared to the dominant arm. Therefore, an online learning method that can adapt to such variations of EMG properties is needed to discriminate the EMG pattern successively for a long-term operation. However, the correct teacher signals cannot be obtained in the operation since it is impossible to directly find the operator's intended motion.

Figure 4. Membership functions for do-nothing operation and suspending motion ($A_1 = 4.0$, $B_1 = 0.5$, $A_2 = 8.0$, $B_2 = 0.7$)

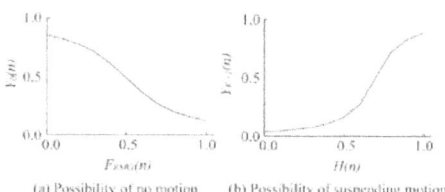

(a) Possibility of no motion   (b) Possibility of suspending motion

For that, the replacement of learning data and the relearning of LLGMN are executed according to the reliability of outputs of the LLGMN for the EMG pattern $\mathbf{x}(n)$, that is, the entropy $H(n)$ given in (14). If the entropy $H(n)$ is less than a given threshold H_o, the EMG pattern $\mathbf{x}(n)$ is replaced with the oldest pattern in the set of the stored learning data. The weights of LLGMN are then updated using the new set of the learning data only when the energy function J is decreased by the relearning procedure to avoid incorrect learning.

Bio-Mimetic Impedance Control

Generally speaking, a human forearm is compliant when holding a soft object, while it stiffens when holding a hard or heavy one. Such dynamic properties of human movements can be represented by the mechanical impedance parameters: stiffness, viscosity, and inertia (Tsuji et al., 1995). If the human impedance characteristics of the forearm can be applied to control the robotic manipulator, it is possible to realize natural movements like a human forearm. This system tries to realize natural motions of the end-effectors by using the human impedance characteristics estimated from EMG signals (Fukuda et al., 2002).

The dynamic equation of the jth joint of the prosthetic forearm under impedance control is defined as

$$I_j \ddot{\theta}_j + B_j(\alpha_j)\dot{\theta}_j + K_j(\alpha_j)(\theta_j - \theta_j^e) = \tau_j^{ex}, \tag{18}$$

$$\theta_j^e = \frac{\alpha_j \tau_{jk}^{max}}{K_j(\alpha_j)}, \tag{19}$$

where I_j, $B_j(\alpha_j)$, and $K_j(\alpha_j)$ are the inertia, viscosity, and stiffness. The viscosity and the stiffness are related to the muscular contraction ratio α_j represented by a non-linear model using α_j (Fukuda et al., 2002). θ_j and θ_j^e are the measured and equilibrium angles of the jth joint, and τ_j^{ex} and τ_{jk}^{max} are the external torque and the prespecified maximal torque for the motion k.

The driven joint j is selected according to determination result k in the motion determination part. The muscular contraction ratio α_j is defined using $F_{EMG}(n)$ as

$$\alpha_j(n) = \frac{F_{EMG}(n)}{EMG_k^{max}}, \tag{20}$$

where EMG_k^{max} is the mean value of F_{EMG} while keeping the maximum voluntary contraction (MVC) for motion k ($k = 1,2,\cdots,K$). If a discriminated motion is determined as the suspending motion, the motion keeps the last motion as $\tau_j(n) = \tau_j(n-1)$.

The desired joint angles are calculated in the impedance filter part, and they are controlled using the tracking control part as illustrated in Figure 5, where K_p, K_i, K_v are the gain parameters for a PID control method. This method realizes a natural feeling of control similar to that of the original limb, if the impedance parameters are set to similar values of the human arm. In this system, the impedance parameters are updated to suitable values according to the task state estimated by a task model.

Upper Arm Control Part

The upper arm control part uses a 3-D position sensor (ISOTRACK II: POLHEMUS, Inc.) as an input device for the control signal. The operator

Figure 5. Block diagram of a biomimetic impedance control part

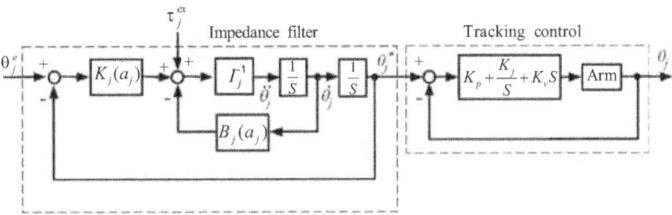

attaches this sensor at his or her wrist, and the desired joint angles of the forearm $(\theta_{1w}, \theta_{2w}, \theta_{3w})$ are calculated from the measured operator's wrist position. The motion of each joint is controlled by the PID control method. The system adopts the non-contact impedance control (Tsuji & Kaneko, 1999) to adjust dynamic characteristics of the dual-arm according to the relative movements between them.

Figure 6 schematically represents the non-contact impedance control. Consider the case in which an object (the left end-effector) approaches the right manipulator, and set a virtual sphere with radius r at the center of the end-effector. When the object enters the virtual sphere, the normal vector from the surface of the sphere to the object $dX_0 \in \Re^l$ can be represented as

$$dX_o = X_r - rn, \tag{21}$$

$$n = \begin{cases} \dfrac{X_r}{|X_r|} & (X_r \neq 0) \\ 0 & (X_r = 0) \end{cases}. \tag{22}$$

When the object is in the virtual sphere $(|X_r| < r)$, the virtual impedance works between the end-effector and the object so that the virtual external force $F_0 \in \Re^l$ is exerted on the end-effector by

$$F_o = \begin{cases} M_o d\ddot{X}_o + B_o d\dot{X}_o + K_o dX_o & (|X_r| \leq r) \\ 0 & (|X_r| > r) \end{cases}, \tag{23}$$

where M_o, B_o, and $K_o \in \Re^{l \times l}$ represent the virtual inertia, viscosity, and stiffness matrices. Note that $F_o = 0$ when the object is outside the virtual sphere or at the center of the sphere. Thus, the dynamic equation of the end-effector for non-contact impedance control can be expressed with (22) and (23) as

$$M_e d\ddot{X} + B_e d\dot{X} + K_e dX = F_{int} + F_0. \tag{24}$$

Because of the virtual sphere defined at the end-effector, a virtual external force F_0 is exerted on an end-effector of the manipulators, so that the robot can be

Figure 6. Schematic representation of a non-contact impedance control. One arm has virtual sphere, while the other arm does not have it.

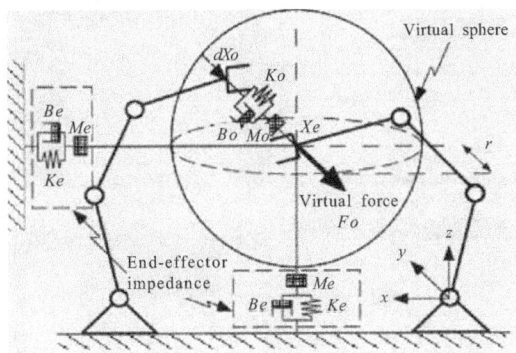

controlled before contact with the environment. Also, the existence and radius of the virtual spheres and virtual impedance parameters can be suitably changed by a task model during tasks.

Feedback Part

Before the operation is started, an operator has to check whether the EMG signals are measured by using the graphical feedback display, shown in Figure 7(a). After calculating $\overline{EMG}_i^{st}$ and EMG_i^{max} (Figure 7(b)), the EMG pattern is extracted for each motion to collect teacher vectors (Figure 7 (c)). The LLGMN is then trained with the teacher vectors (Figure 7(d)). Finally, the operator checks the motion-discriminated results (Figure 7(e)). If the discrimination results are improper, the teacher vectors are measured again for the learning of LLGMN.

The operator controls two manipulators by watching a set of monitors placed in front of him or her. The image sequence is captured by a pair of cameras as shown in Figure 8(a), and the computer graphics of the task environment are provided as feedback to the operator in Figure 8(b). Camera A is set up at the back of the manipulators, and Camera B is set up at the side of the right arm. Camera B uses Nu-View (3D.com, Inc.) to construct a 3-D perspective image, so that the operator can find three-dimensional information of the virtual environment by wearing LCD shutter glasses.

Figure 7. Graphical display for the myoelectric teleoperation

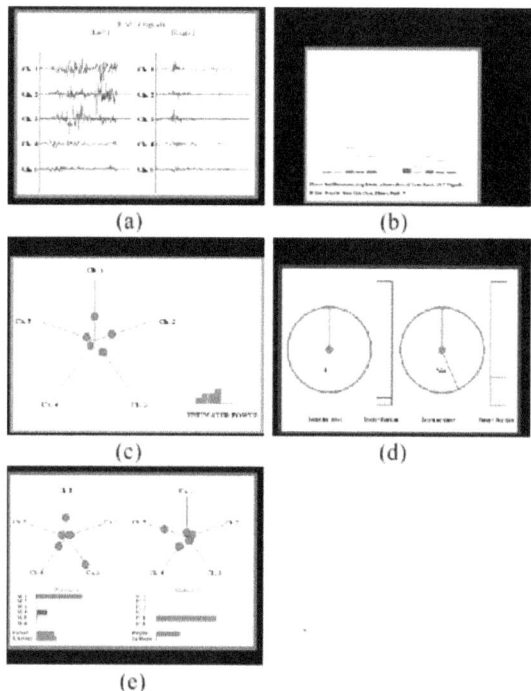

Figure 8. An operator maneuvering the teleoperation system via feedback displays

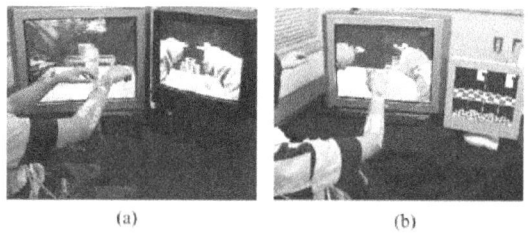

Figure 9. Experimental apparatus of the task environment in the remote place

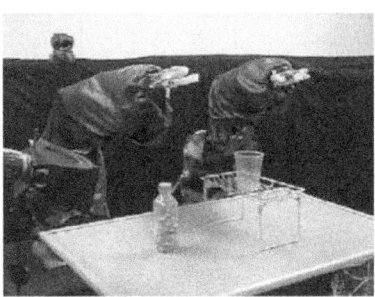

Experiments

Experiments were conducted with four male subjects (graduate students, 23-25 years old; Subjects A, B, and C: right handers; Subject D: left hander) to demonstrate the verification of the developed dual-arm manipulator system.

Operation of Dual-Arm Manipulator

A subject was asked to perform a given task including subtasks: grasp a bottle with the right hand, remove the bottle cap with the left hand, and pour from the bottle into a cup. Figure 9 shows the robot manipulators and task environment established in the remote place. Table 2 represents the eight task states and the eight primitive motions of the dual-arm manipulator prepared for the given task, while Figure 10 shows the designed task model using Petri nets in this chapter.

In the experiment, three pairs of electrodes (ch.1, 2, 3) were set at muscles of the operator's forearm, and two pairs of electrodes at muscles of the operator's upper arm (ch. 4, 5). Six motions are discriminated as a primitive hand motion (hand opening, hand closing, hand closing and pronation, hand opening and pronation, pronation, and supination). The control parameters in (13) and (15) were set as $(A_1, A_2, B_1, B_2) = (4.0, 4.0, 0.2, 0.3)$ for the right manipulator and $(4.0, 4.0, 0.15, 0.3)$ for the left manipulator.

Figure 11 shows a typical scene of teleoperation of the dual-arm system for the given cooperation task by subject A. In each task state, a left photo gives operator's motion while a right one shows the dual-arm robot's motion teleoperated

Table 2. Places and transitions

(a) Places

p_0	Standby	p_5	Grasping a tube
p_1	Grasping a bottle	p_6	Grasping a tube and cup
p_2	Opening the cap	p_7	Pouring into a cup
p_3	Grasping a bottle and cup	p_8	Grasping a cup
p_4	Pouring into a cup		

(b) Transitions

t_0	Open	t_5	Grasp (left hand)
t_1	Grasp (right hand)	t_6	Grasp (right hand)
t_2	Grasp (left hand)	t_7	Pronation and Grasp (left hand)
t_3	Grasp (left hand)	t_8	Open (right hand)
t_4	Pronation (right hand)		

Figure 10. Task model used in experiments

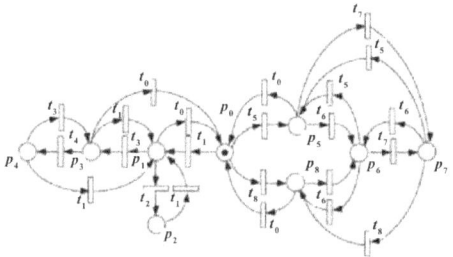

by the subject. Figure 12 represents time profiles of the EMG signals measured from the right and left arms, the estimated forces and discriminated motions of the right and left arms, and the estimated task states using Petri nets, in order from the top, during the operation shown in Figure 11. Since the motion discrimination is performed well, it can be seen that the subject can operate the proposed system properly by remote control using EMG signals to achieve the given task.

Motion-Discrimination with Adaptive Learning

The effectiveness of adaptive learning of neural networks for motion discrimination was examined using long-term (5-day) experiments. Subjects were asked to perform the same six motions as the ones in the previous subsection at regular intervals for 120 minutes; they executed almost 1,440 motions in this experiment.

Figure 11. An example of the dual-arm control

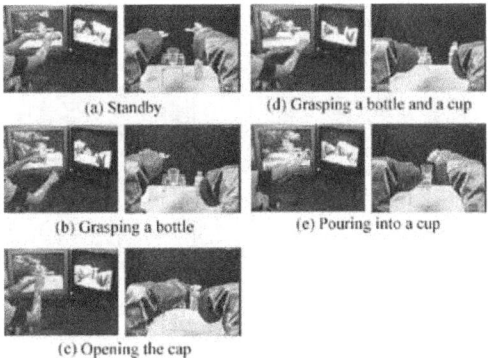

(a) Standby

(d) Grasping a bottle and a cup

(b) Grasping a bottle

(e) Pouring into a cup

(c) Opening the cap

Figure 12. An example of the experimental results by subject A

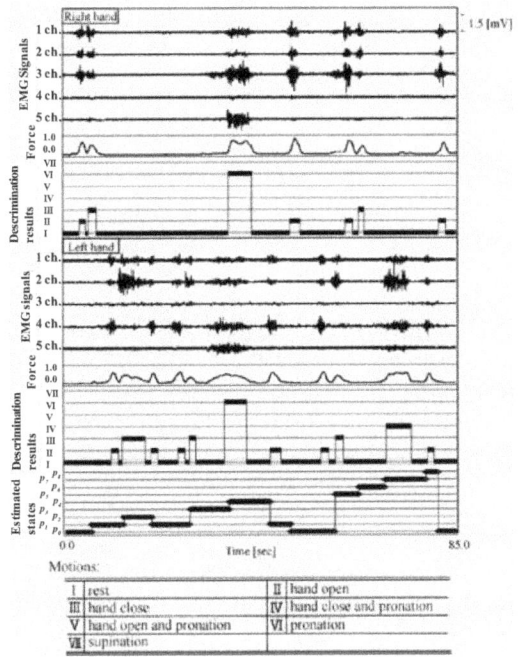

Figure 13. Effect of adaptive learning on the motion discrimination ability by subject A who is right-handed

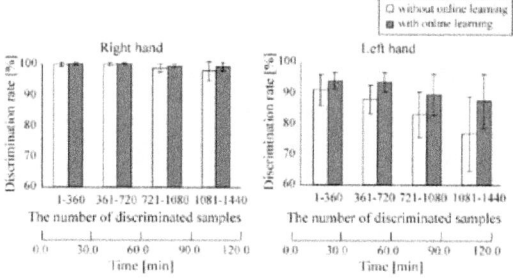

Figure 14. Experimental results of hand motion discrimination for four subjects

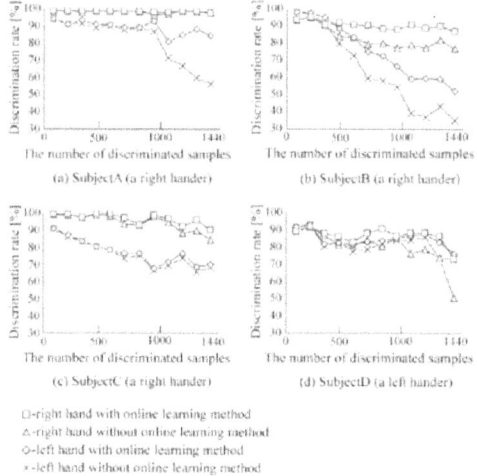

□-right hand with online learning method
△-right hand without online learning method
○-left hand with online learning method
×-left hand without online learning method

The adaptive learning of neural networks was carried out by setting the number of learning data at $N = 120$ and the learning thresholds H_o at 0.2. The subjects were not informed of the discrimination result to exclude intentional changes of EMG patterns during the experiment. Also, each element of the modifying vector $(\gamma_{m0}, \cdots, \gamma_{m9K=1})$ was set at 1.0.

Figure 13 shows the averages and standard deviations of discrimination rates by subject A, in which the discrimination rates were calculated every 360 motions. The discrimination rate without the online learning method decreased with time because of the variation of EMG patterns caused by fatigue and/or sweat. It should be noted that the effectiveness of the online learning method can be observed clearly from the discrimination rates of the non-dominant hand.

Figure 14 presents the discrimination rates of all subjects calculated every 120 motions for one day. The discrimination rates of all subjects are high at the beginning of the experiment and tended to decrease as the operation continued. However, it can be seen that the rates are maintained at a sufficiently high level by using the online learning method.

Conclusion

This chapter has described a novel teleoperation technique using neural networks for a dual-arm manipulator system teleoperated by EMG signals. In the developed system, an operator is not physically constrained by a control device like the traditional master arm, so that he or she can control the manipulators by using bioelectric signals as hoped. The system utilizes an event-driven task model and non-contact impedance control to achieve skilled movements such as coordinated tasks by dual arms, and high discrimination performance can be attained by adapting the variation of EMG signals caused by individual differences, electrode locations, physical fatigue, sweat, and operator's posture.

The experimental results demonstrated that coordinated tasks can be performed with the proposed cybernetic control of the dual-arm system and that the high accuracy of motion discrimination can be maintained by the proposed adaptive learning method of neural networks even after the operator has controlled the manipulators for a long period of time.

The teleoperation system using EMG signals has enough potential as an operational interface to maneuver robotic manipulators by remote control intuitively. In future research, we would like to establish a task model with learning ability and feedback enhancement. We also plan to expand the developed dual-arm manipulator using EMG signals into a human-assisting system for the handicapped, such as an amputee and the aged (Fukuda et al., 2003).

Acknowledgments

The authors would like to thank Dr. O. Fukuda of National Institute of Advanced Industrial Science and Technology (AIST). This research work was supported in part by a Grant-in-Aid for Scientific Research from the Japanese Ministry of

Education, Science and Culture (11555113, 15360226, and 16760203). The support from New Energy and Industrial Technology Development Organization (NEDO) of Japan is also much appreciated.

References

Englehart, K., & Hudgins, B. (2003, July). A robust, real-time control scheme for multifunction myoelectric control. *IEEE Transactions on Biomedical Engineering, 50*(7), 848-854.

Farry, K. A., Walker, I. D., & Baraniuk, R. G. (1996). Myoelectric teleoperation of a complex robotic hand. *IEEE Transactions on Robotics and Automation, 12*(5), 775-788.

Fukuda, O., Tsuji, T., Kaneko, M., & Otsuka, A. (2003, April). A human-assisting manipulator teleoperated by EMG signals and arm motions. *IEEE Transactions on Robotics and Automation, 19*(2), 210-222.

Fukuda, O., Tsuji, T., Takahashi, K., & Kaneko, M. (2002). Skill assistance for myoelectric control using an event-driven task model. *Proceedings of the 2002 IEEE/RSJ International Conference on Intelligent Robots and Systems (IROS2002)*, 1445-1450.

Goertz, R. C. (1954). Manipulator systems development at ANL. *Proceedings of the 12th Conference on Remote Systems Technology* (pp. 117-136). American Nuclear Society.

Kim, K. -Y., Kim, D. -H., Jeong, Y., Kim, K., & Park, J. -O. (2001). A biological man-machine interface for teleoperation. *Proceedings of the 32nd International Symposium on Robotics*, 574-579.

Mobasser, F., Hashtrudi-Zaadand, K., & Salcudean, S. E. (2003). Impedance reflecting rate mode teleoperation. *Proceedings of the 2003 IEEE International Conference on Robotics and Automation (ICRA2003)*, 3296-3302.

Reisig, W. (1988). *Petri nets.* Springer-Verlag.

Sheridan, T.B. (1992). *Telerobotics, automation and human supervisory control.* MIT Press.

Shimamoto, M.S. (1992). Teleoperator/telepresence system (TOPS) concept verification model (CVM) development. *Recent Advances in Marine Science and Technology*, 97-104.

Suryanarayanan, S., & Reddy, N.P. (1997). EMG based interface for position tracking and control in VR environments and teleoperation. *Teleoperators and Virtual Environments, 6*(3), 282-291.

Tsuji, T., Fukuda, O., Ichinobe, H., & Kaneko, M. (1999, February). A log-linearized Gaussian mixture network and its application to EEG pattern classification. *IEEE Transactions on System, Man and Cybernetics, Part C, Applications and Reviews, 29*(1), 60-72.

Tsuji, T., Ishinobe, H., & Makoto, M. (1994). A proposal of the feedforward neural network based on the Gaussian mixture model and the log-linear model (in Japanese). *The Transactions of the Institute of Electronics, Information and Communication Engineers, J77-D-II*(10), 2093-2100.

Tsuji, T., & Kaneko, M. (1999). Non-contact impedance control for redundant manipulators. *IEEE Transactions on Systems, Man, and Cybernetics, Part A, Systems and Humans, 29*(2), 184-193.

Tsuji, T., Morasso, P. G., Goto, K., & Ito, K. (1995). Human hand impedance characteristics during maintained posture. *Biological Cybernetics, 72*, 457-485.

Tsujiuchi, N., Koizumi, T., & Yoneda, M. (2004). Manipulation of a robot by EMG signals using linear multiple regression model. *Proceedings of the 2004 IEEE/RSJ International Conference on Intelligent Robots and Systems (IROS2004)*, 1991-1996.

Ueda, J., & Yoshikawa, T. (2004, June). Force-reflecting bilateral teleoperation with time delay by signal filtering. *IEEE Transactions on Robotics and Automation, 20*(3), 613-619.

Wolpaw, J. R., Ramoser, H., McFarland, D. J., & Pfurtscheller, G. (1998). EEG-based communication: Improved accuracy by response verification. *IEEE Transactions on Rehabilitation Engineering, 6*, 326-333.

Yokokohji, Y., & Yoshikawa, T. (1994). Bilateral control of master-slave manipulators for ideal kinesthetic coupling. *IEEE Transactions on Robotics and Automation, 10*, 605-620.

Yoon, W. -K., Goshozono, T., Kawabe, H., Kinami, M., Tsumaki, Y., Uchiyama, M., Oda, M., & Doi, T. (2001). Model-based teleoperation of a space robot on ETS-VII using a Haptic Interface. *Proceedings of the 2001 IEEE International Conference on Robotics and Automation (ICRA2001)*, 407-412.

Section IV

Electroencephalography and Evoked Potentials

Chapter VIII

Artificial Neural Networks in EEG Analysis

Markad V. Kamath, McMaster University, Canada

Adrian R. Upton, McMaster University, Canada

Jie Wu, McMaster University, Canada

Harjeet S. Bajaj, McMaster University, Canada

Skip Poehlman, McMaster University, Canada

Robert Spaziani, McMaster University, Canada

Abstract

The artificial neural networks (ANNs) are regularly employed in EEG signal processing because of their effectiveness as pattern classifiers. In this chapter, four specific applications will be studied: On a day to day basis, ANNs can assist in identifying abnormal EEG activity in patients with neurological diseases such as epilepsy, Huntington's disease, and Alzheimer's disease. The ANNs can reduce the time taken for interpretation of physiological signals such as EEG, respiration, and ECG recorded during sleep. During an invasive surgical procedure, the ANNs can provide objective parameters derived from the EEG to help determine the depth of anesthesia. The ANNs have made significant contributions toward extracting embedded signals within the EEG which can be used to control external devices. This rapidly developing field, which is called brain-computer interface, has a large number of applications in empowering handicapped individuals to independently operate appliances, neuroprosthesis, or orthosis.

Introduction

The *electroencephalogram* (EEG), generally recorded on the scalp from a number of electrodes, is the result of asynchronous firing of billions of neurons within the nervous system. Digital signal processing of the EEG has been a major domain of research in biomedical engineering for many years. Development of *artificial neural networks* for EEG analysis is a natural evolution of bringing better engineering and analytical methods to medicine in general and to neurology in particular. Artificial neural networks (ANNs) can be used as part of a primary pattern recognition system to assist the physician. In the 1970s and 1980s when computers were centrally located, applications were based on understanding the frequency composition of EEG. Specifically, the frequency analysis of the EEG into delta (0-4 Hz), theta (5-7 Hz), alpha (8-13 Hz), and beta (13-18 Hz) bands was the most widely used tool as a source of critical information for diagnosis.

With widespread use of personal computers, analysis of EEG signals has been approached by both linear and non-linear (chaos) methods. If the data can be structured suitably, then ANNs can potentially enhance the quality of pattern identification and assist the user. The ANNs also learn from experience, have fault tolerance capabilities, and can create complex decision surfaces for classification. The ANNs provide a greater depth of technological innovation and have generated novel paradigms of pattern recognition. For example, the *brain-computer interface* (BCI) can enable physically disabled subjects to interact with the computer and consequently the external environment. The BCI has given rise to a number of technologies which can make life easier for such individuals. In this chapter, we summarize the state-of-the-art of applying ANNs in EEG analysis during neurological diagnosis, monitoring the depth of *anesthesia*, automated *sleep* scoring, and toward enhancing the BCI, among a myriad of applications of ANNs.

Background

Research on applications of ANNs in EEG signal analysis is based on the principle that the cortical EEG signal contains embedded information about ongoing physiological and cognitive processes. Further, through a combination of mathematical modeling and efficient training of the ANN, one can employ EEG signals to understand the underlying pathology, identify sleep stages, measure the depth of anesthesia, or activate external mechanical devices. The technology of EEG signal acquisition, signal characterization, sampling, and filtering is well documented in the literature and is not the subject of this chapter. We review some salient applications of ANNs which are employed for EEG analysis, diagnosis of pathological conditions, sleep stage interpretation, and monitoring and regulation of anesthesia. Finally, we will identify some recent developments within the emerging field of brain-computer interface where the EEG can be used to regulate an external device.

Artificial Neural Networks during EEG Analysis and Neurological Diagnosis

The electrodiagnostic laboratory of a neurology department employs a considerable amount of personnel and computational resources to acquire diagnostic EEG from each patient. An acute EEG recording lasts approximately 30 to 45 minutes and generates a large amount (several megabytes) of digital data. Although paper traces were used until recently, most laboratories now display stored EEG records on a computer screen, for the physician to view off-line. A neurophysician is trained to identify segments containing abnormal patterns within the record and combine such information with a physical examination to arrive at an accurate diagnosis of the underlying pathology. The ANNs can be trained to review the EEG, either online or offline and optimize the time a neurophysician spends identifying the critical information relevant to diagnosis (Robert et al., 2002a). Because of space limitations, we will review research where ANNs have been employed in three specific pathologies: *epilepsy*, *Huntington's disease*, and *Alzheimer's disease*.

Epilepsy and Seizure Detection

Epilepsy is characterized by sudden recurrent and transient disturbances of mental function and/or movement of the body that result from excessive discharging of groups of brain cells. Patients who are suspected of having epileptogenic foci are subjected to an EEG recording in the neurophysiology laboratory. In clinical neurological practice, detection of abnormal EEG plays an important role in the diagnosis of epilepsy. Spikes or spike discharges are transient waveforms present in the human EEG and have a high correlation with seizure occurrence. Therefore, identification and scoring of spikes in the EEG signal contributes relevant information toward determining a diagnosis of epilepsy. Epileptic EEG contains a combination of spikes (which lasts 20-70 ms), sharp waves (lasting 70-200 ms but not as sharply contoured as a spike), spike and wave complex (a spike followed by a slow wave, which may occur below 3 Hz), and polyspikes combined with slow waves. While experts may disagree on a precise definition of each of these waveform complexes, there is general agreement that automated spike detection is a well recognized task for an ANN in a neurodiagnostic laboratory. Automatic detection of spikes and seizures has engaged a number of research groups over the years (Gotman, 1982; Iasemidis, 2003; Wilson & Emerson, 2002). The objective of such an exercise is to identify waveforms during or before the onset of an epileptic seizure. Gotman and his colleagues have developed a number of algorithms with clinically useful results (Gotman et al., 1997; Qu & Gotman, 1997). Recently, Webber et al. (1996), Tarassenko et al. (1998), and Ozdamar and Kalayci (1998) have all presented well documented algorithms using backpropagation architecture that detects spikes and seizures. Ozdamar and Kalayci have shown that a three layer feedforward backpropagation (BP) network trained with raw EEG can also yield respectable results. Petrosian et al. (2000) considered raw EEG recorded from scalp and intracranial electrodes of two epileptic patients, as input to discrete-time recurrent multilayer perceptrons. They conclude that intracranial recordings provide better results in identifying spikes. Pang et al. (2003) compared the performance of four backpropagation based classifiers using features derived from algorithms developed by Tarassenko, Webber, and Kalyaci. It was concluded that ANNs trained with features selected using any one of the above algorithms, as well as raw EEG signal fed directly to the ANN, all yield similar results with accuracies ranging from 82.83%-86.61%. In contrast to these methods, Pradhan et al. (1996) used learning vector quantization (LVQ) neural network for detecting seizure activity. They used a two layer network: the first layer, called competitive layer, learns to classify the input vectors, and the second linear layer transforms the output of the first layer to user defined target classes. The network is trained with sampled EEG segments, and Kohonen's rule is used for learning. Once trained on the EEG containing epileptiform discharges from one subject, the LVQ based network can generalize the learning process and detect spikes from other subjects. When tested on the EEG recorded from four subjects containing seizure activity, the LVQ based system accurately identified 91% of the epochs containing seizure activity.

More recently, it has been possible to combine preseizure and seizure EEG detection using ANN with neurostimulation for responsive control of seizures. The most important development has been the implantation of miniaturized systems in the body or the skull. Such systems are already in clinical trials (Tcheng et al., 2004; Vossler et al., 2004).

Diagnosis of Huntington's Disease

Huntington's disease (HD) is an autosomal dominant neurodegenerative illness characterized by disorders of movement, cognition, behavior, and functional capacity (De Tommaso et al., 2003). All offspring of an affected individual begin life at a 50% risk of developing the disease. Clinical manifestations typically begin in the fourth decade of life and are characterized by inexorable, progressive deterioration in functional capacity. The EEG of HD shows a substantial reduction of alpha rhythm (Bylsma et al., 1994). De Tommaso et al. (2003) recently studied 13 confirmed HD patients, 7 gene carriers (considered high risk for HD), and 13 healthy controls. In order to determine whether EEG abnormalities were linked to functional changes preceding the onset of the disease, artifact-free epochs were selected and analyzed through fast Fourier transform. Features derived from power spectra of the EEG were tested using Fisher's linear discriminant (FLD) function, a likelihood ratio method (LRM) and an ANN classifier. They employed a multilayered perceptron of 13 input neurons, a hidden layer with a variable number of units (2-10) and an output neuron trained to register one when the EEG of a patient with HD was presented to the neural network (and a zero otherwise). It was found that the absolute alpha power was not correlated with cognitive decline. The pereceptron based classifier yielded superior performance compared to FLD and LRM. The ANN correctly classified 11 of 13 patients and 12 of 13 normal subjects. Further, for high risk patients, scores obtained from ANN were correlated with expected time before the onset of HD.

Diagnosis of Alzheimer's Disease (AD)

As many as 4.5 million Americans suffer from Alzheimer's disease, according to National Institute of Aging, U.S.A. (http://www.alzheimers.org/pubs/adfact.html). The disease usually begins after age 60, and the risk of AD goes up with age so that about 5% of men and women between ages 65-74 have AD, and nearly half of those who are age 85 and older may have the disease. However, AD is not a normal part of aging. EEG signal analysis of patients with AD reveals abnormal frequency signatures (Bennys et al., 2001; Jonkman, 1997;

Moretti et al., 2004). Compared to normal subjects, AD patients are known to have "slowing" of the EEG, namely, an increase of the delta (0.5-4 Hz) and theta (4-8 Hz) power along with a decrease of the alpha power (8-13 Hz). EEG rhythms and the power in the alpha band are highly correlated with dementia severity and disease progression from the earliest stages of AD. EEG analysis can contribute to an accurate diagnosis of AD and compares well with imaging tools in terms of sensitivity and specificity (Bennys et al., 2001; Jonkman, 1997). Petrosian et al. (2001) recorded continuous EEGs (as well as their wavelet-filtered subbands) from parieto-occipital channels of 10 early AD patients and 10 healthy controls. The EEG was used as input into recurrent neural networks (RNNs) for training and testing purposes. The RNNs were chosen for the classification task because they can implement non-linear decision boundaries and possess memory of the state. The best training/testing results were achieved using a three-layer RNN on left parietal channel using level 4 high-pass wavelet sub-bands. The classification procedure reported by Petrosian et al. (2001) had 80% sensitivity at 100% specificity. Features derived from wavelet analysis combined with the RNN approach may be useful in analyzing long-term continuous EEGs for early recognition of AD.

Analysis and Scoring of Sleep EEGs

The objective of a sleep study in a clinical laboratory is to chart the progress of the sleep through various stages and identify abnormal/pathological transitions between sleep states or physiological conditions (e.g., sleep apnea and hypoxia). Analysis of physiological data recorded during sleep, called polysomnography (PSG), is a time consuming task. It requires a sleep technologist to identify various stages of sleep and assign an appropriate class to each segment of PSG tracings and report observations to the physician. Physiological variables such as the EEG, ECG, EMG, EOG, measures of respiration, and arterial oxygen saturation (by pulse oximetry) are recorded during a typical PSG session. These signals result in large amounts of raw digital data (Agarwal & Gotman, 2001; Bock & Gough, 1998; Penzel & Conradt, 2000). Broadly speaking, awake, light sleep, deep sleep, and rapid eye movement sleep stages are identified by the technologist using a classification originally described by Rechtschaffen and Kales (1968), called *R&K classification*. While the original *R&K classification* predates digital computers in a sleep laboratory, researchers since the 1970s have tried to automate the task of sleep stage identification through computerized signal processing and classification. Power in delta, theta, and alpha bands of the EEG, occurrence of specific patterns such as K-complexes, sleep spindles, and vertex sharp waves are typical features used in sleep scoring. From the EOG, patterns such as rapid and slow eye movements are obtained. Such processing also rejects artifacts due to ECG, EOG, EMG, body movement, electrode movement, or sweating. Combinations of above features are fed into ANNs to determine sleep stages (Robert et al., 1998).

Schaltenbrand et al. (1993) trained their ANN-based sleep scoring system on the basis of twelve night recordings and tested it on eleven other datasets. There was an 80.6% agreement between visual scoring and the computerized system, with lowest agreement for sleep stage 1 and 3. A second publication by the same group reports a study in 60 subjects with expert–machine agreement of 82.3% (Schaltenbrand et al., 1996). By adding expert supervision for ambiguous and unknown epochs, the automatic/expert agreement grew from 82.3% to 90% even with a supervision over only 20% of the night. Agarwal and Gotman have employed cluster analysis to identify naturally occurring clusters in features derived from the PSG recording (Agarwal & Gotman, 2001, 2002). Compared to manual scoring, there was a concurrence of 80.6% between the physician and automated methods. Maximum error was found while identifying stage 1 sleep which was misclassified as either stage 2 or awake.

Estimation of the Depth of Anesthesia

Determination of appropriate level of anesthetic medication and the depth of anesthesia reached for a specific patient during surgery is a daily clinical challenge faced by an anaesthesiologist. Anaesthetic agents are often a combination of pharmacological agents that obey pharmacokinetic and pharmacodynamic laws and alter the normal functioning of the peripheral, central, and autonomic nervous systems. An appropriately administered anesthetic agent makes the patient unconscious, analgesic (pain free), and amnesic (has no memory of operating procedure) with inhibition of automatic muscular tonuses. Further, only a small amount of anesthetic agent is administered to the patient during the course of a surgical procedure, which may last several hours. The issue of which parameters derived from physiological variables would yield a robust measure of the depth of anesthesia, has intrigued pharamacologists, anesthesiologists, surgeons, and, more recently, the engineering/computer science community (Senhadji et al., 2002). Of several anesthetic agents which have been employed during surgery, studies using ANNs to determine the depth of anesthesia have been reported on enflurane, propofol, halothane, thiopental, and isoflurane (Robert et al., 2002b; Van Gils et al., 2002). An investigator who wishes to develop an ANN-based system for monitoring the depth of anesthesia must take into consideration the type of physiological signal/signals employed, the specific anesthetic agent used, and, finally, the feature or combination of features to be used to quantify the depth of anesthesia.

Features Used by the Physician to Measure the Depth of Anesthesia

Both amplitude and frequency of the EEG are affected by the dosage and the nature of the anesthetic agent. Autospectral and bispectral features derived from the EEG have gained acceptance in the surgical suite as a method to assess the depth of anesthesia. Other features include minimum alveolar concentration (MAC) of the inhalational agent, latencies, and amplitudes of mid-latency auditory evoked potentials (MLAEPs) in the range of 10-60 ms, along with blood pressure and heart rate (Eger et al., 1965; Van Gils et al., 2002). Peak latencies of MLAEPs reflect the hypnotic component of anesthesia while amplitudes reflect the analgesic component. The anesthetist observes continuous traces of heart rate, systolic and diastolic blood pressure, pupil size, lacrimation, muscular movement, and sweating to maintain the level of anesthesia.

Features for ANNs to Estimate the Depth of Anesthesia

In order to provide more quantitative information to the surgical team about the depth of anesthesia, designers have employed ANNs for measuring the depth of anesthesia (Krkic et al., 1996; Robert et al., 2002b). The variety of features for quantifying the state of consciousness and effectiveness of anesthesia is rather broad. They include the traditional EEG measures (power in delta, theta, alpha, and beta bands), features derived from bispectra, mutual information, and non-linear dynamics (chaos) models of the EEG signal (Ortolani et al., 2002; Zhang et al., 2001; Zhang & Roy, 2001). Krkic et al. (1996) employed spectral entropy of the EEG derived from complexity analysis as a feature. Jeleazcov et al. (2004) recently developed a backpropagation ANN with 22 inputs, 8 hidden, and 4 output neurons and tested it with EEG data recorded during surgery. They obtained sensitivity ranging from 72-90% and specificity from 80-92%. Huang et al. (2003) present an approach based on mutual information (MI) to predict response during isoflurane anesthesia. In their studies, the MI between EEG recorded from four cortical electrodes was computed from 98 consenting patients prior to incision during isoflurane anesthesia of different levels. The system was able to correctly classify purposeful response with an average accuracy of 91.84% of the cases.

Brain-Computer Interface

Brain-computer interface operates on the principle that non-invasively recorded cortical EEG signals contain information about an impending task and that such information can be identified by an ANN. Consequently, it is imperative that the intent of the subject is translated into some external control signal (Blanchard & Blankertz, 2004). From a computer scientist's point of view, the BCI is a translational algorithm which converts electrophysiological signals into an output that controls an external device (Vaughn et al., 2003). A BCI system comprises of EEG amplifiers, a feature extractor, a pattern recognition system, and a mechanical interface to achieve the motor component of the task. It is necessary that the sensors (electrodes) used to pick up EEG are easy to handle and mount. Software for feature extraction and recognition must be optimized for rapid response, and the mechanical device coupled to a BCI is easy to operate.

It is anticipated that BCI may become a medium for paralyzed patients to control a motorized device (e.g., a wheel chair, an appliance at home) or perform computer-related tasks (e.g., move a mouse or slow typing), operate a neuroprosthesis, or orthosis. Information transfer rate currently achieved is still a modest ~25 bits/min (Schalk et al., 2004). Patients with cerebral palsy, amyotrophic lateral sclerosis, or brainstem stroke may be trained to operate and would therefore benefit from BCI driven devices. The research on BCI involves several disciplines including mathematics, engineering, computer science, medicine, physical rehabilitation, and has engaged an increasingly larger number of investigators in the recent past. Key groups in this rapidly advancing field have met regularly either at workshops or through publication media in order to arrive at standards, common vocabulary, and consensus regarding procedures, software, training, ergonomics, and to discuss ethical issues (Vaughn et al., 2003). These meetings and interactions have provided forums for developing international cooperation and for preparation of detailed specification of standards (Mason & Birch, 2003; Pfurtscheller et al., 2003; Schalk et al., 2004). Several innovative designs have been offered in the public domain (Mason & Birch, 2003). Such openness provides criteria for objective comparison between various designs.

Types of BCI

There are mainly two types of BCI systems: In synchronous BCI, brain signals are analyzed in cue- or stimulus-triggered time windows, either by recognizing changes in EPs or slow cortical potential shifts or EEG components. In an asynchronous BCI, a continuous analysis of brain signals is performed either with the purpose of detecting event-related potentials or transient changes in EEG components (Pfurtscheller et al., 2003). Asynchronous mode of BCI is "noncue-based", and ongoing brain signals have to be analyzed and classified continuously. Mental events have to be detected and discriminated (from noise and non-events) and transformed into a control signal as quickly and accurately as possible.

Usually, a physiological mechanism and its use as a medium of control underscores the development of BCI. For example, volitional control can be exerted over 8-12 Hz (μ-rhythms) and 18-26 Hz frequency bands (β-rhythms) through training. Such learning ability has been the source of BCI instruments for controlling the location of a cursor on a computer screen (Schalk et al., 2004).

Functional Architecture for BCI

In order to standardize devices, instrumentation and systems, terminology, functional criteria, and end user friendliness, Mason and Birch (2003) describe a framework for the design of BCI. For BCI to be effective, the response time of the system should be low (< 1 second), have a high accuracy, and a low false positive rate. The display device is often the source of feedback for the user. In order to encourage research in BCI, Schalk et al. (2004) offer executable files, source code, and documentation of a BCI at http://www.bci2000.org, at no charge. The BCI 2000, as it is called, contains modules for data acquisition, storage, signal processing, user application, and user interface. These modules communicate through a protocol based on TCP/IP. The instrument has a number of important features such as real time capability, use of multiple programming languages, and flexibility to interface with hardware from different vendors. The BCI2000 is programmed with paradigms capable of running real time control of the screen through slow cortical potentials, evoked potentials, and μ/β rhythms, contained within the EEG. An imaginative implementation of BCI2000 employs the cortical potential found around 300 ms (called P300 wave). The P300 is generated following an odd-ball stimulation and is often used for a spelling task. With BCI2000, one can rapidly prototype applications suitable for the end-user, that is, the patient. While the framework for this instrument is not exclusively based on the ANN, feature extraction and signal conditioning are amply provided for. An user-defined command sequence can initiate classifier strategies on EEG/EP signals, including neural network classifiers (Schalk et al., 2004). In general, artificial neural networks form a crucial part of all BCI systems. Lal et al. (2004) have used a support vector machine (SVM) based on ANN for objectively identifying suitable channels of EEG for a motor imagery paradigm. Peters et al. (1998) initially compute EEG-based feature vectors using a large number (n =30) of multilayer perceptrons, one for each channel of the EEG.

Following training, the ANNs were pruned until a generalized estimate of the error to perform a motor task was minimized. Peters et al. report that their classifier achieves an accuracy of 92% on one second segments of EEG. Kaper et al. (2004) use a three-step approach to identify P300 event-related signals in the EEG. First, the data from selected channels were bandpass filtered (0-30 Hz). An SVM-based classifier was trained on a labeled training set. Classification accuracy was tested on an unlabeled test set. Kaper et al. obtained an accuracy of 84.5% for separation of EEG containing P300 potentials from epochs containing no P300 waveforms.

Types of Applications

While much of the current research focuses on various algorithms that translate the EEG, evoked potentials (EPs), and slower potentials, some institutions have embarked on developing specific instruments and devices that can be actuated with a BCI. Controlling a keyboard, non-invasive brain-actuated mobile robot, and manipulation of hand orthosis are some novel designs that are being investigated (Mason & Birch, 2003; Pfurtscheller et al., 2003).

Issues, Controversies, and Problems

We have discussed four major areas where artificial neural networks (ANNs) have contributed to our increasing knowledge of how the brain embeds information within the EEG. While only a small part of the brain's function is represented by EEG, the surface EEG signal is quite rich with information. Scientists have a great deal of work to do, as they explore, identify, and employ the most relevant and pertinent information. We list below some of the controversies and open problems in the field:

1. Even with the progress of computer and information technology in all its varied forms, including hardware with ever-increasing speed, development of sophisticated algorithms, and parallel computing, it would be simplistic to state that the application-oriented software described herein can match the accuracy of an expert in the field, as yet.

2. Selection of optimum features for performing pattern classification of EEG is still inadequately understood. Pang et al. (2003) compared four algorithms for detecting spikes in the EEG and found that the sampled raw EEG fed into the ANN for training gives as good a performance as mathemati-

cally derived features. Garrett et al. (2003) found that non-linear classification methods, such as support vector machine, offer only a marginal advantage over linear discriminant classifiers while classifying EEG during five mental tasks. Garrett et al. (2003) suggest that since the EEG is high dimensional and noisy, any advantage of non-linear classification methods over linear ones is limited.

3. Sleep staging and identification of wakefulness is still a subjective task. Some form of human input is necessary for identification of such events.

4. During anesthesia monitoring, features used by both the physician and the ANNs are quite varied, and there is an ongoing controversy on feature selection.

5. It is humanly not possible to verify if the anaesthetic is adequate at the time of surgery because one cannot ask the patient during the sedated state.

6. In spite of considerable research, monitoring the effects of different types of surgical procedures and anaesthetic agents is still dependent on the training of the attending anesthesiologist.

7. Different anaesthetic agents and their effects on depth of anesthesia have to be tuned to individual ANN designs.

8. It is conceivable that the same BCI can be used across a group of subjects. Toward this end, the designers have to incorporate facilities to tune the software for individualized use. Recent publications and designs address some of these concerns (Schalk et al., 2004).

9. BCIs require some degree of normal functioning of the brain and sensory input. Individual users fitted with BCI must be able to generate neurophysiological signals required to activate the BCI.

10. Most BCI employ scalp EEG which contains noise and artifacts with a concomitant reduction in signal-to-noise ratio.

Solutions and Recommendations

Evaluation of various types of ANNs, especially those with the most promising results, by independent assessors, is necessary to benchmark their results. Such studies may assist in solving issues related to quality control and reliability of software packages. In sleep studies, the role of computers as storage and display devices is rather mundane, and the diagnostic use of computer software, especially using ANNs, is underutilized. Sleep laboratories have a role to play in establishing rigorous standards for identifying sleep stages based on EEG and other physiological signals. Measurement of pain during surgery is not easy; and therefore, other variables arising out of autonomic nervous system, such as heart rate variability and its power spectra, may enhance the quality of decision making (Van Gils et al., 2002). In the area of brain-computer interface, the field is still young. The process of transferring BCI technology from a laboratory bench to a disabled patient requires some thought and would include personalized tuning, ongoing maintenance, and education of both the caregiver and the patient. Currently, ethical issues such as who gets priority (of use) following the development of a BCI device have not arisen in the laboratory and may become relevant with the progression of technology.

Suggestions for Future Work

For those applications described in this chapter, it would be a step forward if a common data pool consisting of appropriate physiological signals was available for evaluation by various groups. Future work in BCI may involve innovative types of biofeedback combined with BCI to reach larger groups of patients with psychological and cognitive disorders such as depression, dyslexia, and attention deficit disorders. The increase of information transfer rate in BCI is an issue that needs attention. It is therefore necessary to refine procedures and algorithms that extend the type and quality of analysis of the scalp EEG. Methodological issues, such as how to safely access EEG signals using cortical implants over long periods of time (several months to years), have to be addressed. It is likely that basic building blocks, such as VLSI/ASIC chips, specialized hardware platforms incorporating algorithms designed specifically for applications described in this chapter, will emerge in the near future.

Summary

Analysis of EEG signals using artificial neural networks has yielded a number of tangible benefits. Of several applications reported in the literature, we examined four important areas related to diagnosis of diseases, sleep scoring, assessment of the depth of anesthesia, and building a brain-computer interface. Integration of these technologies to solve clinical problems will require cooperation between various laboratories and professionals.

Acknowledgment

Dr.Kamath and Dr. Upton received support from DeGroote Foundation for their research. Dr. Kamath and Dr. Poehlman acknowledge the grant support from Natural Sciences and Engineering Research Council of Canada.

References

Agarwal, R., & Gotman, J. (2001). Computer assisted sleep staging. *IEEE Transactions on Biomedical Engineering, 48*(12), 1412-1423.

Agarwal, R., & Gotman, J. (2002). Digital tools in polysomnography. *Journal of Clinical Neurophysiology, 19*(2), 136-143.

Bennys, K., Rondouin, G., Vergnes, C., & Touchon, J. (2001). Diagnostic value of quantitative EEG in Alzheimer's disease. *Neurophysiologie Clinique, 31*(3), 153-160.

Blanchard, G., & Blankertz, B.(2004). BCI Competition 2003—Data set IIa: Spatial patterns of self-controlled brain rhythm modulations. *IEEE Transactions on Biomedical Engineering, 51*(6), 1062-1066.

Bock, J., & Gough, D.A. (1998). Toward prediction of physiological state signals in sleep apnea. *IEEE Transactions on Biomedical Engineering, 45*(11), 1332-1341.

Bylsma, F. W., Peyser, C., Folstein, S. E., Folstein, M. F., Ross, C., & Brandt, J. (1994). EEG power spectra in Huntington's disease: Clinical and neuropsychological correlates. *Neuropsychologia, 32*(2), 137-150.

de Tommaso, M., De Carlo, F., Difruscolo, O., Massafra, R., Sciruicchio, V., & Bellotti, R. (2003). Detection of subclinical brain electrical activity changes in Huntington's disease using artificial neural networks. *Clinical Neurophysiology, 114*(7), 1237-1245.

Eger, E. I., Saidman, L. J., & Brandstater, B. (1965). Minimum aleveolar anaesthetic concentration. A standard of anaesthetic potency. *Anaesthesiology, 26*(6), 756-763.

Garrett, D., Peterson, D. A., Anderson, C. W., & Thaut, M. H. (2003). Comparison of linear, nonlinear, and feature selection methods for EEG signal classification. *IEEE Transactions on Neural Systems and Rehabilitation Engineering, 11*(2), 141-144.

Gotman, J. (1982). Automatic recognition of epileptic seizures in the EEG. *Electroencephalography and Clinical Neurophysiology, 54*(5), 530-540.

Gotman, J., Flanagan, D., Zhang, J., & Rosenblatt, B. (1997). Automatic seizure recognition in the newborn: Methods and initial evaluation. *Electroencephalography and Clinical Neurophysiology, 103*(3), 356-362.

Huang, L., Yu, P., Ju, F., & Cheng, J. (2003). Prediction of response to incision using the mutual information of electroencephalograms during anesthesia. *Medical Engineering & Physics, 25*, 321-327.

Iasemidis, L. D. (2003). Epileptic seizure prediction and control. *IEEE Transactions on Biomedical Engineering, 50*(5), 549-558.

Jeleazcov, C., Egner, S., Bremer, F., & Schwilden, H. (2004). Automated EEG preprocessing during anesthesia: New aspects using artificial neural networks. *Biomedizinische Technik, 49*(5), 125-131.

Jonkman, E. J. (1997). The role of the electroencephalogram in the diagnosis of dementia of the Alzheimer type: An attempt at technology assessment. *Clinical Neurophysiology, 27*(3), 211-219.

Kaper, M., Meinicke, P., Grosskathoefer, Lingner, T., & Ritter, H. (2004). BCI competition 2003—Data set b: Support vector machines for P300 speller paradigm. *IEEE Transactions on Biomedical Engineering, 51*(6), 1073-1076.

Krkic, M., Roberts, S. J., Rezek, I., & Jordan, C. (1996, April). EEG-based assessment of anaesthetic depth using neural networks. *Proceedings of the IEE Colloquium on AI Methods in Biosignal Analysis,* London.

Lal, T. N., Schröder, M., Hinterberger, T., Weston, J., Bogdan, M., Birbaumer, N., & Schölkopf, R. (2004). Support vector channel selection in BCI. *IEEE Transactions on Biomedical Engineering, 51*(6), 1003-1010.

Mason, S. G., & Birch, G. E. (2003). A general framework for brain-computer interface design. *IEEE Transactions on Neural Systems and Rehabilitation Engineering, 11*, 70-85.

Moretti, D.V., Babiloni, C., Binetti, G., Cassetta, E., Dal Forno, G., Ferreri, F., Ferri, R., Lanuzza, B., Miniussi, C., Nobili, F., Rodriguez, G., Salinari, S., & Rossini, P. M. (2004). Individual analysis of EEG frequency and band power in mild Alzheimer's disease. *Clinical Neurophysiology, 115*(2), 299-308.

Ortolani, O., Conti, A., Di Filippo, A., Adembri, C., Moraldi, E., et al. (2002). EEG signal processing in anesthesia. Use of a neural network technique for monitoring depth of anesthesia. *British Journal of Anesthesia, 88*(5), 644-648.

Ozdamar, O., & Kalayci, T. (1998). Detection of spikes with artificial neural networks using raw EEG. *Computers and Biomedical Research, 31*(2), 122-142.

Pang, C. C. C., Upton, A. R. M., Shine, G., & Kamath, M. V. (2003). A comparison of algorithms for detection of spikes in the electroencephalogram. *IEEE Transactions on Biomedical Engineering, 50*(4), 521-526.

Penzel, T., & Conradt, R. (2000). Computer based sleep recording and analysis. *Sleep Medicine Reviews, 4*(2), 131-148.

Peters, B. O., Pfurtscheller, G., & Flyvbjerg, H. (1998). Mining multi-channel EEG for information content: An ANN based method for brain computer interface. *Neural Networks, 11*(7-8), 1429-1433.

Petrosian, A. A., Prokhorov, D., Homan, R., Dasheiff, R., & Wunsch, D. C. (2000). Recurrent neural network based prediction of epileptic seizures in intra- and extracranial EEG. *Neurocomputing, 30*(1-4), 201-218.

Petrosian, A. A., Prokhorov, D. V., Lajara-Nanson, W., & Schiffer, R. B. (2001). Recurrent neural network-based approach for early recognition of Alzheimer's disease in EEG. *Clinical Neurophysiology, 112*(8), 1378-1387.

Pfurtscheller, G., Neuper, C., Muller, G. R., Obermaier, B., Krausz, G., Schlögl, A., et al. (2003). Graz-BCI: State of the art and clinical applications. *IEEE Transactions on Neural System and Rehabilitation Engineering, 11*(2), 177-180.

Pradhan, N., Sadasivan, P. K., & Arunodaya. (1996). Detection of seizure activity in EEG by an artificial neural network: A preliminary study. *Computers and Biomedical Research, 29*(4), 303-313.

Qu, H., & Gotman, J. (1997). A patient specific algorithm for the detection of seizure onset in long term EEG monitoring: Possible use as a warning device. *IEEE Transactions on Biomedical Engineering, 44*(2), 115-122.

Rechtschaffen, A., & Kales, A. (1968). *A manual of standardized terminology, techniques, and scoring system for sleep stages of human subjects* (NIH Publication No. 204). Washington, DC: Public Health Service, US Government Printing Office.

Robert, C., Gaudy, J., & Limoge, A. (2002a). Electroencephalogram processing using neural networks. *Clinical Neurophysiology, 113*(5), 694-701.

Robert, C., Guilpin, C., & Limoge, A. (1998). Review of neural network applications in sleep research. *Journal of Neuroscience Methods, 79*(2), 187-193.

Robert, C., Karasinski, P., Arreto, C. D., & Gaudy, J. F. (2002b). Monitoring anesthesia using neural networks: A survey. *Journal of Clinical Monitoring and Computing, 17*(3-4), 259-267.

Schalk, G., McFarland, D. J., Hinterberger, T., Birbaumer, N., & Wolpaw, J.R. (2004). BCI2000: A general-purpose brain-computer interface (BCI) system. *IEEE Transactions on Biomedical Engineering, 51*(6), 1034-1043.

Schaltenbrand, N., Lengelle, R., & Macher, J. P. (1993). Neural network model: Application to automatic analysis of human sleep. *Computers and Bio-medical Research, 26*(2), 157-171.

Schaltenbrand, N., Lengelle, R., Toussaint, M., Luthringer, R., Carelli, G., Jacqmin, A., et al. (1996). Sleep stage scoring using the neural network model: Comparison between visual and automatic analysis in normal subjects and patients. *Sleep, 19*(1), 26-35.

Senhadji, L., Wodey, E., & Claude, E. (2002). Monitoring approaches in general anesthesia: A survey. *Critical Reviews in Biomedical Engineering, 30*(1-3), 85-97.

Tarassenko, L., Khan, Y. U., & Holt, M. R. G. (1998). Identification of inter-ictal spikes in the EEG using neural network analysis. *IEE Proceedings of Science, Measurement and Technology, 145*(6), 270-278.

Tcheng, T., Esteller, R., & Echauz, J. (2004). Suppression of epileptiform activity by responsive electrical stimulation in epileptic patients. *Proceedings of the 58th Annual Conference of American Epilepsy Society,* New Orleans, LA.

Van Gils, M., Korhonen, I., & Yli-Hankala, A. (2002). Methods for assessing adequacy of anesthesia. *Critical Reviews in Biomedical Engineering, 30*(1-3), 99-130.

Vaughan, T. M., Heetderks, W. J., Trejo, L. J., Rymer, W. Z., Weinrich, M., Moore, M. M., et al. (2003). Brain-computer interface technology: A review of the Second International Meeting. *IEEE Transactions on Neural Systems & Rehabilitation Engineering, 11*(2), 94-109.

Vossler, D., Doherty, M., Goodman, R., Hirsch, L., Young, J., & Kraemer, D. (2004, December). Early safety experience with a fully implanted intracranial responsive neurostimulator for epilepsy. *Proceedings of the 58th Annual Conference of American Epilepsy Society,* New Orleans, Louisiana.

Webber, W. R. S., Lesser, R. P., Richardson, R. T., & Wilson, K. (1996). An approach to seizure detection using an artificial neural network (ANN). *Electroencephalography and Clinical Neurophysiology, 98*(4), 250-272.

Wilson, S. B., & Emerson, R. (2002). Spike detection: A review and comparison of algorithms. *Clinical Neurophysiology, 113*(12), 1873-1881.

Zhang, X. S., & Roy, R. J. (2001). Derived fuzzy knowledge model for estimating the depth of anesthesia. *IEEE Transactions on Biomedical Engineering, 48*(3), 312-323.

Zhang, X. S., Roy, R. J., Schwender, D., & Daunderer, M. (2001). Discrimination of anesthetic states using mid-latency auditory evoked potentials and artificial neural networks. *Annals of Biomedical Engineering, 29*(5), 446-453.

Chapter IX

The Use of Artificial Neural Networks for Objective Determination of Hearing Threshold Using the Auditory Brainstem Response

Robert T. Davey, City University, London, UK

Paul J. McCullagh, University of Ulster, Northern Ireland

H. Gerry McAllister, University of Ulster, Northern Ireland

H. Glen Houston, Royal Victoria Hospital, Northern Ireland

Abstract

We have analyzed high and low level auditory brainstem response data (550 waveforms over a large age range; 126 were repeated sessions used in correlation analysis), by extracting time, frequency, and phase features and using these as inputs to ANN and decision tree classifiers. A two stage process is used. For responses with a high poststimulus to prestimulus power ratio indicative of high level responses, a classification accuracy of

98% has been achieved. These responses are easily classified by the human expert. For lower level responses appropriate to hearing threshold, additional features from time, frequency, and phase have been used for classification, providing accuracies between 65% and 82%. These used a dataset with repeated recordings so that correlation could be employed. To increase classification accuracy, it may be necessary to combine the relevant features in a hybrid model.

Introduction

The recording of an evoked response is a standard noninvasive procedure, which is routine in many audiology and neurology clinics. The auditory brainstem response (ABR) provides an objective method of assessing the integrity of the auditory pathway and hence of assessing an individual's hearing level. Labeling and interpreting ABR data is a time consuming process and has depended on access to expert opinion. Interpretation requires a subjective analysis of the ABR waveform data, and human experts are not always in agreement, especially as the stimulation intensity decreases toward threshold level. Artificial intelligence techniques can be applied to assist with the interpretation, further adding to the objectivity of the assessment.

In this chapter, we review the approaches previously adopted and assess the methods on a clinical dataset which contains both high and low stimulus responses. In general, the higher stimulus levels produce clearer responses which should be easier to detect, whereas the lower stimulus intensities produce responses with much lower signal to noise ratios, requiring more complex analysis. Most research studies to date have used features extracted from ABR time waveform, simulating the interpretative work of the trained audiologist (for example, see Boston, 1989; Gronfors, 1993; Habraken et al., 1993; Herrmann et al., 1995). However, additional information is available from the frequency domain. In particular, the power spectrum and phase data provide an alternative view and possibly some complementary information. The cross-correlation function has been used with time domain data, to assess the repeatability of the waveform and extracted features. This approach can also be applied to the frequency domain data.

Our objective is to classify both high level and low level ABRs by evaluating features derived from both time and frequency domain, and employing the cross-correlation technique with both sources. We assess classification performance using two alternative approaches: the artificial neural network and the decision tree algorithm. It is likely that by combining the results of individual classifiers, a greater degree of accuracy can be achieved than from any one of the individual sources, and this provides potential for future research.

Literature Review

The first electrophysiological recordings from the human brain were made in 1924 by Hans Berger. The term *electroencephalogram (EEG)* (Berger, 1969) is used to describe the brain potentials he recorded. Using electrodes placed on the surface of the scalp, the EEGs he produced also showed a change in their rhythm when he either dropped a steel ball into a dish or exploded a firecracker to produce a sudden loud noise. This resultant change in rhythm in the EEG is known as an evoked response.

Evoked responses can be recorded using acoustic, visual, and somatosensory stimuli. A computer can be used to record and display this brain electrical activity. Electrodes are placed on the surface of the scalp, and after amplifying and filtering, the analogue signals from the brain are then sampled using an analogue to digital converter. The computer not only displays the data in graphic form, but also allows the data to be manipulated and investigated further.

To record auditory evoked responses, electrodes are commonly placed on the vertex, ipsilateral and contralateral mastoids. Click stimuli are applied to one or both ears. The auditory brainstem response appears within 10ms from the onset of the stimulus, and its amplitude is typically less than 1µVolt. The amplitude of the ABR in a single sweep, however is very small and consequently is masked by the ongoing brain electrical activity (50-100 µVolt). The measurement and interpretation of an ABR is therefore difficult, time consuming, error prone and hence expensive.

The traditional method of isolating the evoked response from the other ongoing brain activity has been the use of the averaging (McGillem & Aunon, 1987) technique. As successive sweeps are averaged together, the response potentials, time locked to the stimuli, remain constant while the other ongoing brain activity tends to cancel toward zero. Using this technique alone, several thousand sweeps of data will need to be obtained and averaged to elicit a clear response from an ABR recording.

When the stimulus level is high and the subject's hearing pathways are normal, the evoked response will usually take the shape of a five-peak waveform, known as the Jewett waveform (Jewett, 1970). The ABR can be used as an objective assessment of hearing ability. Such a test is useful where a subjective response is difficult to obtain, for example, in young children. Because the ABR waves emanate from anatomical structures (Starr & Don, 1988), the test assists with the localization of auditory lesions to within several millimeters. The ABR can help in the diagnosis of acoustic neuromas, intrinsic brainstem lesions (including multiple sclerosis), brainstem infarctions, brainstem gliomas, and various degenerative disorders of the central nervous system.

An ABR hearing test is performed by making successive recordings, while applying stimuli of varying intensity to each ear, until the threshold level of hearing is determined. The resulting data, though showing a familiar trend in most cases, do not fit a standard template and are a function of numerous recording factors such as electrode placement, filtering ranges, intensity levels, and ear used. Waveforms are also dependent on individual patient characteristics such as head shape. For interpretation, it has thus depended on access to expert opinion. The human expert, in making an interpretation, checks the latencies of waves I, III, and V; examines the overall morphology of the waveform; and evaluates how consistent the subaverages are.

In this way, the human expert classifies the waveform as to whether a response is present or not. When the stimulus level is high, for example, around 70dBnHL (normal hearing level), and the subject's hearing pathways are normal, the five peak Jewett waveform would normally be present (Figure 1), waves IV and V can often merge.

When the stimulus level is reduced to about 30dBnHL, which is the approximate hearing threshold of a person with normal hearing level, waves I, II, III, and IV have usually reduced below the background EEG levels, and only wave V and its following negative-going slope remain (Figure 2).

The process, therefore, of identifying this wave V and its following negative-going slope from the background EEG activity, is central to classifying the waveform as to whether a response is present or not, and so also to determining the hearing threshold level.

Alpsan and Ozdamar (1992a) compared human expert and neural network classification accuracies and found that three human experts had about 80%

Figure 1. Jewett waveform illustrating waves I-V in response to 70dBnHL

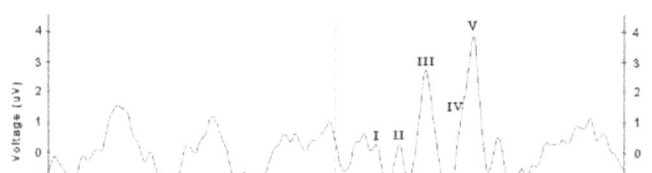

Figure 2. Response to 30dBnHL, illustrating wave V with its characteristic slope

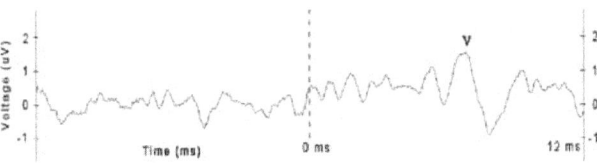

agreement on the recordings, but this was reduced to about 70% when intensity or both intensity and amplitude clues were removed using scaled and normalized classification tasks. Pratt et al. (1995) reported observations for repeated evaluations of ABR waveforms in judging for presence or absence of waves I, III, and V. Agreement between pairs of judges ranged from 86% to 100% for the same waveforms. Intra-judge agreement for repeated reviews of the waveforms was 87% to 95%.

Classification of the ABR waveform can be difficult, especially near the threshold level of hearing. There can also be inconsistency between judges, and even for the same judge when recordings are reviewed after a period of time. The process is time consuming due to the number of sweeps that must be averaged together and the time required by the audiologist to inspect recordings and manually overlay waveforms to confirm their similarity.

Feature extraction (McGillem & Aunon, 1987) is a necessary but difficult step in analyzing the recorded and averaged event-related potential (ERP) data. Heuristic feature extraction usually consists of measuring the latency and amplitude of the major peaks and valleys. As this involves subjective judgment, automated peak measuring procedures have been devised for this purpose. Statistical methods (Gevins, 1987) of feature extraction such as principal component analysis (PCA) allow an investigator to compare large sets of averaged evoked response potentials by producing a set of "principal components" that are common to all of the potentials considered. The major drawback, however, is that the small amount of residual variance unaccounted for by the major components might be crucial in distinguishing the clinical or experimental categories studied.

Automated Classification

Automated systems have also been developed to assist in the interpretation of the ABR data. The ALGO-I infant hearing screener (Herrmann et al., 1995) had the single purpose of identifying hearing loss in infants in order to optimize the design and for effective control of the test factors. The screener calculates the likelihood of a response using a weighted-binary template-matching algorithm. However, a standard template cannot be used with the response data obtained from a wide age range. There may be a familiar trend in the data, but the response is a function of numerous recording factors and is also dependent on individual patient characteristics.

The use of artificial neural networks to classify the time domain waveform has had some success. Alpsan and Ozdamar (1992b) reported 78.7% accuracy, and McCullagh and King (1996), 73.7% accuracy. No rules or knowledge base was needed, and the features selected and represented by ANNs resembled the features used by experts in making their classification. The accuracies obtained were similar to those of the expert, when the expert did not have access to contextual information such as stimulus intensity and relative amplitude. However, the neural network accuracy would drop significantly when the stimulus was reduced to near threshold level. Habraken et al. (1993) combined ANNs with an algorithmic approach to create a feature extractor for determining the latency of wave V peak. For the real data waveforms, this feature extractor generated results that complied with the opinion of a human expert in $80 \pm 6\%$ of cases. It should be remembered that these feature extractors were used on data recorded at a high stimulus level, and accuracy would probably drop significantly when the stimulus level is reduced to near threshold level.

Delgado and Ozdamar (1994) reported a complete automated system for ABR identification and waveform recognition. Spectral analysis, filtering, and modeling of ABR data was used to develop filters that would detect the positions of the various peaks of a response. They identified three primary frequency components of approximately 200, 500, and 900 Hz in the ABR waveform, supporting previous research (Boston, 1981; Pratt et al., 1989; Suzuki, 1982). The system could label peaks and generate latency-intensity curves and showed at least a 50:1 improvement ratio over the time taken by a human expert. Accuracy ranged from 86.7% to 94%. Ozdamar et al. (1994) reported a less complex system which returned just the threshold level of hearing. This method used the cross-correlation function on consecutive averages that had been recorded with the same stimulus level. The thresholds derived from use of this sliding window methodology agreed with expert-derived thresholds, within ±10dB, over 96% of the time.

Gronfors (1994) devised a multistage process for automatic ABR peak detection using the pedestal peak method (Gronfors, 1993; Urbach & Pratt, 1986) and advanced pattern recognition. Using 212 waveforms for 32 subjects, the author reported 86% accuracy with 90dB stimulation and 76% accuracy with 70dB stimulation for a group of waveforms where almost all peaks were present. For other auditory responses which did not display the classical Jewett waveform morphology, typically, only peak V was identifiable. With 90dB stimulation intensity, the accuracy was 76%, and with 70dB stimulation intensity, 56% accuracy was obtained.

Vannier et al. (2002) describe a detection method in the time domain based on supervised pattern recognition. A previously used pattern recognition technique, relying on cross-correlation with a template, was modified in order to include *a priori* information, thus increasing detection accuracy. While there have been previous peak identification methods employed, neural networks (Popescu et al., 1999; Tian et al., 1997; van Gils & Cluitmans, 1994), syntactic pattern recognition (Madhavan et al., 1986), expert system design (Boston, 1989), or band pass filtering (Delgado & Ozdamar, 1994; Gronfors, 1994; Pratt et al., 1989) show good performance when applied to waveforms obtained from normal subjects at high stimulation intensity. The difficulty arises with waveforms obtained at low stimulus intensity because it can be difficult to distinguish a small wave V peak from another peak that is part of the background noise. The accuracy of detection obtained by Vannier was better than 90%, and the average accuracy of threshold determination was 5dB. The approach depends, however, on recordings made at reducing intensity levels to enable the generation of a latency-intensity curve. The disadvantage is the time required for recording several ABRs instead of one, which can be a limitation for universal screening.

Aoyagi and Harada (1988) concluded that there were three peaks in the power spectrum of the ABR, at a sufficient level of stimulation. When the stimulation is reduced below approximately 50dB, the power above 600Hz is decreased. The phase variance [var{$\varphi(m)$}] of each Fourier component among 10 averaged waveforms was computed. 1-var{$\varphi(m)$} was named the component synchrony measure (CSM) and varied from 0 to 1. Averaged CSM values were found to have three peaks at 80-50dB stimulation intensity and two peaks at 40-20dB. At 10dB, which is the threshold of ABR, only one peak could be observed within a frequency range of 100-300Hz. Highest accuracy was obtained when this one frequency range was the basis of the criterion used for ABR threshold detection. The threshold levels obtained by the system coincided with human experts 75% of the time.

Davey et al. (2003) obtained a similar result when using software modeling to classify selected data from the time and frequency domains of ABR waveforms. A greater accuracy was obtained with the models that used the frequency domain waveform data, especially when restricted frequency ranges, around 200Hz and 500Hz, were selected.

Concluding this review of previous work, it is obvious that time domain features are important but that the amplitude or power spectrum and phase angle information obtained from ABR waveforms can provide useful information for classification, especially when the 200, 500, and 900Hz frequency ranges are selected. The cross-correlation function has been used with time domain data, but not with the frequency domain data.

Data Description

The data used in this research were recorded by the Audiology Department of the Royal Group of Hospitals in Northern Ireland. It comprised a total of 550 waveforms from both male and female patients at various stimulation levels down to threshold, an age range from 1 month to 70 years, and patients with both normal and abnormal hearing. Each of the 550 ABR waveforms was classified by an audiologist as a Yes response or a No response. The total number of ears tested by the recordings was 175, and many of these recordings were "repeat sessions", used by an audiologist to provide confirmation in difficult cases, especially when near the threshold level of hearing. The repeat sessions, 360 in total, were used by this research to cross-correlate waveforms, inspired by and replicating, the visual comparison that an audiologist makes on a computer monitor.

Further, the set of 550 waveforms contained 396 recordings with a Yes response and 154 with a No response. Consequently, the data were partitioned at times, according to the need for repeat sessions, and also to provide a balance of yes and no responses in the data subset. The content of each subset created is detailed when the relevant tests are discussed.

Each waveform consisted of 480 sample points acquired over 24msec, the stimulus applied at the halfway point. This gave a 12msec prestimulus period with 240 data points, where a response was never present, and a 12msec poststimulus period with 240 data points, where a response may be present. Before sampling, the signal was band limited by an analogue filter with pass-band 100-3000Hz. The sampling frequency (20kHz) is therefore more than twice the highest frequency component (3kHz) present in the signal. Between 1,000-2,000 ensembles were then averaged together to make one subaveraged ABR waveform before saving the data to file.

At the 70dBnHL stimulus level, the response was often clear enough for the audiologist, but at the 30dBnHL stimulus level, there was uncertainty, and so a repeat recording at this stimulus level was taken, so that the audiologist could visually correlate the two recordings on the screen and make sure that what seemed to be a wave V peak and associated negative-going slope was consistent in both waveforms. This lack of repeat recordings at the higher stimulus levels gave rise eventually to the partitioning of the dataset so that different detection methods were applied to data where a large response is present and data where the response is not so clear, reflecting in some measure, how the audiologist handles this classification process.

Feature Extraction

Sanchez et al. (1995) used artificial neural network (ANN) classification models with the raw time domain data and also with selected features. The results of the raw data models indicated that restricted portions of the ABR waveform (from about peak I to peak V) contain the information useful for classification. But the feature based models outperformed the raw data models. Extraction of features, therefore, from all the ABR waveforms was considered to be a prerequisite for classification. Consequently, various features were extracted from the raw time and frequency domain data, and the software classifiers were allowed to select those which would be of importance in the classification process.

Visual comparison of ABR waveforms with one another, and of the poststimulus section with the prestimulus section, gave the qualitative impression of a power increase in the poststimulus section whenever a response was present. It was noted that a sustained increase in amplitude, for the duration of the poststimulus activity, contributed to at least a doubling of the waveform power. It was therefore possible that a threshold value based on relative power could be used as a simple detector of a response. As the algorithm was refined, the whole of the prestimulus section was used, but only part of the poststimulus waveform, from 1.5-9.5msec, where waves I-V are usually found, as this was found to be less prone to artifact. This feature was named TDpost/prePwr.

Cross-correlation values were calculated for those ABR waveforms which had a repeat session at the same stimulus level. Four feature values were extracted from each pair of time domain waveforms by finding the cross-correlation coefficient for these four different time periods in the waveforms: (1) the whole of both prestimulus periods, (2) the whole of both poststimulus periods, (3) only the 1.5-9.5msec poststimulus period of both waveforms where waves I-V would be found, and (4) only the 5.5-9.5msec poststimulus period of both waveforms where wave V would be found. These four features were named, TDPreCCR, TDpostCCR, TDw1to5CCR, and TDwave5CCR, respectively.

The cross-correlation coefficient value for both prestimulus waveform periods was also calculated so this could be used in a comparison with the poststimulus value. It was thought that the ratio or difference of the two coefficient values might be meaningful. Evaluation of the importance of all these features was left for the software classification models to show.

Aoyagi and Harada (1988) looked at four uses of the FFT data in the analysis of the ABR waveform: digital filtering, power spectral analysis, cross-correlation function, and phase spectral analysis. In the analysis of the power spectrum, their data showed three peaks with troughs at 300-450Hz, 600-800Hz, and 1200-1500Hz. The peaks therefore occur within the ranges of 0-300Hz, 450-600Hz, and 800-1200Hz. At near threshold intensities, the frequency components above 600 Hz are greatly decreased. Figure 3 concurs with these findings and shows peaks at approximately 200, 500, and 900Hz, with a stimulation intensity of 70dBnHL, but only peaks at 200 and 500Hz for 30dBnHL stimulation intensity.

Features of the phase information were also extracted. A summary table of the extracted features with their names and a short description is provided in Table 1.

Results

The raw data waveforms were first preprocessed by digital filtering using the wavelet transform multiresolution decomposition method. These filtered wave-

Figure 3. Relative amplitude vs. frequency (Hz) for 70dB and 30dB stimulation intensities (1 μV peak sine wave is equivalent to 250, and the value varies proportionately)

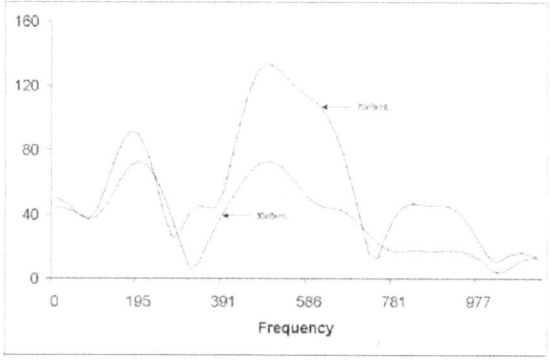

Table 1. List of features extracted from time, frequency, and phase

Feature name	Domain	Description
TDpost/prePwr	Time	Ratio of mean poststimulus to mean prestimulus power
TDPreCCR	Time	Cross-correlation coefficient of whole of both prestimulus waveforms
TDpostCCR	Time	Cross-correlation coefficient of whole of both poststimulus waveforms
TDw1to5CCR	Time	Cross-correlation coefficient of both poststimulus waveforms (1.5-9.5msec)
TDwave5CCR	Time	Cross-correlation coefficient of both poststimulus waveforms (5.5-9.5msec)
FFTpostCCR	Frequency	Cross-correlation coefficient of both poststimulus FFT waveforms (0-1100Hz)
FFTpreCCR	Frequency	Cross-correlation coefficient of both prestimulus waveforms (0-1100Hz)
FFTavgCCR	Frequency	Cross-correlation coefficient of post- and prestimulus averaged FFT waveforms
Frequencies e.g. 253.9Hz and 312.5Hz	Frequency	Poststimulus less prestimulus FFT data. See data filename re: negative values
Frequencies e.g. 253.9Hz and 312.5Hz	Frequency	Ratio of post- to prestimulus FFT data (0-1100Hz)
FFTs3pwr100..... FFTs3pwr1000	Frequency	Post-Pre stim FFT power values averaged in a 200Hz moving window (0-1100Hz)
FFTarea200 FFTarea350 FFTarea500 FFTarea700 FFTarea900	Frequency	Poststimulus less prestimulus FFT data used. Area under peaks at 200, 500, and 900Hz, and troughs at 350 and 700Hz, calculated by adding amplitude values
PHpost100..... PHpost1000	Phase	Cross-correlation of poststimulus phase values in 200Hz window (0-1100Hz)
PHpostpre100.... PHpostpre1000	Phase	Post- and prestimulus phase values cross-correlated in 200Hz window (0-1100Hz)

forms were then normalized and any dc offset removed. Time domain features were extracted and output to a text file for use by the time domain software models. The FFT data of the time domain waveforms were then obtained. From this, frequency and phase features were extracted and also output to a text file to be used by the frequency and phase software models. The individual time, frequency, and phase software models used artificial neural networks and decision trees to classify the data.

The Clementine data mining software system (http://www.spss.com) provides two machine learning technologies, rule induction, and neural networks. Neural networks are powerful general function estimators. They usually perform prediction tasks at least as well as other techniques, and sometimes perform significantly better. They also require minimal statistical or mathematical knowledge to train or apply. Clementine incorporates several features to avoid some of the common pitfalls of neural networks, including sensitivity analysis to aid in interpretation of the network, pruning and validation to prevent overtraining, and dynamic networks to automatically find an appropriate network architecture. In this study, we chose many of the default options provided by Clementine, allowing the package to choose the network topology, using the Quick option. Prevent Overtraining was switched off to permit the networks to be trained on all the data given to it.

The neural network models created used the backpropagation algorithm (Rumelhart et al., 1986) and the rule induction models used the standard C5.0 algorithm (Quinlan, 1986). The backpropagation training algorithm for neural networks has been widely used in the field of pattern recognition, and Habraken et al. (1993) have demonstrated that it has led to good results in a variety of fields such as time-domain signal processing and signal classification (Gorman & Sejnowski, 1988; Waibel et al., 1989). A decision tree uses a set of training data to look for underlying relationships and features in the data, creating a model that can be later used for prediction. The dataset or subset of data within each node is split depending on the value of a variable, associating rules with nodes and creating a tree of rules that classifies the data. The tree's structure, and therefore the reasoning behind the classification process, is open and explicit and can be viewed. The method will automatically include in the rules only those factors that really matter in making a decision; the others will be discarded. This can be a useful process for reducing the data to features that are important before training a neural network because a neural network cannot handle a large number of inputs as effectively as a decision tree can. These individual models looked at the morphology of the time domain data, the power spectrum, and the phase spectrum of the frequency domain data and the correlation of subaverages.

The results presented employed feature extraction before classification, cross validation techniques to verify the results obtained, and used a dataset with a 50:50 balance of Yes and No responses.

Five time domain features were used with the software models: TDpost/prePwr, TDPreCCR, TDpostCCR, TDw1to5CCR, and TDwave5CCR. A provisional training and test set of 50 records each were used for the purpose of exploring the usefulness of these features. The rule set generated for the decision tree model showed that the most important feature was TDpost/prePwr, and the next most important was TDwave5CCR. The inputs to the neural network models were then varied by removing some of these five features and training and testing repeatedly. Highest accuracies were obtained again when TDpost/prePwr and TDwave5CCR were used as inputs, the former having the greatest influence on accuracy.

Having discovered the importance of the TDpost/prePwr feature, this was then used as the sole criterion for classification, using the complete dataset of 550 records. This ratio of poststimulus power (1.5-9.5msec) to the prestimulus power (-12msec to 0 msec) was then computed. Manual analysis was carried out using different threshold values for the TDpost/prePwr feature. Using an initial threshold value of 2, there were 322 recordings that satisfied the criterion, with 305 classified as "response" and 17 classified as "no response", yielding an accuracy of 94.7%. The results of this are provided in Table 2.

The threshold value of 5 was chosen because it gave a 98.6% accuracy with only 2 false positives out of 148 waveforms analyzed. This first classification stage has been shown to provide a high degree of accuracy with the application of such a simple rule.

Of the 550 total waveforms available, 148 were filtered out by the first classification stage, leaving 402 waveforms with a poststimulus to prestimulus power ratio less than 5. Obviously, the brainstem response would be less evident in these 402 waveforms and also would be more difficult to detect by both the software classification models and an audiologist. The second stage of classification made use of cross-correlation between waveforms, just as an audiologist would, and consequently needed repeat recordings using the same stimulus level on the same ear. Of these remaining 402 waveforms, there were 150 that could not be used because they did not have a repeat recording for cross-correlation purposes. Consequently, the dataset for the second stage of classification comprised the remaining 252 recordings, that is, 126 repeat recordings, and this dataset was balanced with 50% Yes responses and 50% No responses.

Time Domain Correlation Results

Training and test sets, of 63 records each, were created and the four time domain features, TDPreCCR, TDpostCCR, TDw1to5CCR, and TDwave5CCR, were used as input to decision tree classification models only. Inspection of the rule sets created by the decision trees showed that TDwave5CCR and TDpostCCR were almost always the only features used. Consequently, a series of tests was run using the 126 repeat recordings dataset, with 6-fold cross validation to verify the results. Each training set used 105 records and each test set used 21 records, and records in both sets were interleaved with Yes and No response records. TDwave5CCR and TDpostCCR were used as input features for the classification models, and in further tests, TDpost/prePwr and the stimulus level value were also used as input features. The results of these tests are found in Table 3.

Table 2. Classification accuracy using only TDpost/prePwr feature value

Threshold	Records > threshold	Response = Yes	Response = No	Accuracy %
2	322	305	17	94.7
3	258	252	6	97.7
4	189	185	4	97.9
5	148	146	2	98.6

Table 3. Time domain classification accuracy using 6-fold cross validation

Features used	Only TDwave5CCR and TDpostCCR		Also TDpost/prePwr and stimulus level	
Test	C5.0	NN	C5.0	NN
1	80.95	76.19	80.95	80.95
2	76.19	76.19	76.19	71.43
3	80.95	76.19	80.95	80.95
4	80.95	80.95	80.95	80.95
5	80.95	85.71	80.95	85.71
6	95.24	90.48	90.48	95.24
Average	82.54	80.95	81.75	82.54

The C5.0 classification models for the 6-fold testing showed almost the same accuracy whether only two features were used (TDwave5CCR and TDpostCCR) or four were used (TDwave5CCR, TDpostCCR, TDpost/prePwr, and stimulus level). When the C5.0 rule sets for the six tests were inspected, they used TDwave5CCR and TDpostCCR so that TDpost/prePwr and stimulus level made almost no difference to the classification process. The exception to this was for a small number of records that appeared in Test 6 of the 6-fold process, which confirms the use of n-fold validation and averaging. This testing was part of the second stage classification process which used waveforms where TDpost/prePwr < 5, and the post- to prestimulus power ratio was small and made little impact on the classification decisions. Stimulus level made little impact also because the other features were using cross-correlation values where the comparison of one subaverage waveform with another had a much higher importance than evaluating the stimulus level. Conversely, the NN used stimulus level to reach its highest classification accuracy of 95.4%. The highest average accuracy of 82.54% was obtained by decision tree models when only two features were used, and by neural network models when all four features were used. Decision tree models were only able to provide a symbolic output of Yes or No, whereas neural network models were able to provide an output variable between 0 and 1, which could then be used as a confidence figure.

FFT Correlation Results

Cross-correlation features were also extracted from the frequency domain data. FFTpostCCR compared the poststimulus FFT data of two subaverage wave-forms, FFTpreCCR compared the prestimulus FFT data of the two subaverage waveforms, and FFTavgCCR compared the poststimulus with the prestimulus FFT data of the averaged waveforms. Again, the dataset, which contained 126 repeat recordings, was used to enable the cross-correlation calculations between these repeat FFT data waveforms. Table 4 shows the results from tests carried out using

Table 4. Frequency domain correlation feature results

Features used	FFTpostCCR, FFTpreCCR, FFTavgCCR		FFTpostCCR, FFTpreCCR FFTavgCCR, Stim Level	
Test	C5.0	NN	C5.0	NN
1	80.95	71.43	80.95	57.14
2	61.90	66.67	66.67	61.90
3	61.90	61.90	61.90	71.43
4	80.95	80.95	80.95	71.43
5	76.19	76.19	76.19	80.95
6	68.42	63.16	68.42	57.89
Average	*71.72*	*70.05*	*72.51*	*66.79*

the above three FFT cross-correlation features and 6-fold cross validation. The stimulus level was also used as an additional feature in one set of tests.

Examination of the rule sets created by the decision tree models showed that FFTpostCCR was the most useful feature for classification and that adding the stimulus level gave inconclusive results.

The C5.0 rule sets almost ignored the stimulus level, possibly, because the other features were cross-correlation ones. But the stimulus level must have been useful with a small number of records that appeared in Test 2. The cause of this sensitivity is worthy of further investigation but has not been addressed in this study. The n-fold cross validation process averages out such discrepancies across the dataset.

Average Power Results

When a response is present in the poststimulus waveform, three FFT data peaks are often found at approximately 200, 500, and 900 Hz. These are generally quite wide peaks though, spread over many frequency components. A 200Hz moving window was used as a way of gauging the FFT power across several frequency components, from 39-1100 Hz. The features FFTs3pwr100.....FFTs3pwr1000 are the average power values of each 200Hz-wide window, with the number representing the center frequency of the window. The 126 repeat records dataset was again used without requiring cross-correlation calculations, so the repeat subaveraged waveforms were averaged together before calculating the FFT power spectrum values and the average window powers. Prestimulus FFT power values were subtracted from their respective poststimulus power values, and for some tests, FFT data were normalized and any negative FFT power values zeroed.

Table 5. Classification using average power in a 200Hz-wide moving window

	No Stimulus Level		Use Stimulus Level	
200Hz-wide moving window	C5.0	NN	C5.0	NN
200, 500, 900Hz windows FFT data were normalized Negative FFTs not zeroed	66.67	73.02	68.26	75.40

Table 5 shows the accuracy where peaks were expected, at 200, 500, and 900 Hz, when the FFT data were first normalized, when the negative FFT data values were not zeroed, and also when the stimulus level was included. The figures are the averaged accuracies after using 6-fold cross validation.

Phase Modeling Results

The features PHpost100.....PHpost1000 used cross-correlation to compare the poststimulus phase information of two subaverage waveforms. A 200Hz window was moved across the frequency spectrum from 0-1100 Hz with a 50% overlap each time the window was moved. The phase components within each window were cross-correlated. The aim was to see if there was a higher cross-correlation at certain frequency ranges, especially at 200, 500, and 900 Hz, which could indicate a response was present. The features PHpostpre100....PHpostpre1000 used a similar technique to measure the cross-correlation values between the poststimulus and prestimulus phase information of the combined subaverage waveforms. The 126 repeat records dataset was again used. The results in Table 6 were the averaged accuracies using 6-fold cross validation.

The best accuracy obtained using phase feature extraction was not as high as with frequency or time domain feature extraction, and the results did not show an increase in accuracy as the features used were restricted to the 200, 500, and 900 Hz ranges. The results that related to cross-correlation of the poststimulus and the prestimulus sections of the waveforms showed a very low accuracy, which was expected.

Table 6. Classification using correlation of phase

Features used	C5.0	NN
PHpost100.....PHpost1000	70.64	65.08
PHpost200, PHpost500, PHpost900	68.26	65.87
PHpostpre100....PHpostpre1000	47.62	43.65

Discussion and Future Trends

A review of previous studies indicates that ABRs may be classified based on time and frequency domain features. Correlation measures and standard templates have also been used. High level responses have been classified with reported accuracies, generally greater than 70%, but this falls off when lower level responses closer to hearing threshold are included. Approaches become more complex and sometimes require *a priori* information for successful classification.

This study assesses the classification accuracy using ANNs and the C5.0 decision tree algorithm. The dataset comprises high and low level ABRs from a wide age range. High level responses can be classified in a straightforward manner using a poststimulus to prestimulus power ratio (TDpost/prePwr). It was understood that a higher mean power value in the poststimulus section could be due to factors other than a response being present. A low frequency wave superimposed on the ABR waveform could distort this measurement. The use of band-pass wavelet filtering, as a preprocessing technique, was shown to limit this distortion. Stimulus, ocular and other muscular artifacts, could also contribute to a high mean poststimulus power value. Visual inspection of ABR waveforms showed that these artifacts tended to be found, either within the first millisecond after the stimulus onset or in the last few milliseconds of the poststimulus period. By restricting calculation of poststimulus mean power to the 1.5-9.5msec period, these artifact amplitudes tended then to get excluded from the calculation.

Normal ongoing background EEG activity could also cause a higher poststimulus to prestimulus mean power ratio. However, this background EEG activity causes small changes in the Post/Pre Power Ratio value. Setting a threshold value for the Post/Pre Power Ratio feature is a suitable way of making allowance for the variability in the background EEG power levels.

For responses with a TDpost/prePwr < 5, additional features have been used for classification. These used a dataset with repeated recordings so that correlation could be used for both time and frequency and phase features. This adopts the approach favored by the expert, when interpreting lower stimulus recordings.

For correlation based on time domain features, highest average accuracy of 82.54% was obtained (TDwave5CCR and TDpostCCR). For correlation based on frequency domain features, examination of the rule sets created by the decision tree models showed that FFTpostCCR was the most useful feature for classification. Accuracies of 66.79% to 72.51% were obtained. Features which measure the 200, 500, and 900 Hz components (FFTs3pwr200, FFTs3pwr500, and FFTs3pwr900) have also been used. An accuracy of 75.4% was obtained by use of four features, the average power in 200Hz-wide windows centered on

200, 500, and 900 Hz, and the stimulus level. The best accuracy obtained using phase feature extraction (65.87%-70.64%) was not as high as with frequency or time domain feature extraction, and the results did not show an increase in accuracy as the features used were restricted to the 200, 500, and 900 Hz ranges.

In order to increase classification accuracy further, it will be necessary to combine the models using a further stage of processing which combines the best features from time, frequency, and possibly phase, in a hybrid model. One possible approach uses the Dempster-Shafer (Shafer, 1990) discounting factor, to achieve accuracy higher than that achieved with individual models. This assumes that the individual sources of evidence provide complementary information. In particular, the frequency and phase parameters may provide morphology information, which permits an expert to make the subjective judgment that a low level ABR should be classified as a response. The ANN classification models discussed in this chapter could provide inputs to any further stage of processing, and the output in the range 0-1 can be considered a confidence value. While decision trees provide a clearer explanation of "decisions", their outputs cannot accommodate further processing in the same way.

References

Alpsan, D., & Ozdamar, O. (1992a). Auditory brainstem evoked potential classification for threshold detection by neural networks. 1. Network design, similarities between human-expert and network classification, feasibility. *Automedica, 15*, 67-82.

Alpsan, D., & Ozdamar, O. (1992b). Auditory brainstem evoked potential classification for threshold detection by neural networks. 2. Effects of input coding, training set size, and composition and network size on performance. *Automedica, 15*, 83-93.

Aoyagi, M., & Harada, J. (1988). Application of fast Fourier transform to auditory evoked brainstem response. *Med. Inform., 13*(3), 211-220.

Berger, H. (1969). On the electroencephalogram of man (P. Gloor, Trans.). *Electroencephalography and Clinical Neurophysiology, 28*(Suppl.), 267-287. Elsevier.

Boston, J. R. (1989). Automated interpretation of brainstem auditory evoked potentials: A prototype system. *IEEE Transactions on Biomedical Engineering, 36*, 528-532.

Boston, R. (1981). Spectra of auditory brainstem responses and spontaneous EEG. *IEEE Transactions on Biomedical Engineering, 28*, 334-341.

Davey, R. T., McCullagh, P. J., et al. (2003). Modeling of the brainstem evoked response for objective automated interpretation. *Proceedings of ITAB 2003, 4th International IEEE EMBS Special Topic Conference on Information Technology Applications in Biomedicine,* Birmingham, UK.

Delgado, R. E., & Ozdamar, O. (1994). Automated auditory brainstem response interpretation. *IEEE Engineering in Medicine and Biology,* 227-237.

Gevins, A. S., & Redmond, A. (Eds.). (1987). Overview of computer analysis in handbook of electroencephalography and clinical neurophysiology: Methods of analysis of brain electrical and magnetic s*ignals, 1,* 64.

Gorman, R. P., & Sejnowski, T. J. (1988). Learned classification of sonar targets using a massively parallel network. *IEEE Transactions Acoust. Speech Signal Process, 36,* 1135.

Gronfors, T. K. (1993). Peak identification of auditory brainstem responses with multifilters and attributed automaton. *Comput. Methods Progr. Biomed., 40,* 83-87.

Gronfors, T. K. (1994). Computer analysis of auditory brainstem responses by using advanced pattern recognition. *Journal of Medical Systems, 18*(4), 191-199.

Habraken, J. B. A., van Gils, M. J., et al. (1993). Identification of peak V in brainstem auditory evoked potentials with neural networks. *Computers in Biology and Medicine, 23*(5), 369-380.

Herrmann, B. S., Thornton, A. R., et al. (1995). Automated infant hearing screening using the ABR: Development and validation. *American Journal of Audiology, 4*(2), 6-14.

Jewett, D. L. (1970). Volume conducted potentials in response to auditory stimuli as detected by averaging in the cat. *Electroencephalography and Clinical Neurophysiology, 28*(Suppl.), 609-618.

Madhavan, G. P., de Bruin, H., et al. (1986). Classification of brainstem auditory evoked potentials by syntactic methods. *Electroenceph. Clin. Neurophysiol., 65,* 289-296.

McCullagh, P. J., King, G., et al. (1996). Classification of brainstem auditory evoked potentials using artificial neural networks. In J. Brender, J. P. Christensen, J. R. Scherrer, & P. McNair (Eds.), *Medical informatics Europe '96* (pp. 547-550). Amsterdam: IOS Press.

McGillem, C.D., & Aunon, J.I. (1987). Analysis of event-related potentials. In A.S. Gevins & A. Remond (Eds.), *Handbook of electroencephalography and clinical neurophysiology: Methods of analysis of brain electrical and magnetic signals* (Vol. 1, pp. 143-145). Elsevier.

Ozdamar, O., Delgado, R. E., et al. (1994). Automated electrophysiologic hearing testing using a threshold-seeking algorithm. *J Am Acad Audiol, 5*, 77-88.

Popescu, M., Papadimitriou, S., et al. (1999). Adaptive denoising and multiscale detection of the V wave in brainstem auditory evoked potentials. *Audiol Neurootol, 4*, 38-50.

Pratt, H., Urbach, D., et al. (1989). Auditory brainstem evoked potentials peak identification by finite impulse response digital filters. *Audiology, 28*, 272-283.

Pratt, T. L., Olsen, W. O., et al. (1995). Four-channel ABR recordings: Consistency in interpretation. *American Journal of Audiology, 4*(2), 47-54.

Quinlan, J. R. (1986). Induction of decision trees. *Machine Learning, 1*, 81-106.

Rumelhart, D. E., Hinton, G. E., et al. (1986). *Learning internal representations by error propagation. in parallel distributed processing: Explorations in the microstructure of cognition* (Vol. 1, p. 318). Cambridge, MA: MIT Press.

Sanchez, R., Riquenes, A., et al. (1995). Automatic detection of auditory brainstem responses using feature vectors. *International Journal of Bio-Medical Computing, 39*, 287-297.

Shafer, G. (1990). Perspectives on the theory and practice of belief functions. *International Journal of Approximate Reasoning, 3*, 1-40.

Starr, A., & Don, M. (1988). Brain potentials evoked by acoustic stimuli. In E. W. Picton (Ed.), *Handbook of electroencephalography and clinical neurophysiology: Human event-related potentials* (Vol. 3, p. 128). Elsevier.

Suzuki, T. (1982). Power spectral analysis of auditory brainstem responses to pure tone stimuli. *Scand Audiol, 11*, 25-30.

Tian, J., Juhola, M., et al. (1997). Latency estimation of auditory brainstem response by neural networks. *Artificial Intelligence in Medicine, 10*, 115-128.

Urbach, D., & Pratt, H. (1986). Application of finite impulse response digital filters to auditory brainstem evoked potentials. *Electroenceph. Clin. Neurophysiol., 64*, 269-273.

Van Gils, M. J., & Cluitmans, P. J. M. (1994). Automatic peak identification in auditory evoked potentials with the use of artificial neural networks. *Proceedings of the 16th Annual International Conference, IEEE-EMBS*, IEEE Press.

Vannier, E., Adam, O., et al. (2002). Objective detection of brainstem auditory evoked potentials with a priori information from higher presentation levels. *Artificial Intelligence in Medicine, 25*, 283-301.

Waibel, A., Hanazawa, T., et al. (1989). Phoneme recognition using time-delay neural networks. *IEEE Transactions on Acoust. Speech Signal Process, 37*, 328.

Section V

Applications in Selected Areas

Chapter X

Movement Pattern Recognition Using Neural Networks

Rezaul Begg, Victoria University, Australia

Joarder Kamruzzaman, Monash University, Australia

Ruhul Sarker, University of New South Wales, Australia

Abstract

This chapter provides an overview of artificial neural network applications for the detection and classification of various gaits based on their typical characteristics. Gait analysis is routinely used for detecting abnormality in the lower limbs and also for evaluating the progress of various treatments. Neural networks have been shown to perform better compared to statistical techniques in some gait classification tasks. Various studies undertaken in this area are discussed with a particular focus on neural network's potential in gait diagnostics. Examples are presented to demonstrate the suitability of neural networks for automated recognition of gait changes due to aging from their respective gait patterns and their potential for identification of at-risk or non-functional gait.

Introduction

Neural networks have been shown to be successful in a variety of applications, including solving problems in biomedical, financial, and engineering areas. Recently, there has been particularly rapid growth in biomedical and health-related applications because of better predictive abilities and non-linear modeling capabilities compared to traditional statistical techniques. Specifically, recognition of movement patterns, especially gait, has benefited as a result of neural network usages. The aim of this chapter is to provide an overview of neural network applications in movement pattern identification for possible use of neural networks as a diagnostic tool. A brief overview of gait analysis is first provided followed by neural network applications in various gait studies.

Gait Analysis

Gait analysis is the analysis of various aspects of human walking and running patterns, the most common forms of human locomotion. Winter (1991) describes it as one of the most complex and totally integrated human movements involving coordinated processes of the neural and musculoskeletal systems. Many studies have investigated human gait to understand the process of movement control and to quantify the changes due to various diseases and with aging. Gait is periodic in that the normal gait cycle starts with the heel contact or foot contact and finishes with the next heel or foot contact of the same foot. The gait cycle time is generally calculated as the time interval between two successive events (e.g., heel contact) of the same foot (Figure 1). It is characterized by a stance phase (~60% of the total gait cycle) and a swing phase (~40%). The stance phase includes, among many events, the main events of heel contact, foot flat, midstance, heel off, and toe off. The swing phase starts from toe off, through midswing and ends with the heel contact of the same foot (see Figure 1). While performing gait analysis, deviations or abnormalities in gait are frequently referred to these events (Perry, 1992).

Instrumentation used to study gait ranges from the least sophisticated approaches to complicated and expensive devices (Begg et al., 1989). Researchers have extracted hundreds of parameters from the gait cycle to characterize aspects of the gait pattern. Most of the gait parameters may be grouped under the following main headings:

- Basic time-distance measures such as cadence, walking velocity, stride lengths, stance/swing times;

Figure 1. Stick figure representation showing the positions of the trunk and lower limb segments (thigh, shank, and foot) during different phases and events of a gait cycle (right heel contact to right heel contact). HC = heel contact, FF = foot flat, MSt = midstance, HO = heel off, TO = toe off, MSw = midswing.

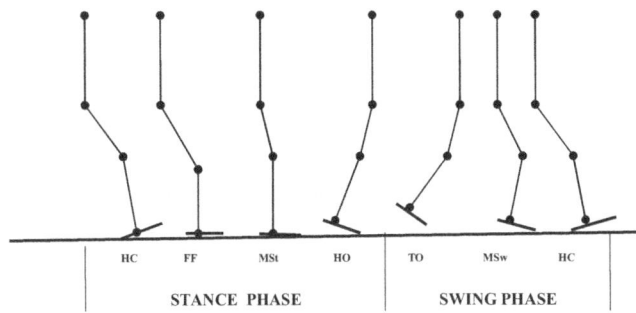

- Kinematic measures such as joint/segment angles and angular range of motion (ROM), toe clearance, velocity/accelerations of body segments, and so forth;

- Kinetic measures that include force and pressure distribution under the foot, joint/muscle moments;

- Electromyographic data which are electrical activity measures (timing and amplitude) of the contracting muscles;

- Energy states (potential and kinetic) of the limb segments and the whole body.

Consequently, many hundreds of papers have emerged in the scientific literature documenting their usefulness in many applications, including clinical, rehabilitation, health, and sports (Begg & Sparrow, 2000; Schieb, 1986; Whittle, 1991; Winter, 1991).

Gait, Aging, and Health

With age, gait functions reflected in the walking pattern measures degenerate and can affect the balance control mechanisms of the locomotor system. The reported declines in the gait measures include basic spatial-temporal parameters such as stride length, walking speed, stance/swing times (Hageman & Blanke, 1986; Winter, 1991); joint angular excursions at the hip, knee, and ankle joints (Öberg et al., 1994); and kinetic parameters as reflected in the foot-to-ground reaction force-time data such as the vertical and horizontal peak forces (Judge et al., 1996). Gait analysis has been recommended by many investigators to identify individuals with a decline in performance of the locomotor system. Recently, extensive research has been undertaken describing age-related changes to gait. The main objective of such analysis is to develop diagnostic techniques based on the affected gait features to identify individuals at risk of sustaining falls and injuries.

Falls in the older population, and the resulting injuries and other related consequences, are a major public health issue in the community due to frequency, morbidity, mortality, and costs. For example, in Australia, costs to the community associated with falls have been estimated to be about $2.4 billion per annum (Fildes, 1994). Epidemiological studies have shown that approximately 30% of people aged 65 years or more, and approximately 50% in individuals over the age of 75 years, sustain a fall at least once a year sufficiently serious enough to cause injury (Snow, 1999). Furthermore, recent statistics on future population projections indicate that by the year 2035, Australia will have 22% of its population over the age of 65 years, compared to 12% in 2005 (*The Australian*, 2005). Hence, with increase in the aging population, the incidence of falls and the associated costs are expected to rise unless effective preventative techniques are implemented.

Neural Networks in Gait

Many computational intelligence techniques such as neural networks, fuzzy logic, evolutionary computing, and support vector machines have been applied to recognize gait from their parameters (Begg & Kamruzzaman, 2005a; Chau, 2001; Schöllhorn, 2004). Among these techniques, applications involving neural networks are most widespread with most of these applications including gait data modeling (Sepulveda et al., 1993) and gait pattern classification (e.g., Barton & Lees, 1997). Specifically, a number of studies have used neural networks for automatic recognition of gait types, and the success of such discrimination abilities could lead to many applications. For example, neural networks could be used as a tool for the diagnosis of gait abnormalities based on the respective kinematic and kinetic gait characteristics or evaluation of improvement (or otherwise) as a result of various intervention schemes.

Neural Networks in the Recognition of Simulated and Pathological Gait

Joint angular measures over the gait cycle and their corresponding transformed Fourier coefficients have been used by Barton and Lees (1997) to simulate various gait types (e.g., leg length discrepancy). Gait data were collected from 5 male and 3 female subjects via four reflective markers located at the neck, hip, knee, and ankle joint positions, and this information was used to determine the hip and knee angles over one stride. Each of the knee and hip angle data were normalized to 128 time intervals, and the corresponding fast-Fourier transformed (FFT) coefficients were determined. Of all the Fourier coefficients, the first 8 real and 7 imaginary (excluding the zero term) were used in neural network training and testing for recognition of simulated gait types and classification. The network was trained with backpropagation learning, and it consisted of four layers (input layer with 30 nodes taking both hip and knee angle data; two hidden layers with 5 and 4 nodes, respectively; and output layer with 3 output nodes, one for each of the three gait classifications). The training set included 6 subjects' data, and the test set had 2 subjects' data. Although the sample size was low, the results (correct assignment ratio by the neural network to be 83.3%) demonstrate that simulated gait types can change the gait kinematics (joint angle) to the extent that these changes can be effectively categorized by the use of neural networks.

Several studies have been reported concerning the application of neural networks in recognizing normal and pathological gait. Holzreiter and Kohle (1993) applied neural networks to distinguish between healthy and pathological gait using two force plates to measure the vertical force components of two consecutive foot strikes during normal walking. The experiment used a sample size of 225, including 131 patients of different etiology and 94 healthy persons. Of the foot strikes, the vertical force information was normalized into 128 constant time intervals, and all force components were normalized to the test subjects' body weight. The resulting data were fast-Fourier transformed (FFT), and the lower 30 real and imaginary coefficients were used as inputs to the neural networks. A three-layer feedforward neural network topology was used: 30 input nodes and a single classification output node corresponding to healthy or pathological class. The network was trained 80 times with the backpropagation algorithm with different random weight initialization and using a different proportion of the dataset (20 to 80%). The remaining data were used to test the performance of the network. The maximum trainability of the networks was consistently higher for larger training sets; the maximum success rate in analyzing and categorizing gaits was 95% for a training set size of 80% of total data. Wu et al. (2000) also used foot-ground reaction force measures during gait to differentiate between gait patterns of patients with ankle arthrodesis and normal subjects using neural networks. Begg et al. (2005) applied neural networks to recognize healthy and fall-prone (balance-impaired) gaits using minimum toe clearance (MTC) variables during the swing phase of the gait cycle. MTC data were quite effective in diagnosing the at-risk (trip-related falls) individuals by the neural networks with 91.7% accuracy. Neural networks have also been shown to perform better than statistical predictions for gait recognition. For example, using force platform gait data in a group of normal and pathological populations, Wu et al. (1998) demonstrated that the gait class prediction rates of neural networks were better than a statistical (e.g., linear discriminant analysis, LDA) based classifier (98.7% vs. 91.5%).

These research outcomes demonstrate neural network's potential for use as a gait diagnostic tool from various gait variables. Further details of related studies concerned with gait recognition and classification applications using neural networks may be found in a number of review articles (e.g., Chau, 2001; Schöllhorn, 2004; Uthmann & Dauscher, 2005).

Aging Gait Recognition Using Neural Networks

As reported earlier, gait changes occur across the lifespan, and these changes are reflected in the various gait recordings. Some of these changes in the older populations might be detrimental due to the fact that these changes can affect their balance control mechanisms and may lead to injuries during locomotion. Past research has indicated that machine-learning approaches (e.g., support vector machines) are effective in discriminating young and aged gait patterns (Begg & Kamruzzaman, 2005a). These research outcomes also highlight that gait features extracted from ground reaction forces and joint angular excursion range-of-motion (ROM) measures carry useful information regarding the quality and functional status of the gait. Therefore, these characteristics might be used to detect the declines in gait performance due to aging or pathology. Neural networks have the potential to play a significant role in such applications as well, by being able to recognize a faulty or defective gait pattern. Thus, a neural network could be used for early identification of an at-risk or faulty gait, which might lead to appropriate measures for corrective intervention and gait rehabilitation.

For the recognition of age effects on gait patterns, a neural network classifier was applied with three well-known algorithms: standard backpropagation (BP), scaled conjugate gradient (SCG), and Bayesian regularization (BR). The steps

Figure 2. Main steps in a gait classification task using neural networks

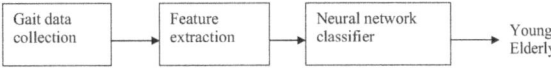

that are followed in a gait classification task can be shown in a flow diagram as depicted in Figure 2. These classifiers were trained and tested using standard gait measures collected during normal locomotion (Begg & Kamruzzaman, 2005a). Subsequently, we compared their relative suitability for gait pattern recognition tasks using accuracy rates and measures of the receiver operating characteristics (ROC) curves such as sensitivity, specificity, and area under the ROC plots to evaluate performance of the classifiers.

Motion Analysis and Extraction of Gait Features

For testing the potentials of neural networks in gait pattern recognition, gait analysis was conducted on 12 healthy young adults (mean age: 28 years) and 12 healthy older adults (mean age: 69 years). The subjects had no known injuries or abnormalities that would affect their gait. Gait recordings were carried out during normal walking on the laboratory walkway. Gait characteristics were captured using an AMTI force platform and a PEAK 2D Motion Analysis system (Peak Performance Inc, USA). Gait features were extracted from the gait data describing lower limb joint motion and foot-ground reaction force-time characteristics, and used for training and testing the gait classifiers. The gait features in this study included stride cycle time-distance data (walking speed, stance, swing and double-stance times and their corresponding normalized data, and stride length); lower limb joint angles and angular ROM data. Movement of the lower limb was recorded using the PEAK motion analysis system and reflective markers attached to lower limb joints and segments (hip, knee, ankle, heel, and toe). The angular data included knee and ankle joint angles at key events (heel contact and toe-off); joint ROM during the stance, swing, and stance-to-swing transition phases of the gait cycle; and characteristics of the foot-to-ground reaction forces (GRF). Foot-ground reaction forces along vertical and anterior-posterior directions were recorded using one force-sensing platform. Peak forces during key phases of the gait cycle were normalized to body weight; these included vertical peak forces during weight acceptance, midstance, and push-off phases, and horizontal peak forces during braking and propulsive phases. These gait measures have been shown to be useful indicators of aging in a number of

Figure 3. A multilayer feedforward neural network architecture showing inputs (x₁), outputs (y₁), hidden layer (h₁), and the connection weights (w) between the neurons

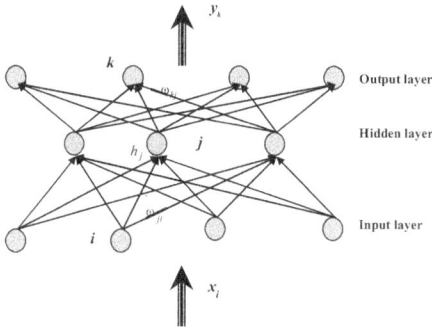

investigations (Begg et al., 1998; Begg et al., 2003; Judge et al., 1996; Nigg et al., 1994).

Neural Network Algorithms

Artificial neural networks learn the underlying relationships between the inputs and outputs by way of repeated presentation of examples. This is especially useful when the exact relationship between inputs and outputs is unknown or is very complex to quantify using mathematical formulation. Neural networks have found applications in numerous areas as a powerful classifier (cf. Fogel & Robinson, 2003; Schöllhorn, 2004; White & Racine, 2001). Here we apply artificial neural networks for the analysis of human gait and to build a model between the gait types (young and elderly) and the associated gait features. The performance of the different neural network learning algorithms was investigated in relation to this particular problem of aging gait recognition.

Figure 3 illustrates the architecture of a multilayer feedforward neural network (MFNN), which is one of the most commonly used neural networks. It consists of an input layer, an output layer, and one or more intermediate layers called the hidden layers. All the nodes in each layer are connected to each node at the upper layer by interconnection strength, called weights. All the interconnecting weights between the layers are initialized to small random values at the beginning. During training phase, the input features are presented at the input layer, and the associated target outputs are presented at the output layer. A training algorithm is used to attain a set of weights that minimizes the difference between the target output and actual output produced by the network.

Many algorithms are proposed in the literature to train an MFNN network. There exists a theoretical framework that focuses on estimating the generalization ability of a network as a function of architecture and training set. The region of weight space is considered consistent with the training set; a particular learning rule might favor some regions over others (Hetrz et al., 1991). The suitability of a training algorithm in producing good generalization ability, in relation to a particular application, is, however, usually determined by experiments. In this study, we experimented using three commonly applied neural network learning algorithms, namely, standard backpropagation (BP), scaled conjugate gradient algorithm (SCG), and backpropagation with Bayesian regularization (BR) in order to find the best suited algorithm for detecting human gait pattern changes. In the following, we provide a brief description of the three algorithms.

Standard Backpropagation (BP)

Backpropagation updates the weights iteratively to map a set of input vectors $\{x_1, x_2, ..., x_p\}$ to a set of corresponding output vectors $\{y_1, y_2, ..., y_p\}$. The algorithm uses gradient descent technique to adjust the connection weights between the neurons. The input x_p is presented to the network and multiplied by the weights. All the weighted inputs to each unit of the upper layer are summed and produce an output governed by the following equations.

$$y_p = f(W_o h_p + \theta_o), \tag{1}$$

$$h_p = f(W_h x_p + \theta_h), \tag{2}$$

where W_o and W_h are the output and hidden layer weight matrices; h_p is the vector denoting the response of hidden layer for pattern p; θ_o and θ_h are the output and hidden layer bias vectors, respectively; and $f(.)$ is the sigmoid activation function.

The error function to be minimized in standard BP is the sum of squared error, defined as

$$E = \frac{1}{2} \sum_p (t_p - y_p)^T (t_p - y_p) \tag{3}$$

where $\mathbf{t}_p$ is the target output vector for pattern p. The algorithm uses gradient descent technique to adjust the connection weights between neurons. Denoting the fan-in weights to a single neuron by a weight vector $\mathbf{w}$, its update in the t-th epoch is governed by the following equation.

$$\Delta\mathbf{w}_t = -\eta\,\nabla E\,(\mathbf{w})\big|_{\mathbf{w}=\mathbf{w}_t} + \alpha\,\Delta\mathbf{w}_{t-1} \tag{4}$$

The parameters η and α are the learning rate and the momentum factor, respectively. The learning rate parameter controls the step size used for the individual iteration. For a large-scale problem, the backpropagtion learning becomes very slow, and its convergence largely depends on the choice of suitable values of η and α by the user.

Scaled Conjugate Gradient (SCG)

The backpropagation algorithm has the drawback of slow convergence; it iterates successive steps in the direction of negative gradient of the error surface. The error surface may contain long ravines with sharp curvature and gently sloping floor, which cause slow convergence. In conjugate gradient methods, a search is performed along conjugate directions, which produces generally faster convergence than steepest descent directions (Hagan et al., 1996). In steepest descent search, a new direction is perpendicular to the old direction. This approach to the minimum is a zig-zag path, and one step can be mostly undone by the next. In conjugate gradient methods, a new search direction spoils as little as possible the minimization achieved by the previous direction, and the step size is adjusted during every iteration. The general procedure to determine the new search direction is to combine the new steepest descent direction with the previous search direction so that the current and previous search directions are conjugate. Conjugate gradient techniques are based on the assumption that, for a general non-quadratic error function, error in the neighborhood of a given point is locally quadratic. The weight changes in successive steps are given by the following equations.

$$\mathbf{w}_{t+1} = \mathbf{w}_t + \alpha_t\mathbf{d}_t \tag{5}$$

$$\mathbf{d}_t = -\mathbf{g}_t + \beta_t\mathbf{d}_{t-1} \tag{6}$$

with

$$\mathbf{g}_t \equiv \nabla E(\mathbf{w})\big|_{\mathbf{w} = \mathbf{w}_t} \tag{7}$$

$$\beta_t = \frac{\mathbf{g}_t^T \mathbf{g}_t}{\mathbf{g}_{t-1}^T \mathbf{g}_{t-1}} \quad \text{or} \quad \beta_t = \frac{\Delta \mathbf{g}_{t-1}^T \mathbf{g}_t}{\mathbf{g}_{t-1}^T \mathbf{d}_{t-1}} \quad \text{or} \quad \beta_t = \frac{\Delta \mathbf{g}_{t-1}^T \mathbf{g}_t}{\mathbf{g}_{t-1}^T \mathbf{g}_{t-1}} \tag{8}$$

where $\mathbf{d}_t$ and $\mathbf{d}_{t-1}$ are the conjugate directions in successive iterations. The step size is governed by the coefficient α_t and the search direction is determined by β_t. In scaled conjugate gradient, the step size α_t is calculated by the following equations.

$$\alpha_t = -\frac{\mathbf{d}_t^T \mathbf{g}_t}{\delta_t} \tag{9}$$

$$\delta_t = \mathbf{d}_t^T \mathbf{H}_t \mathbf{d}_t + \lambda_t \|\mathbf{d}_t\|^2 \tag{10}$$

where λ_t is the scaling coefficient and $\mathbf{H}_t$ is the Hessian matrix at iteration t. λ is added because, in case of non-quadratic error function, the Hessian matrix need not be positive definite. In this case, without λ, δ may become negative and weight update may lead to an increase of error function. With sufficiently large λ, the modified Hessian is guaranteed to be positive ($\delta > 0$). However, for large values of λ, step size will be small. If the error function is not quadratic or $\delta < 0$, λ can be increased to make $\delta > 0$. In case of $\delta < 0$, Moller (1993) suggested the appropriate scale coefficient $\bar{\lambda}_t$ to be

$$\bar{\lambda}_t = 2\left(\lambda_t - \frac{\delta_t}{\|\mathbf{d}_t\|^2} \right) \tag{11}$$

Rescaled value $\bar{\delta}_t$ of δ_t is then expressed as

$$\bar{\delta}_t = \delta_t + (\bar{\lambda}_t - \lambda_t)\|\mathbf{d}_t\|^2 \tag{12}$$

In addition to the increase in λ_t to ensure $\bar{\delta}_t$ is positive, the scaled coefficient needs adjustment to validate the local quadratic approximation. The measure of quadratic approximation accuracy, Δ_t is expressed by

$$\Delta_t = \frac{2\{E(\mathbf{w}_t) - E(\mathbf{w}_t + \alpha_t \mathbf{d}_t)\}}{\alpha_t \mathbf{d}_t^T \mathbf{g}_t} \tag{13}$$

If Δ_t is close to 1, then the approximation is a good one and the value of λ_t can be decreased (Bishop, 1995). On the contrary, if Δ_t is small, the value of λ_t has to be increased. Some prescribed values suggested in Moller (1993) are as follows:

For $\Delta_t > 0.75$, $1_{t+1} = 1/2$

For $\Delta_t < 0.25$, $1_{t+1} = 4 1_t$

Otherwise, $1_{t+1} = 1_t$

If $\Delta_t < 0$, the step will lead to an increase in error and the weights are not updated. λ_t is then increased according to the above criteria, and Δ_t is reevaluated.

Bayesian Reguralization (BR)

A desired neural network model should produce small error not only on the training data but also on the test data. To produce a network with better generalization ability, Mackay (1992) proposed a method to constrain the size of network parameters by regularization. Regularization forces the network to settle to a set of weights and biases having smaller values. This causes the network response to be smoother and less likely to overfit (Hagan et al., 1996) and capture noise. In the regularization technique, the cost function F is defined as

$$F = \gamma E_D + (1 - \gamma) E_W \tag{14}$$

where E_D equals E defined in Equation (3), $E_w = \|\mathbf{w}\|^2 / 2$ is the sum of squares of the network parameters, and γ (<1.0) is the performance ratio parameter, the magnitude of which dictates the emphasis of the training on regularization. A large γ will drive the error E_D to small value whereas a small γ will emphasize parameter size reduction at the expense of error and yield smoother network response. One approach of determining optimum regularization parameter automatically is the Bayesian framework (Mackay, 1992). This method allows the parameter to be selected using only the training data, without having to use separate training and validation data. The Bayesian framework considers a probability distribution over the weight space, representing the relative degrees of belief in different values for the weights. The weight space is initially assigned some prior distribution. Let D = {$\mathbf{x}_m$, $\mathbf{t}_m$} be the dataset of the input-target pair, m be a label running over the pair, and M be a particular NN model. After the data are taken, the posterior probability distribution for the weight $p(\mathbf{w}|D,\gamma,M)$ is given according to the Bayesian rule.

$$p(\mathbf{w}\,|D,\gamma\,,M)=\frac{p(D\,|\,\mathbf{w},\gamma\,,M)p(\mathbf{w}\,|\,\gamma\,,M)}{p(D\,|\,\gamma\,,M)} \tag{15}$$

where $p(\mathbf{w}|\gamma,M)$ is the prior distribution, $p(D|\mathbf{w},\gamma,M)$ is the likelihood function, and $p(D|\gamma,M)$ is a normalization factor, which guarantees the total probability is 1. In the Bayesian framework, the optimal weight should maximize the posterior probability $p(\mathbf{w}|D,\gamma,M)$, which is equivalent to minimizing the function in Equation (14). The performance ratio parameter is optimized by applying the Bayes' rule:

$$p(\gamma\,|D,M)=\frac{p(D\,|\,\gamma\,,M)p(\gamma\,|\,M)}{p(D\,|\,M)} \tag{16}$$

If we assume a uniform prior distribution $p(\gamma|M)$ for the regularization parameter γ, then maximizing the posterior probability is achieved by maximizing the likelihood function $p(D|\gamma,M)$. Since all probabilities have a Gaussian form, it can be expressed as

$$p(D\,|\,\gamma\,,M)=(\pi\,/\gamma\,)^{-N/2}[\pi\,/(1-\gamma\,)]^{-L/2}Z_F(\gamma) \tag{17}$$

where L is the total number of parameters in the NN. Supposing that F has a single minimum as a function of $\mathbf{w}$ at $\mathbf{w}^*$ and has the shape of a quadratic function in a small area surrounding that point, Z_F is approximated as (Mackay, 1992),

$$Z_F \approx (2\pi)^{L/2} \det^{-1/2} H^* \exp(-F(\mathbf{w}^*)) \tag{18}$$

where $H = \gamma \nabla^2 E_D + (1-\gamma)\nabla^2 E_W$ is the Hessian matrix of the objective function. Using Equation (18) into Equation (17), the optimum value of γ at the minimum point can be determined.

Foresee and Hagan (1997) propose to apply Gauss-Newton approximation to estimate the Hessian matrix, which can be conveniently implemented if the Lebenberg-Marquart optimization algorithm (More, 1977) is used to locate the minimum point. This minimizes the additional computation required for regularization.

Cross-Validation Tests

Models were developed for recognizing aging effects, that is, classification between young and old using the three algorithms. Each neural network model had an input layer consisting of 24 input neurons corresponding to the input features, one hidden layer, and an output layer unit representing the gait types (young and elderly). All features were normalized using their equivalent z-scores to have unity variance.

For relatively small datasets, cross validation (k-fold) tests are recommended. In this test, the input dataset is divided into a number of equal segments. In this experiment, all subjects' data were divided into six segments; five segments were used to train the classifier whereas the remaining segment was used to test the accuracy of prediction. This was then repeated until all subjects' data appeared in the test sample. All neural network architectures were developed, trained, and tested using routines written in Matlab toolbox 6.12 (The MathWorks, Natick, MA).

Experimental Results

Accuracy of Gait Recognition

The neural networks were trained using three different algorithms: Standard BP, SCG, and BR, and each algorithm was tested 20 times. The average and maximum accuracy rates of the cross validation tests are shown in Table 1. While there were small differences among the three classifiers with regard to average classification accuracy, presumably due to variation of initial weights (Kecman, 2002), the maximum accuracy rate was the same for all classifiers

Table 1. Percentage gait classification accuracy (maximum accuracy in bracket), sensitivity, and specificity results by neural networks to differentiate young/elderly gait patterns

Algorithms	Accuracy	Sensitivity	Specificity	ROC Area
Standard BP	79.4 (83.3)	85.0	74.2	.82
Scaled Conjugate Gradient	79.6 (83.3)	86.3	73.3	.84
Bayesian Regularization	82.7 (83.3)	91.3	74.2	.90

(83.3%). While previous research has supported neural network's ability to differentiate between normal and pathological gait from respective force platform recordings (Holzreiter & Kohle, 1993), this research suggests that neural network can also be equally effective in detecting gait changes due to aging. Such automatic gait classification capability has many potential benefits including, monitoring gait deterioration due to aging, identifying at-risk or faulty gait, and evaluation of intervention outcomes.

Sensitivity, Specificity, and ROC Plots

In addition to accuracy results, classifier performance is frequently evaluated in terms of its *Sensitivity*, *Specificity*, and *Receiver Operating Characteristic* or *ROC* plots. ROC plots have been used in many investigations (cf. Chan et al., 2002) to gauge the predictive ability of a classifier over a wide range of threshold values in order to obtain a more complete picture of the classification performance. The predicted output of a classifier in response to an unknown gait pattern commonly results in an output between -1.0 and 1.0. A threshold value chosen other than 0 is likely to provide different outcomes in the corresponding accuracy measures for young and elderly gaits. An output above the threshold would be assigned into a young category whereas a value equal to or below the threshold would be assigned into an elderly category. In regard to aging gait classification, *Sensitivity* can be defined as a measure of the ability of the classifier to identify an older gait, whereas *Specificity* is a measure of the classifier to detect young gait characteristics. ROC areas were calculated numerically to compare the three classifiers quantitatively.

BR showed greater sensitivity and specificity rates (see Table 1). ROC area was higher for the BR compared to the other two classifiers. The larger the area under the ROC curves, the better the classification performance. The results suggest that, out of the three algorithms, BR had the best performance in separating the age groups.

Figure 4. 3D scatter plot showing young/elderly data using the three selected key features (feature numbers 6, 14, and 19) and a hyper-plane separating the two age groups

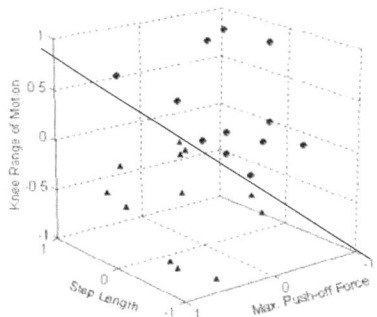

Effect of Feature Selection on Gait Recognition

The performance of a pattern recognition task will depend on the features used to separate the classes. Past research (Begg & Kamruzzaman, 2005a; Chan et al., 2002) involving the influence of input features on classification outcomes has demonstrated that there can be two types of features. There are useful or good features that tend to separate the classes or groups, but there are also some features that could negatively affect the classification accuracy. In the feature selection method, a feature is added one at a time that provides the maximum classification performance or results in the least reduction in performance. A forward feature selection algorithm was applied to the aging gait separation problem, and it was found that the performance of the aging gait classifier was also dependent on the number of features used to train and test the classifier. It is interesting to note that the percentage accuracy rate was higher with a few selected features compared to that obtained when trained with all the features. In aging gait, the features selected to achieve maximum classification included *knee range of motion* from the kinematic data groups, *maximum horizontal (anterior-posterior) push-off force* from the kinetic data group, and *step length* from the basic gait data (Begg & Kamruzzaman, 2005b). A 3D scatter diagram of the three selected features has been illustrated in Figure 4, which demonstrates that, in this case, the two age groups are linearly separated in the 3D space. The two age groups would be perfectly separated (100% classification accuracy) if these three features were selected in advance and then used as inputs to the classification process. However, the maximum classification was 91.7% if all the features were used as inputs to the classifier.

Concluding Remarks and Future Directions

In this chapter, we have reviewed gait pattern recognition and classification abilities of neural networks and explored the performance of three neural networks algorithms (standard backpropagation, scaled conjugate gradient, and Bayesian regularization) with respect to aging gait recognition tasks. Gait features used for training and testing the neural networks are usually extracted from gait recording data using standard techniques and instrumentation. The gait features employed in various studies are extensive and include basic descriptors of the gait cycle, kinematic, kinetic, and electromyography variables. Previous findings from many experiments support the use of neural networks for recognizing healthy, pathological, or aging gaits. Neural networks based on the aforementioned three well-known learning algorithms provided promising classification outcomes for recognizing young and old gait. The Bayesian regularization proved to be superior in performance measured both in accuracy rates and in ROC plots (ROC area, sensitivity, and specificity measures). Gait recognition performance was significantly enhanced when a subset of selected features was used to train the classifiers. Therefore, feature selection appears to be an important consideration while dealing with gait pattern recognition. There can also be some further advantages by selecting a small number of features. For example, a small number of features would help to reduce the dimensionality of the input data and, hence, less computational complexity.

It is clear that neural networks can offer plenty of benefits in gait data modeling and gait pattern prediction tasks. In most of these applications, the reported classification accuracy is quite high (>90%) which suggests excellent prediction abilities by the neural networks as well as their suitability in modeling the underlying structures in gait data. Furthermore, it has been shown, by studies undertaken on healthy and pathological gait recognition, to offer superior performance outcomes compared to an LDA-based classifier (Wu et al., 1998); this might suggest the importance of non-linear approaches to model relationships between disease or aging effects and the associated gait characteristics.

Future research in this area may gain profitably by:

- Applying neural network algorithms for recognition of gait changes due to falling behavior and various pathologies;

- Incorporating other feature selection algorithms, such as backward elimination techniques (Chan et al., 2002) and genetic algorithms (Yom-Tov & Inbar, 2002) that may be applied for separating the relevant and irrelevant features in order to improve the effectiveness of gait detection and classification tasks;

- Incorporating more than one artificial intelligence technique (i.e., hybridization) that might lead to further improvement in the performance of the classification process. Some examples might include combining a neural network with fuzzy logic (neuro-fuzzy scheme) or evolutionary algorithms (Yao, 1999; Yao & Liu, 2004), or developing Fuzzy Controller based Genetic Algorithm (Haque et al., 2003).

Great progress has been made over the past decade or so on the applications of neural networks in recognizing gait and establishing neural networks as a valuable tool in this area. Clearly, much more research efforts are needed in this area before they are available in clinical and rehabilitation settings as routine healthcare diagnostic tools. The future looks promising in the applications of neural networks and other related artificial intelligence techniques for gait diagnostics in aging and pathological populations.

References

Australian, The. (2005, March 30). Higher education supplement. The Australian Newspaper.

Barton, J. G., & Lees, A. (1997). An application of neural networks for distinguishing gait patterns on the basis of hip-knee joint angle diagrams. Gait and Posture, 5, 28-33.

Begg, R. K., Hasan, R., Taylor, S., & Palaniswami, M. (2005, January). Artificial neural network models in the diagnosis of balance impairments. Proceedings of the Second International Conference on Intelligent Sensing and Information Processing, Chennai, India.

Begg, R. K., & Kamruzzaman, J. (2005a). A machine learning approach for automated recognition of movement patterns using basic, kinetic and kinematic gait data. Journal of Biomechanics, 38(3), 401-408.

Begg, R. K., & Kamruzzaman, J. (2005b). Artificial neural networks for detection and classification of walking pattern changes. Submitted.

Begg, R. K., Kamruzzaman, J., & Zayegh, A. (2003). An application of support vector machines for recognizing young-old gait patterns. *Proceedings of the World Congress on Medical Physics & Biomedical Engineering,* Sydney, Australia.

Begg, R. K., & Sparrow, W. A. (2000). Gait characteristics of young and older individuals negotiating a raised surface: Implications for the prevention of falls. *Journal of Gerontology: Medical Sciences, 55A,* 147-154.

Begg, R. K., Sparrow, W. A., & Lythgo, N. D. (1998). Time-domain analysis of foot-ground reaction forces in negotiating obstacles. *Gait and Posture, 7,* 99-109.

Begg, R. K., Wytch, R., & Major, R. E. (1989). Instrumentation used in clinical gait analysis: A review. *Journal of Medical Engineering and Technology, 13,* 290-295.

Bishop, C. M. (1995). *Neural network for pattern recognition.* New York: Oxford University Press.

Chan, K., Lee, T. W., Sample, P. A, Goldbaum, M. H, Weinreb, R. N., & Sejnowski, T. J. (2002). Comparison of machine learning and traditional classifiers in glaucoma diagnosis. *IEEE Transaction on Biomedical Engineering, 49,* 963-974.

Chau, T. (2001). A review of analytical techniques for gait data. Part 2: Neural network and wavelet methods. *Gait and Posture, 13,* 102-120.

Fildes, B. (1994). *Injuries among older people: Falls at home and pedestrian accidents.* Melbourne: Dove Publications.

Fogel, D. B., & Robinson, C. J. (2003). *Computational intelligence.* IEEE Press.

Foresee, F.D., & Hagan, M.T. (1997). Gauss-Newton approximation to Bayesian learning. *Proceedings of IEEE International Conference on Neural Networks, 3,* 1930-1935.

Hagan, M. T., Demuth, H. B., & Beale, M. H. (1996). *Neural network design.* Boston: PWS Publishing.

Hageman, P. A., & Blanke, D. J. (1986). Comparison of gait of young women and elderly women. *Physical Therapy, 66,* 1382-1387.

Haque, S. A., Kabir, Z., & Sarker, R. (2003). Optimization model for opportunistic replacement policy using GA with fuzzy logic controller. *Proceeding of IEEE 2003 International Congress on Evolutionary Computation,* Canberra, Australia (pp. 2837-2843).

Hetrz, J., Krogh, A., & Palmer, R.G. (1991). *Introduction to the theory of neural computation.* Redwood, CA: Addison-Wesley.

Holzreiter, S. H., & Kohle, M. E. (1993). Assessment of gait pattern using neural networks. *Journal of Biomechanics, 26,* 645-651.

Judge, J. O., Davis, R. B., & Ounpuu, S. (1996). Step length reductions in advanced age: The role of ankle and hip kinetics. *Journal of Gerontology Medical Science, 51*, 303-312.

Kecman, V. (2002) *Learning and soft computing: Support vector machines, neural networks and fuzzy logic models.* NJ: IEEE.

Mackay, D. J. C. (1992). A practical Bayesian framework for backpropagation networks. *Neural Computation, 4*, 415-447.

Moller, A. F. (1993). A scaled conjugate gradient algorithm for fast supervised learning. *Neural Network, 6*, 525-533.

More, J. J. (1977). The Levenberg-Marquart algorithm: Implementation and theory. In G. A. Watson (Ed.), *Numerical analysis. Lecture notes in mathematics 630* (pp. 105-116). London: Springer-Verlag.

Nigg, B. M., Fisher, V., & Ronsky, J. L. (1994). Gait characteristics as a function of age and gender. *Gait and Posture, 2*, 213-220.

Öberg, T., Karsznia, A., & Öberg, K. (1994). Joint angle parameters in gait: Reference data for normal subjects, 10-79 years of age. *Journal of Rehabilitation Research and Development, 31*, 199-213.

Perry, J. (1992). *Gait analysis: Normal & pathological function.* Thorofare, NJ.

Reich, Y., & Barai, S. V. (1999). Evaluating machine learning models for engineering problems. *Artificial Intelligence Engineering, 13*, 257-272.

Schieb, D. A. (1986). Kinematic accommodation of novice treadmill runners. *Research Quarterly for Exercise & Sport, 57*, 1-7.

Schöllhorn, W. I. (2004). Applications of artificial neural nets in clinical biomechanics. *Clinical Biomechanics, 19*, 876-898.

Sepulveda, F., Wells, D., & Vaughan, C. L. (1993). A neural network representation of electromyography and joint dynamics in human gait. *Journal of Biomechanics, 26*, 101-109.

Snow, C. M. (1999). Exercise effects on falls in frail elderly: Focus on strength. *Journal of Applied Biomechanics, 15*, 84-91.

Uthmann, T., & Dauscher, P. (2005). Analysis of motor control and behavior in multi agent systems by means of artificial neural networks. *Clinical Biomechanics, 20*(2), 119-125.

White, H., & Racine, J. (2001). Statistical inference, the bootstrap, and neural-network modelling with application to foreign exchange rates. *IEEE Transactions on Neural Networks, 12*, 657-673.

Whittle, M. (1991). *Gait analysis: An introduction.* Oxford: Butterworth Heinemann.

Winter, D. A. (1991). *The biomechanics and motor control of human gait: Normal, elderly and pathological.* Waterloo: University of Waterloo Press.

Wu, W. L., Su, F. C., & Chou, C. K. (1998). Potential of the back propagation neural networks in the assessment of gait patterns in ankle arthrodesis. In E. C. Ifeachor, A. Sperduti, & A. Starita (Eds.), *Neural networks and expert systems in medicine and health care* (pp. 92-100). Singapore: World Scientific Publishing.

Wu, W. L., Su, F. C., & Chou, C. K. (2000). Potential of the back propagation neural networks in the assessment of gait patterns in ankle arthrodesis. *Clinical Biomechanics, 15*, 143-145.

Yao, X. (1999, September). Evolving artificial neural networks. *Proceedings of the IEEE, 87*(9), 1423-1447.

Yao, X., & Liu, Y. (2004). Evolving neural network ensembles by minimization of mutual information. *International Journal of Hybrid Intelligent Systems, 1*(1), 12-21.

Yom-Tov, E., & Inbar, G.F. (2002). Feature selection for the classification of movements from single movement-related potentials. *IEEE Transactions on Neural Systems, 10*, 170-177.

Chapter XI

Neural and Kernel Methods for Therapeutic Drug Monitoring

G. Camps-Valls, Universitat de València, Spain

J. D. Martín-Guerrero, Universitat de València, Spain

Abstract

Recently, important advances in dosage formulations, therapeutic drug monitoring (TDM), and the emerging role of combined therapies have resulted in a substantial improvement in patients' quality of life. Nevertheless, the increasing amounts of collected data and the non-linear nature of the underlying pharmacokinetic processes justify the development of mathematical models capable of predicting concentrations of a given administered drug and then adjusting the optimal dosage. Physical models of drug absorption and distribution and Bayesian forecasting have been used to predict blood concentrations, but their performance is not optimal and has given rise to the appearance of neural and kernel methods that could improve it. In this chapter, we present a complete review of neural and kernel models for TDM. All presented methods are theoretically motivated, and illustrative examples in real clinical problems are included.

Introduction

In clinical practice, the collection of patient concentration-time data along with clinically relevant factors, such as anthropometrical, biochemical, or haematological parameters and the dosing history are routinely conducted as part of therapeutic monitoring for a variety of drugs. Over the last few years, numerous studies have shown that therapeutic drug monitoring (TDM) is an efficient tool for controlling the toxicity of therapeutic drugs. The adoption of a consistent, robust, and accurate TDM protocol has contributed, for example, to the improvement of cancer chemotherapy and the monitoring of transplant recipients and patients in periodic haemodialysis, in terms of the patient's quality of life (QoL) and survival.

The administered dose is commonly adjusted individually using either *a priori* or *a posteriori* methods. *A priori* methods allow the computation of the first dose based on biometrical, biological, or clinical data. *A posteriori* methods use plasma drug concentrations to adjust the subsequent doses. In this context, nomograms allowing dose adjustment on the basis of blood concentrations are commonly used. Multiple regression models have also been developed to predict a single exposure variable, such as the area under the concentration-time curve (AUC) or blood concentrations. These models take advantage of a small number of plasma concentrations obtained at predetermined times after a standard dose. Bayesian estimation offers more flexibility in blood sampling times and accuracy. Unlike other *a posteriori* methods, Bayesian estimation is based on population pharmacokinetic (PK) studies. Pharmacokinetics (PK) defines the quantitative study of the concentration-time profile of the drug in the body including the absorption, distribution, metabolism, and excretion of the drug (Evans et al., 1992). Bayesian estimators can take into account the effects of different individual factors on the pharmacokinetics of the drug and have been widely used to determine maximum tolerated systemic exposure thresholds, as well as for the routine monitoring of drugs, which are characterized by high inter- and intra-individual pharmacokinetic variability. Recently, a number of population modeling programs have become available. Among these, the NONMEM program was the first developed and has been used most extensively in the analysis of actual clinical pharmacokinetic data. Building a population pharmacokinetic model requires understanding and selection of various mathematical/statistical submodels that include a pharmacokinetic structure model relating dose, sampling time, and pharmacokinetic parameters to plasma drug levels, regression models for relationships between patient characteristics and the pharmacokinetic parameters, a population model for inter-subject variability, and a variance model for random residual variation in the data (intra-patient variability). This process can be tedious and time-consuming, and thus developing mathematical models for concentration prediction that do not need *a priori* knowledge about the problem seems necessary. In this context, artificial neural networks (ANNs) have demonstrated good capabilities for prediction of blood concentrations of a given drug based on patient follow-up. Recently, kernel-based methods have also demonstrated good robustness and accuracy capabilities in this field of application.

In this chapter, we present a complete review of neural and kernel models for TDM. All presented methods are theoretically motivated, and illustrative examples in real clinical problems are included, such as (1) monitoring of kidney recipients, (2) monitoring of patients receiving periodic haemodialysis, and (3) prediction of morbidity associated with long-term treatment of cardiac diseases. We provide some discussion on the clinical aspects of each application and the limitations and possible extensions of these works.

Literature Review on Neural Networks for TDM

Clinical decision support systems have used Artificial Intelligence (AI) methods since the end of the 1950s (Ledley & Lusted, 1959). Nevertheless, it was only during the 1990s that decision support systems were routinely used in clinical practice on a significant scale. For instance, by 1995, more than 1,000 citations of neural networks could be found in biomedical literature (Baxt, 1995), whereas now, a search on a database such as PUBMED offers more than 9,000 results. However, this number is substantially lower when the search also involves the term "drug monitoring." In fact, a PUBMED search involving "neural networks" and "drug monitoring" only offers 37 results, all very recent. As we will demonstrate later, these recent works show that the application of neural networks and kernel methods have emerged as a suitable tool for TDM, becoming a promising and expanding field from both the theoretical and practical point of view.

One of the first relevant studies involving ANNs and TDM was carried out by Gray et al. (1991). In this work, an ANN-based drug interaction warning system was developed with a computerized real-time entry medical records system. The aim of the study was to provide physicians with timely warnings of potential drug interactions as therapies were prescribed. In a dialysis unit, physicians and clinical pharmacists defined rules of proper drug therapy, and a neural network was then trained with those rules. When the network was used to review previous therapies on this patient population, a number of inconsistencies were discovered, and medication orders were changed on several patients. Real-time implementation of this monitoring system could provide messages to ensure that drug therapy is consistent and proper, according to rules created by the providers of healthcare, thus preventing the occasional mistakes that arise in drug therapy.

A reference work in this field is found in Brier et al. (1995), in which the capabilities of ANNs and NONMEN are benchmarked. Predictions of steady state peak and trough serum gentamicin concentrations were compared using a traditional population kinetic method and the computer program NONMEM, to an empirical approach using neural networks. Peak serum concentration predictions using neural networks were statistically less biased and showed comparable precision with paired NONMEM predictions. The prediction errors were lower for the neural networks than for NONMEM, and the neural network reproduced the observed multimodal distribution more accurately than NONMEM. It was concluded that neural networks can predict serum drug concentrations of gentamicin, and thus, may be useful in predicting the clinical pharmacokinetics of drugs.

There are a number of applications related to anaesthesia due to the difficult control of its depth. In Nebot et al. (1996), approaches based on ANNs and fuzzy inductive reasoning were proposed to individualize dose, by taking into account common and different characteristics among patients. In Zhang et al. (2002), the authors reviewed various modeling techniques for neuro-monitoring the depth of anaesthesia (DOA). The revision included both *traditional techniques*, such as parametric, predictive, optimal, adaptive, proportional, integral, and derivative modeling, together with *modern techniques* such as bispectral, ANNs, fuzzy logic, and neuro-fuzzy modeling. Specifically, the authors reviewed drug pharmacokinetic/pharmacodynamic (PK/PD) modeling techniques for a balanced total intravenous anaesthesia (TIVA) administration. In addition, they discussed the existing technical problems and clinical challenges, suggesting new techniques necessary for the future development of a DOA monitoring and control system.

In Leistritz et al. (2002), the applicability of generalized dynamic (recurrent) neural networks for the design of a two-valued anaesthetic depth indicator during isoflurane/nitrous oxide anaesthesia was analyzed. The aim of Vefghi and Linkens (1999) was to examine the capabilities of neural network models for dynamic monitoring and control of patient anaesthetic and dose levels. The network models under study were split into two basic groups: static networks and dynamic networks. Static networks were characterized by memory-less equations, while dynamic networks were systems with memory. Additionally, principal components analysis (PCA) was applied as both a preprocessing and postprocessing technique. In the first case, PCA was used to reduce the dimensionality of the data to more manageable intrinsic information. In the second case, PCA was employed to understand how the neurons in the hidden layer separate the data, in order to optimize the network architecture.

Diabetes is also a deeply studied field of research. For instance, Hernando et al. (1996) presented an intelligent decision support system for the analysis of home monitoring data and therapy planning in gestational diabetes. A causal probabilistic network (CPN) was used to represent the qualitative model in order to manage uncertain and missing monitoring data. The so-called DIABNET software receives inputs from the patient's available ambulatory monitoring data, and the output is a dietary and insulin therapy adjustment that includes initiation of insulin therapy, quantitative insulin dose changes, and qualitative diet and schedule modifications. Over periods of up to seven days, monitoring data were analyzed by the CPN to detect any diet or insulin therapy items, which may have required modification. The qualitative insulin demands were then translated into a quantitative proposal in line with the characteristics of the patient and the modification strategies usually used by doctors. In Mougiakakou and Nikita (2000), a neural network approach for insulin regime and dose adjustment in type 1 diabetes was proposed. The system consisted of two feedforward neural networks, trained with the backpropagation algorithm with a momentum term. The input to the system consisted of the patient's glucose levels, insulin intake, and observed hypoglycaemia symptoms over a short time period. The output of the first neural network provided the insulin regime, which was applied as input to the second neural network to estimate the appropriate insulin dosage for a short time period. The system's ability to recommend an insulin regime was excellent, while its performance in adjusting the insulin dosages for a specific patient was highly dependent on the dataset used during the training procedure.

In Trajanoski et al. (1998), closed-loop control of glucose using subcutaneous tissue glucose measurement and infusion of monomeric insulin was developed and evaluated in a simulation study. The proposed control strategy was a combination of a neural network and a non-linear model predictive control (NPC) technique. A radial basis function neural network (RBFNN) was used for off-line system identification of a Nonlinear Auto-Regressive model with an eXogenous input (NARX) model of the gluco-regulatory system. The explicit NARX model obtained from the off-line identification procedure was then used to predict the effects of future control actions. Numerical studies were carried out using a comprehensive model of glucose regulation.

The approach followed in Bate et al. (1998) is somewhat different. A Bayesian confidence propagation neural network (BCPNN) was developed. This network can manage large datasets, is robust in handling incomplete data, and may be used with complex variables. BCPNN was used for finding adverse drug reactions by analyzing the database of adverse drug reactions held by the Uppsala Monitoring Centre on behalf of the 47 countries of the World Health Organization (WHO). Since this Collaborating Programme for International Drug Monitoring contains nearly 2 million reports, as the largest database of its kind in the world, a powerful data mining technique appeared to be necessary. Using the BCPNN, some time scan examples were given, which showed the power of the technique to find early signals (e.g., *captopril-coughing*) and to avoid false positives where a common drug and adverse drug reactions occur in the database (e.g., *digoxin-acne*; *digoxin-rash*). The same database was used in Lindquist (2000), in order to carry out a retrospective evaluation of a data mining approach to aid the finding of new adverse drug reaction signals. A BPCNN was also used in this work. The first part of this study tested the predictive value of the BCPNN in new signal detection as compared with reference literature sources (*Martindale's Extra Pharmacopoeia* in 1993 and July 2000, and the *Physicians Desk Reference* in July 2000). In the second part of the study, results with the BCPNN method were compared with those of the former signal procedure. The evaluation showed that the BCPNN approach had a high and promising predictive value in identifying early signals of new adverse drug reactions. The work was then extended in Bate et al. (2002) to highlight dependencies in the WHO database. Quantitative, unexpectedly strong relationships in the data were highlighted relative to general reporting of suspected adverse effects. These associations were then clinically assessed.

Neural networks have also been applied to the assessment of HIV immunopathology. In Hatzakis and Tsoukas (2001), a neural network-based model for assessing host dynamics over time was developed and compared to a multiple regression model. Both modeling approaches were applied to the actual, non-filtered clinical observations in 58 HIV-infected individuals treated consistently with Highly Active Anti-Retroviral Therapy (HAART), for a period of more than 52 weeks, resulting in an average of 16 observations *per* patient throughout this time span. Results demonstrated that the neural network was at least as accurate as a multiregression model. The most significant drawback of this work was the small size of the dataset taken into account. Another study related to this topic is Sardari and Sardari (2002).

A data mining study using Bayesian statistics implemented in a neural network architecture was performed in Coulter et al. (2001) to study the relation between antipsychotic drugs and heart muscle disorder. The conclusion was that some antipsychotic drugs seem to be linked to cardiomyopathy and myocarditis. The study showed the potential of Bayesian neural networks in analyzing data on drug safety.

In Takayama et al. (2000), a formulation of a controlled-release tablet containing theophylline was optimized, based on the simultaneous optimization technique in which an ANN was incorporated. A desirable set of release parameters was provided, based on the plasma concentration profiles of theophylline predicted by the pharmacokinetic analysis in humans. The optimization technique incorporating ANNs showed good agreement between observed and predicted results.

Recently, Keijsers et al. (2003) analyzed the effect of long-term use of levodopa by patients with Parkinson's disease, which usually causes dyskinesia. The aim of the study was to use the trained neural networks to extract parameters, which are important in distinguishing between dyskinesia and voluntary movements. Dyskinesia differs from voluntary movements in that dyskinetic movements tend to have lower frequencies than voluntary movements, and also movements of different body segments are not well coordinated. The neural network was able to assess the severity of dyskinesia and could distinguish dyskinesia from voluntary movements in daily life. For the trunk and the leg, the important parameters appeared to be the percentage of time that the trunk or leg was moving and the standard deviation of the segment velocity of the less dyskinetic leg. For the arm, the combination of the percentage of time that the wrist was moving and the percentage of time that a patient sat were important parameters.

Kidney transplantation is of fundamental relevance in today's clinical practice, given the growing need for donors. After transplantation, recipients receive immunosuppressive drugs and are closely monitored in order to avoid organ rejection or patient intoxication. There are a number of recent works involving the use of neural networks for drug delivery in kidney disease:

- A comparison of renal-related adverse drug reactions between rofecoxib and celecoxib, based on the WHO/Uppsala Monitoring Centre safety database, was carried out by Zhao et al. (2001). Disproportionality in the association between a particular drug and renal-related adverse drug reactions was evaluated using a BCPNN method.

- A study of prediction of cyclosporine dosage in patients after kidney transplantation using neural networks and kernel-based methods was carried out in Camps-Valls et al. (2002, 2003). This application will be thoroughly reviewed in the section of applications.

- In Gaweda et al. (2003), a pharmacodynamic population analysis in chronic renal failure patients using ANNs was performed. Such models allow for adjusting the dosing regime.

- Finally, in Martin-Guerrero et al. (2003a,b), the use of kernel-based methods and neural networks was proposed for the optimization of EPO dosage in patients undergoing secondary anaemia to chronic renal failure. This application will also be described in the Applications section.

Advanced Models for TDM

Introduction

In the process of TDM, the healthcare team in the hospital decides the next dose to be administered on a daily basis, by assessment of the patient's factors and progress. The adopted protocols are based on static rules and doctors' previous experience. Nevertheless, from a Signal Theory perspective, adoption of these protocols produces three undesired features in the time series to be processed:

1. *High Variability:* High inter- and intra-subject variability is usually found in pharmacokinetics series (usually measured using the coefficient of variation). This variability commonly depends on the time instant of the patient's follow-up, since in critical periods, it becomes necessary to raise or lower dosage while closely monitoring the patient concentration.

2. *Non-Stationarity:* Therapy tries to keep drug levels in a given therapeutic target range. This forces physicians to adopt certain protocols for drug administration, which in turn provokes the presence of non-stationary processes in the time series, such as local abrupt peaks and dynamics changing in conjunction with global smoothed trends.

3. *Non-Uniform Sampling:* The individualization procedure directly affects the sampling of the time series, which usually becomes unevenly sampled.

To deal with these problems, some issues should be taken into account. On the one hand, the high variability of the time series could be tackled by developing dedicated models to each period of patients' follow-up, or by feeding the model with previous variance of the time series. On the other hand, adaptive and profiled models could treat non-stationarities in the time series efficiently by allowing, for instance, different errors in each period of patients' follow-up. Finally, the problem of non-uniform sampling could be initially addressed using the classical strategy of interpolation and resampling, but this usually produces overoptimistic results. Therefore, in many cases, a good option is to include the temporal information into the model *globally*; that is no time-series differences are thus undertaken. In the following, we review the suitability of neural and kernels methods in pharmacokinetic time series prediction.

From Linear to Non-Linear to Dynamic Models

A common approach to time series prediction is the autoregressive moving average (ARMA) model. However, ARMA models are not suitable for the problem of PK prediction and TDM due to the aforementioned problems of non-linearity, non-uniform sampling, and non-stationarity of the time series. Hence, many researchers have turned to the use of non-linear models, such as neural networks, in which few assumptions must be made. The multilayer perceptron (MLP) is the most commonly used neural network. This network is composed of a layered arrangement of artificial neurons in which each neuron of a given layer feeds all the neurons of the next layer. This model forms a complex mapping from the n-dimensional input to the binary output, $y : R^n \otimes \{0,1\}$, if this model is used for binary classification. For regression purposes, the MLP mapping has the form $y : R^n \otimes R$. However, it is a static mapping; there are no internal dynamics (Weigend & Gershenfeld, 1992). This problem can be addressed by including an array of unit-delay elements, called a tapped-delay line model, to make use of spatially converted temporal patterns. This approximation has been followed in the context of TDM in Brier et al. (1995) and Camps-Valls et al. (2002).

Neural network ARMAX (NNARMAX) modeling is intimately related to the latter approach. In a NNARMAX model (Nörgaard et al., 2001), given a pair of input-output discrete time series, a multilayer perceptron (MLP) is used to perform a mapping between them, in which past inputs, past outputs, and past residuals can be fed into the input layer. Selecting a model structure is much more difficult in the non-linear case than in the linear case (classical ARMA modeling). Not only is it necessary to choose a set of regressors, but a network architecture is also required. Several regression structures are thus available, but the most suited to our interests are NNARMAX2 (the regression vector is formed by past inputs, past outputs, and past residuals), NNSSIF (the regressor is in the form of state space innovations), and NNOE (the regression vector is formed by past inputs and estimations). The use of NNARMAX models in control applications and non-linear system identification has extended in the past few years. Its main advantage is the use of a non-linear regressor (usually an MLP) working on a fully tailored "state" vector (Ljung, 1999). This makes the model particularly well suited to the PK prediction problem because one can design the endowed input state vector to accommodate the non-stationary dynamics. This can be done, for example, by adding more "memory" in the form of error terms. In addition, there are two more approaches for introducing dynamic capabilities into a static neural network:

1. *Synapses as digital filters:* In this approach, the static synaptic weights are substituted by dynamic connections, which are usually linear filters. The

FIR neural network models each synapsis as a finite impulse response (FIR) filter (Wan, 1993). There are striking similarities between this model and the MLP. Notationally, scalars are replaced by vectors, and multiplications by vector products. These simple analogies carry through when comparing standard backpropagation for static networks with *temporal backpropagation* for FIR networks (Wan, 1993). FIR neural networks are appropriate for work in non-stationary environments or when non-linear dynamics are observed in the time series because *time* is treated naturally in the synapsis itself (internal dynamics). In fact, they have demonstrated good results in problems with those characteristics, such as speech enhancement and time series prediction (Wan, 1993).

In addition to the FIR network, the gamma network (de Vries & Principe, 1992) can also offer dynamic capabilities. The Gamma network is a class of Infinite Impulse Response (IIR) filter-based neural network, which includes a local feedback parameter. In this structure, the FIR synapsis that uses the standard delay operator z^{-1} is replaced by the so-called gamma operator

$$G(z) = \frac{\mu}{z - (1 - \mu)}$$

where μ is a real parameter, which controls the memory depth of the filter. As indicated in Principe et al. (1993), gamma filters are theoretically superior to standard FIR filters in terms of number of parameters required to model a given dynamic. The filter is stable if $0 < \mu < 2$ and for $\mu = 1$, $G(z)$ reduces to the usual delay operator. This filter also provides an additional advantage: the number of degrees of freedom (order K) and the memory depth remain decoupled. A proposed measurement of the memory depth of a model, which enables us to quantify the past information retained, is given by K/μ and has units of time. Hence, values of μ lower than the unit increase the memory depth of the filter. The use of the gamma structure in a neural network can be twofold: each scalar weight in an MLP can be substituted with a gamma filter, or a gamma unit delay line used as the first layer of a classical MLP, which yields the so-called *focused gamma network*. The latter approach is simpler and allows scrutinization of the needed memory depth for the problem by analyzing weights of this first layer. In general, the gamma network can deal efficiently with complex dynamics and fewer numbers of network parameters.

2. *Recurrent networks:* These networks are based on constructing loops in the connections between neurons or layers of the network. The Elman's

recurrent network is a simple recurrent model with feedback connections around the hidden layer. In this architecture, in addition to the input, hidden, and output units, there are also context units, which are used only to memorize the previous activations of the hidden units (Elman, 1988). Elman's networks can result in efficient models to both detect and generate time-varying patterns.

Although dynamic neural networks have been extensively used in areas such as signal processing and control, their use in biomedical engineering and medicine in general (and in TDM in particular), has received little attention, despite their theoretical efficiency when dealing with time-varying patterns. This lack of study is due to some serious difficulties in its application to TDM problems. The main limitations in the use of these networks in the context of PK time series prediction are the need for long time series and the unconstrained number of filter parameters through the networks. In addition, using these methods to predict blood concentrations becomes even more tedious since individual rather than population models are preferred, and this imposes *online* learning. This forces a change in the adaptation rules of the network when data coming from a new patient is presented to the networks at each iteration (*epoch*). In these situations, a good option is to update the corresponding internal states (weights or taps) of the network to the same parameters of the patient in the epoch before, and then apply the usual updating rules. This process usually produces oscillation of the training error, which can be alleviated with a correct choice of initialization parameters and, in some cases, by using high values for the momentum term.

From Empirical to Structural Risk Minimization

It is worth mentioning that both static and dynamic neural networks, and other gradient-descent based methods, are trained in order to minimize the *empirical risk*, that is, the error in the training dataset, and they therefore follow the empirical risk minimization (ERM) principle. However, in order to obtain significant results in the validation set ("out-of-sample" dataset), stopping-criteria, regularization, or pruning techniques must be used. Alternatively, support vector machines (SVMs) have been recently proposed as an efficient method for pattern classification and non-linear regression (Vapnik, 1998). Their appeal lies in their strong connection to the underlying statistical learning theory where an SVM is an approximate implementation of the method of *structural risk minimization* (SRM). This principle states that a better solution (in terms of generalization capabilities) can be found by minimizing an upper bound of the generalization error. SVMs have many attractive features. For instance, the solution reduces to solving a quadratic programming (QP) problem, which is globally optimized while, with neural networks, the gradient based training algorithms only guarantee finding a local minima. In addition, SVMs can handle large input spaces, can effectively work with reduced datasets, alleviate overfitting by controlling the margin, and can automatically identify a small subset made up of informative points, namely, *support vectors*.

Support Vector Machines constitute excellent alternatives to the use of ANNs in PK prediction problems. For example, in Camps-Valls et al. (2002), a combined strategy of clustering and support vector regression (SVR) methods was presented to predict Cyclosporine A (CyA) concentration in renal transplant recipients. Clustering combated the high variability and non-stationarity of the time series and reported some information gain in the problem by identifying patient groups. The SVR outperformed other classical neural networks, both static and recurrent models.

In Martin-Guerrero et al. (2003a), the SVR was benchmarked with the classical MLP and the Autoregressive Conditional Heteroskedasticity (ARCH) model. The model was tailored by introducing *a priori* knowledge by relaxing or tightening the e-insensitive region and the penalization parameter depending on the time period of the patient follow-up. The so-called Profile-Dependent SVR (PD-SVR), which was originally presented in Camps (2001), improved results of the standard SVR method and the MLP.

Applications

In the previous section, we reviewed the most useful neural and kernel methods for TDM. Note that either classification or regression approaches can be followed depending on the application. In this section, we illustrate its use in three specific case studies: monitoring of cyclosporine A (time series prediction and classification), prediction of haemoglobin concentration (time series prediction), and discrimination of potentially intoxicated patients treated with digoxin (classification).

Monitoring of Kidney Recipients Treated with Cyclosporine A (CyA)

Cyclosporine A (CyA) is still the drug of choice for immunosuppression in renal transplant recipients. This immunosuppressive drug shortens average hospital stays after kidney transplantation. At present, despite the appearance of new formulations, 90% of therapeutic guidelines are based on CyA, and, consequently, expenses continue to expand year after year. CyA is generally considered to be a critical dose drug. Underdosing may result in graft loss while overdosing causes kidney damage and increases opportunistic infections, systolic and diastolic pressure, and cholesterol. Moreover, the pharmacokinetic behavior of CyA presents a substantial inter- and intra-individual variability, which appears to be particularly evident in the earlier post-transplantation period, when the risk and clinical consequences of acute rejection are higher than in stable renal patients (Lindholm, 1991). Several factors, such as clinical drug interactions and patient compliance, can also significantly alter blood CyA concentrations, and, thus, intensive TDM of CyA is necessary since it influences the patient's QoL and the cost of care.

Consequently, mathematical models capable of predicting the future trough concentration of CyA and then adjusting the optimal dosage become necessary. Population pharmacokinetic models and Bayesian forecasting have been used to predict CyA blood concentrations, but their performance was not optimal (Charpiat et al., 1998; Parke & Charles, 1998). A different approach to TDM of kidney recipients was recently presented in Hirankarn et al. (2000), in which the goal was detection of subtherapeutic and toxic levels. This could aid physicians by providing "alarm signals" on patient progress. Nevertheless, poor results were achieved regarding subtherapeutic level detection, which could lead to dramatic kidney rejection.

In this section, we present novel results on CyA blood concentration prediction. Two main objectives can be distinguished in this work:

- *Prediction of CyA trough levels:* This approach tries to predict values of CyA blood concentration from the previous values by following a time-series methodology (Camps-Valls et al., 2003).

- *Prediction of CyA level class:* Due to the high inter- and intra-subject variability, non-uniform sampling, and non-stationarity of the time series, the prediction task is well known to be difficult. In fact, intensive TDM tries to keep CyA blood levels in the therapeutic range (usually 150-300 ng/mL) making adjustments in the patient's drug regimen. Therefore, an alternative approach to the time-series prediction methodology consists of identifying future toxic (>300 ng/mL) and subtherapeutic levels (<150 ng/mL).

Sixty-seven renal allograft recipients treated in the Nephrology Service of the Dr. Peset University Hospital in València (Spain) were included initially in this study. The exclusion criteria considered patients with serious disorders of other vital organs, active neoplasia or metastasis risk, active infections, presence of HIV virus, presence of urinary or vascular abnormalities, and patients older than 70. In addition, patients who did not fulfill the prescribed posology or who received metabolic inducers or inhibitors were excluded because they modify the pharmacokinetic profile of CyA. Patients received a standard immunosuppressive regimen (triple therapy basis) with a micro-emulsion formulation of CyA (Sandimmun Neoral®), mycophenolate mofetil (2 g/d), and prednisone (0.5-1 mg/kg/d). The initial oral dose of CyA (5 mg/kg b.i.d) was reduced according to the measured CyA blood concentration and the desired target range (150-300 ng/ mL) (Oellerich et al., 1995). Steady state blood samples were drawn 12-14 hours after dose administration. CyA blood levels were measured by a specific monoclonal fluorescence polarization immunoassay (TDx Abbott System Assays, 1999), with inter- and intra-assay variation coefficients of less than 7.5%.

Two thirds of the patients were used to train the models while the remainder were used for their validation using the cross-validation method. The population was randomly assigned to two groups: 39 patients (665 patterns) were used for training the models and 18 patients (427 patterns) for their validation. This process was repeated until three basic conditions were met: (1) variables should have variations in mean and variance between training and validation sets lower than 15%, (2) each subset should contain a similar proportion of male and female patients, and (3) patients monitored over more time were assigned to the validation set. This three-step randomizing methodology ensures balanced datasets to avoid population differences that could bias the models (Kahan et al., 1986).

We developed all neural and kernel methods discussed in the previous section, namely MLP, NNARMAX/NNOE/NNSIF, Elman's, FIR, and Gamma neural networks, along with the standard SVR and the PD-SVR for time series prediction, and MLP and SVM for classification purposes. The criterion used to select a candidate model for the final system was based on the predictive performance in the validation dataset. Bias was measured using the mean error (ME), and the model accuracy was tested by the one-way analysis of variance (ANOVA) method. The root-mean-square error (RMSE) was used as a measure of precision. In addition, we measured blood levels accurately predicted (%BLAP) if an error margin of 20% is fixed, as proposed in Parke and Charles (1998) and Charpiat et al. (1998). We used the mean of the absolute prediction error to compare the precision of the models using one-way ANOVA. Results were also assessed by inspecting the correlation coefficient (r) as a measure of goodness-of-fit.

Despite the fact that the results obtained for the blood concentration prediction were acceptable, they were inferior to those obtained for classification purposes. Nevertheless, its joint consideration could be a valuable help in TDM. The best results for the CyA blood concentration prediction were obtained using the PD-SVR, where an ME of 0.36 ng/mL and an RMSE of 52.01 ng/mL were observed in the validation set. Our results clearly improve a previous study following the time series methodology (Brier, 1995), in which an MLP with lagged inputs was used to predict CyA levels in renal allograft recipients, but the results were not optimal (bias: 25 ng/mL, precision: 74 ng/mL in the test set). From a statistical point of view, there are no significant differences between the neural and kernel models developed in our work. However, from our analysis of model robustness (long-term forecasting accuracy and additive-noise rejection), we can conclude that dynamic neural models give good results, but PD-SVM yields a more robust solution, which is a direct consequence of using a regularized and tailored model.

As regards the classification problem, binary and multiclassification schemes have been attempted and revealed the latter as optimal. Specifically, SVM outperform MLP in classification tasks when analyzing areas under the receiver-operating (AUROC) curves (97.45% for toxic and 87.43% for subtherapeutic levels). We conclude that the joint consideration of these models could be useful for clinicians in designing more robust and stable dosage regimens in order to avoid toxic and subtherapeutic cyclosporine ranges and, in turn, reduce costs to the health care system (HCS).

Based on these outcomes, the application of SVM in the context of TDM can become a clinically useful tool. In this sense, we implemented the best model in an easy-to-use computer program in order to aid the individualization of dosage and pharmacotherapeutic attention, which in turn provides state-of-the-art models to clinicians.

Patients Receiving Periodic Haemodialysis Treated with Recombinant Human Erythropoietin (rHu-EPO)

Anaemia secondary to chronic renal failure (CRF) is a clinical situation which appears to be evident in more than 90% of patients undergoing periodic haemodialysis. This situation increases the rate of hospitalization as well as patient mortality and decreases the patient's QoL. The latter can be attributed to clinical consequences of the chronic anaemia (Lindquist et al., 2000). From this point of view, the accurate diagnosis and treatment of this pathology are of vital importance. A patient is diagnosed with anaemia secondary to CRF when the value of haemoglobin (Hb) is less than 8 g/dl, or rather, when the Hb ranges between 8 and 10 g/dl and the patient shows a clinically important alteration in their QoL (Lindquist et al., 2000). The exogenous administration of recombinant human erythropoietin (rHu-EPO) is currently the chosen treatment for this pathology (Vella et al., 1998), since anaemia develops due to the insufficient synthesis of EPO (Eschbach & Adamson, 1985), and red blood cell transfusions incur a high risk of infection transmission and other complications (Fjornes, 1999). Presently, the objective of EPO treatment is to reach Hb concentrations not less than 11 g/dl in 85% of the patients. However, no recommendation is made to produce monthly increases of Hb greater than 1 g/dl, nor it is advisable to reach values of Hb higher than 14 g/dl. In this way, the patient's QoL is optimized, and the adverse effects attributed to EPO usage, such as hypertension and diverse cardiovascular problems (among which a chance of death rises), are lessened. Generally, EPO treatment is administered subcutaneously in doses ranging between 150 and 900 IU/Kg/week. This wide variability in dosage is due to existing differences between individuals, as well as in pharmacokinetic and pharmacodynamic processes associated with EPO, besides the temporal evolution of the illness. Furthermore, the high economical cost of EPO and the lack of objective methods for dose adjustment justify the efficiency of the dosage individualization process. In this context, the purpose of this work encompasses the attempt to develop a predictive model, which allows for the best dosage individualization of EPO after monitoring the Hb concentration. Few trials have been carried out in this sense (Bellazzi, 1993; Richardson, 2001). In previous works (Martin-Guerrero et al., 2003a,b), we used datasets in which the patients' monitoring visit was monthly, and we performed a one-step ahead prediction. The individualization of the dosage was obtained through the prediction of Hb concentration for the next month, taking into account the two previous values. This is because when dealing with a real-life problem, the usefulness and applicability of the results is more intriguing than obtaining impressive results. Thus, a mathematical model for predicting the Hb level was preferred to a clinician's drug prescribing protocol based on predicting the EPO dose. The objective of individualizing EPO dosage has two direct consequences:

- *To improve patient's QoL:* Patients on EPO treatment have a QoL similar to kidney recipients. However, dangerous side effects associated with the treatment can appear. Upon calculation of the minimal dosage necessary for attaining a determined level of Hb, overdose, which might lead to these consequences, could be avoided.

- *Economic savings to the healthcare system:* Due to the high cost of medication, an individualization of EPO dosage could reduce its usage, and this, in turn, may result in considerable economic savings.

Data were collected for patients with CRF in periodic haemodialysis, who received EPO treatment of two or more administrations per week and dosage of intra-venous iron (IV Fe) less than 650 mg monthly. Those patients with CRF whose etiology showed the presence of kidney cysts were excluded. Also excluded were those patients in whom it was necessary to suspend treatment with EPO and those needing red blood cell transfusions. Those patients showing levels of Hb or a hematocrit (Ht) above the 99% of the highest limits of the prediction interval calculated at the start of the study were also excluded. Additionally, a small set of patients were considered as dropout, due to not being able to complete follow-up visits (some left *exitus*, others received renal transplants, and others changed residence). Every patient was followed up with a monthly visit. For every visit, the following data were collected: age (yr), weight (Kg), Hb concentration (g/dl), hematocrit concentration (%), ferritin (μg/l), dosage of IV Fe (mg/month), number of administrations weekly, and isoform and dosage of EPO (IU/week).

The population was formed of 110 patients, who represented 891 clinical evaluations. Patients belonged to the Dr. Peset University Hospital, in València (Spain). The prediction performance was evaluated through several measures for the Hb concentration prediction: Mean error (ME) as a bias measure and mean absolute error (MAE) and root mean square error (RMSE) as accuracy measures. We compared the bias and the accuracy among the models using one-way ANOVA. In addition, the correlation coefficient (r) between the output offered by the network, and the desired output was also used as a measure of goodness-of-fit. We also computed the percentages of success if we consider a correct prediction (error $\leq$ 0.5 g/dl) and a prediction with a high grade of precision (error $\leq$ 0.25 g/dl). These percentages are usually defined as Blood Levels Accurately Predicted (BLAP % under the margins). For instance, the percentage of predictions with errors lesser than 0.5 g/dl is denoted by BLAP (% $\leq$ 0.5 g/dl). The problem becomes difficult given the high inter- and intra-individual variability computed by the coefficient of variation (48.05 % and 27.83 %, respectively).

A classical model, the ARCH was benchmarked to a static neural model, the familiar MLP trained by the ERA algorithm (Gorse et al., 1997), dynamic neural models (Elman's and FIR networks), and the standard and profile-dependent SVR presented in Camps et al. (2001). Neural models showed an excellent performance in terms of accuracy (RMSE: 0.2081 g/dL), much better than ARCH (0.7726 g/dL), considerably better than SVR (0.2840 g/dL), and slightly worse than PD-SVR (0.1944 g/dL). There were significant errors only when abrupt changes in consecutive tests existed. Since there are usually no large differences between consecutive months, the system's behavior can be considered reliable, except in the case of irregular situations of abrupt trend changes. Due to the excellent outcomes obtained, a software tool to be used as a clinical-decision aid was developed and used in the daily clinical activity. Full details can be obtained in Martin-Guerrero et al. (2003a,b).

Prediction of Morbidity Associated with Patients Treated with Digoxin (DGX)

Digoxin (DGX) is a drug widely used for treating congestive cardiac failure and symptomatic alterations of the heart rate such as auricular fibrillation and paroxysmal supraventricular tachycardia. It improves the effective behavior of the heart, and its immediate consequence is to relax the heartbeat. The main drawback of using this drug is the possibility of intoxication in the patient, due to its narrow therapeutic range, the value of which is usually accepted to be between 0.8 and 2.0 ng/mL (Evans et al., 1992).

Digoxin intoxication is one of the most usual pathologies at Hospital Emergency Services with dangerous consequences for the patient, who sometimes needs to be admitted to an Intensive Care Unit. Thus the development of models for detecting patients with risk of digoxin intoxication is essential. Patients can be classified into two categories: patients with high risk of intoxication (DGX levels >2 ng/mL) and patients with low risk of intoxication (DGX levels <2 ng/mL). The main difficulty in predicting the patients' state appears when plasma DGX concentration not only depends on the externally administered dose but also on the renal activity, the global treatment, and the patient characteristics. Finding a mathematical expression capable of achieving an optimal classification of patients with risk of intoxication is difficult using statistical methods. In fact, logistic regression was the first model attempted but outcomes were not sufficiently accurate (Camps et al., 2000; Jiménez et al., 1999). These limitations propelled us to use more sophisticated tools such as ANNs.

Two hundred and fifty-seven patients, monitored in the Dr. Peset University Hospital in València (Spain), were included in a five-year study. As discriminating information, the collected data was constituted by anthropometrical data of the patient (age, sex, height, and total body weight), renal function parameters (creatinine level and creatinine clearance), indicators of existing interaction with other drugs (treatment with amiodarone), daily dosage and the administration rate (times *per* week).

An MLP trained by the ERA algorithm was used in order to avoid falling into local minima (Gorse et al., 1997). In terms of accuracy and robustness, this approach improved results of the classical backpropagation learning algorithm and of other neural approaches, such as Radial Basis Function Neural Networks (RBFNNs) and One-Class One-Network (OCON) neural networks (Camps et al., 2000). Results obtained by logistic regression were also improved. As in the case of EPO and CyA, an easy-to-use software tool was developed for use by clinicians.

The main limitation encountered in these works was due to the group's location. Since patients were all from the same nephrology or cardiology units, they had a series of characteristics in common. For example, the treatment guidelines and protocol administration for the patients were similar, which means that extrapolations to other centers should be treated with caution. Furthermore, a strict test should be performed before using the application in new situations. This, however, should not prevent the proposed methodology from its use in other nephrology or cardiology units, where they could be implemented, taking into account the local population characteristics and dosing protocols.

Discussion and Concluding Remarks

In this chapter, we have reviewed the field of application of neural networks and support vector machines in TDM and PK time series prediction. The use of these methods is due to the special characteristics of the time series, which are derived from the dose protocol itself. Patients are closely monitored by adjusting dosage according to previous observations of concentration levels. Hence, protocol administration produces time series with difficult characteristics, such as non-stationarities, uneven sampling, and high variability. These are intrinsically difficult situations for any model but can be dramatic for models assuming linear relationships between variables, such as ARMA modeling or a fixed physical model for the underlying system that generated data distribution. Unlike ARMA, neural and kernel methods do not share these limitations and have proven to be efficient methods in this area. The interested reader can visit the Web pages, http://www.imf.es and http://www.oncofarm.com/ where a set of implementation of neural methods for the clinical routine monitoring is provided.

However, development and application of neural networks in a given framework is full of pitfalls and problems, which can become dramatic in TDM. For instance, feature selection is a critical problem because of the high amount of routinely acquired data and because an individual approach, rather than a population one, is commonly carried out. Therefore, removing a variable which is redundant for the whole population on average, could have dramatic consequences for individual prediction in some specific patients. Another interesting problem in the context of blood concentration prediction is the issue of non-uniform sampling. Although there are some useful techniques for dealing with this problem, there are few works in the field of neural networks to tackle the problem efficiently when combined with non-stationary processes. In particular, the issue of applying predictive models to individuals deserves more attention, given that individual dose adjustments require confidence intervals and limits on the provided predictions, something that neural or kernel methods cannot provide directly. Finally, the problems of interpretability, overfitting, and adaptation to changing conditions still remain major concerns in the neural network community and, by extension, in the pharmacotherapeutic community. All these problems should be confronted with a critical spirit, always keeping in mind that an individual patient is not a statistic.

References

Bate, A., Lindquist, M., Edwards, I. R., Olsson, S., Orre, R., Lansner, A., & De Freitas, R. M. (1998). A Bayesian neural network method for adverse drug reaction signal generation. *Eur J Clin Pharmacol, 54*(4), 315-321.

Bate, A., Lindquist, M., Edwards, I. R., & Orre, R. (2002). A data mining approach for signal detection and analysis. *Drug Saf, 25*(6), 393-397.

Baxt, W. G. (1995). Application of neural networks to clinical medicine. *Lancet, 346*(4), 1135-1138.

Bellazzi, R. (1993). Drug delivery optimisation through Bayesian networks: An application to erythropoietin therapy in uremic anemia. *Biomedical Research, 26*, 274-293.

Brier, M. E. (1995). Empirical pharmacokinetic predictions for cyclosporine using a time series neural network. *Pharmaceutical Research, 12*, 363.

Brier, M. E., Zurada, J. M., & Aronoff, G. R. (1995). Neural network predicted peak and trough gentamicin concentrations. *Pharmaceutical Research, 12*(3), 406-412.

Camps, G., Soria, E., & Jiménez, N.V. (2000, July 23-28). Artificial neural networks for the classification of potentially intoxicated patients treated with digoxin. *Proceedings of World Congress on Medical Physics and Biomedical Engineering,* Chicago (p. 1378).

Camps, G., Soria, E., Pérez, J., Artés, A., & Pérez, F. F. A. (2001, December 7). A profile-dependent kernel-based regression for cyclosporine concentration prediction. *Proceedings of NIPS 2001: Workshop on New Directions in Kernel-based Learning Methods,* Vancouver, Canada. Whistler/Blackcomb Resort, BC. Available at http://www.uv.es/gcamps/publications.htm

Camps-Valls, G., Porta-Oltra, B., Soria-Olivas, E., Martin-Guerrero, J. D., Serrano-Lopez, A. J., Perez-Ruixo, J. J., & Jimenez-Torres, N. V. (2003). Prediction of cyclosporine dosage in patients after kidney transplantation using neural networks. *IEEE Transactions on Biomedical Engineering, 50*(4), 442-448.

Camps-Valls, G., Soria-Olivas, E., Perez-Ruixo, J. J., Perez-Cruz, F., Figueiras-Vidal, A. R., & Artes-Rodriguez, A. (2002). Cyclosporine concentration prediction using clustering and support vector regression methods. *IEE Electronics Letters, 12,* 568-570.

Charpiat, B., Falconi, I., Bréant, V., Jellife, R. W., Sab, J. M., Ducerf, C., Fourcade, N., Thomasson, A., & Baulieux, J. (1998). A population pharma-cokinetic model of cyclosporine in the early postoperative phase in patients with liver transplants, and its predictive performance with Bayesian fitting. *Therapeutic Drug Monitoring, 20,* 158-164.

Coulter, D. M., Bate, A., Meyboom, R. H., Lindquist, M., & Edwards, I. R. (2001). Antipsychotic drugs and heart muscle disorder in international pharmacovigilance: Data mining study. *BMJ, 322*(7296), 1207-1209.

de Vries, B., & Principe, J.C. (1992). The Gamma model: A new neural model for temporal processing. *Neural Networks, 5*(4), 565-576.

Elman, J. L. (1988). Finding structure in time. *Cognitive Science, 14,* 179-211.

Eschbach, J. W., & Adamson, J.W. (1985). Anemia of end-stage renal disease (ESRD). *Kidney INTL, 28,* 1-5.

Evans, W., Schentag, J., & Jusko, W. (1992). *Applied pharmacokinetics. Principles of therapeutic drug monitoring. Applied Therapeutics.* Lippincott Williams and Wilkins.

Fjornes, T. (1999). Response and prediction of response to recombinant human erythropoietin in patients with solid tumors and platinum-associated ane-mia. *J Oncol Pharm Practice, 5*(1), 22-31.

Gaweda, A. E., Jacobs, A. A., Brier, M. E., & Zurada, J. M. (2003). Pharma-codynamic population analysis in chronic renal failure using artificial neural networks: A comparative study. *Neural Networks, 16*(5-6), 841-845.

Gorse, D., Sheperd, A. J., & Taylor, J. G. (1997). The new ERA in supervised learning. *Neural Networks, 10*(2), 343-352.

Gray, D. L., Ash, S. R., Jacobi, J., & Michel, A. N. (1991). The training and use of an artificial neural network to monitor use of medication in treatment of complex patients. *J Clin Eng, 16*(4), 331-336.

Hatzakis, G., & Tsoukas, C. (2001). Neural networks in the assessment of HIV immunopathology. *Proceedings AMIA Symposium,* Washington, DC (pp. 249-253).

Hernando, M. E., Gomez, E. J., del Pozo, F., & Corcoy, R. (1996). DIABNET: A qualitative model-based advisory system for therapy planning in gesta-tional diabetes. *Med Inform (Lond), 21*(4), 359-374.

Hirankarn, S., Downs, C., Street, W., & Herman, R. A. (2000, October 31). *Prediction of two ranges of cyclosporine level (subtherapeutic and toxic) using feature subset selection and artificial neural networks.* AAPS Annual Meeting.

Jiménez, N. V., Soria, E., Albert, A., Serrano, A. J., & Camps, G. (1999, December 5-9). Prediction of digoxin plasma potentially toxic levels by using a neural network model. *1999 Midyear Clinical Meeting. ASHP99. American Society of Health-System Pharmacists,* Orlando, FL.

Kahan, B. D., Kramer, W. G., Wideman, C. A., Flechner, S. M., Lorber, M., & van Buren, C. T. (1986). Demographics factors affecting the pharmacokinetics of cyclosporine estimated by radioinmunoassay. *Transplantation, 41*, 459-464.

Keijsers, N. L., Horstink, M. W., & Gielen, S. C. (2003). Movement parameters that distinguish between voluntary movements and levodopa-induced dyskinesia in Parkinson's disease. *Hum Mov Sci, 22*(1), 67-89.

Ledley, R. S., & Lusted, L. B. (1959). Reasoning foundations of medical diagnosis. *Science, 130*, 9-21.

Leistritz, L., Kochs, E., Galicki, M., & Witte, H. (2002). Prediction of movement following noxious stimulation during 1 minimum alveolar anesthetic concentration isoflurane/nitrous oxide anesthesia by means of middle latency auditory evoked responses. *Clin Neurophysiol, 113*(6), 930-935.

Lindholm, A. (1991). Factors influencing the pharmacokinetics of cyclosporine in Man. *Therapeutic Drug Monitoring, 13*(6), 465-477.

Lindquist, M., Stahl, M., Bate, A., Edwards, I. R., & Meyboom, R. H. (2000). A retrospective evaluation of a data mining approach to aid finding new adverse drug reaction signals in the WHO international database. *Drug Saf, 23*(6), 533-542.

Ljung, L. (1999). *System identification. Theory for the user.* Upper Saddle River, NJ: Prentice Hall.

Manual Analitique. (1999). France: Rundix Cedex, Laboratories ABBOTT, Division Diagnostic.

Martin-Guerrero, J. D., Camps-Valls, G., Soria-Olivas, E., Serrano-Lopez, A. J., Perez-Ruixo, J. J., & Jimenez-Torres, N. V. (2003a). Dosage individualization of erythropoietin using a profile-dependent support vector regression. *IEEE Transactions on Biomedical Engineering, 50*(10), 1136-1142.

Martin-Guerrero, J. D., Olivas, E. S., Valls, G. C., Serrano Lopez, A. J., Perez Ruixo, J. J., & Torres, N. V. (2003b). Use of neural networks for dosage individualisation of erythropoietin in patients with secondary anemia to chronic renal failure. *Comput Biol Med, 33*(4), 361-373.

Mougiakakou, S. G., & Nikita, K. S. (2000). A neural network approach for insulin regime and dose adjustment in type 1 diabetes. *Diabetes Technol Ther, 2*(3), 381-389.

Nebot, A., Cellier, F. E., & Linkens, D. A. (1996). Synthesis of an anaesthetic agent administration system using fuzzy inductive reasoning. *Artificial Intelligence in Medicine, 8*(2), 147-166.

Nörgaard, M., Ravn, O., & Poulsen, N. K. (2001). NNSYSID & NNCTRL: Tools for system identification and control with neural networks. *IEEE Computing & Control Engineering Journal, 12*(1), 29-36.

Oellerich, M., Armstrong, V. W., Kahan, B., Shaw, L., Holt, D. W., Yatscoff, R., et al. (1995). Lake Louise consensus conference on cyclosporin monitoring in organ transplantation: Report of the consensus panel. *Therapeutic Drug Monitoring, 17*, 642-654.

Parke, J., & Charles, B. G. (1998). NONMEM population pharmacokinetic modeling of orally administered cyclosporine from routine drug monitoring data after heart transplantation. *Therapeutic Drug Monitoring, 20*(3), 284-293.

Principe, J. C., deVries, B., & Oliveira, P. G. (1993). The gamma filter: A new class of adaptive IIR filters with restricted feedback. *IEEE Transactions on Signal Processing, 41*(2), 649-656.

Richardson, D. (2001). Optimizing erythropoietin therapy in hemodialysis patients. *American Journal of Kidney Diseases, 38*(1), 109-117.

Sardari, S., & Sardari, D. (2002). Applications of artificial neural network in AIDS research and therapy. *Curr Pharm Des, 8*(8), 659-670.

Takayama, K., Morva, A., Fujikawa, M., Hattori, Y., Obata, Y., & Nagai, T. (2000). Formula optimization of theophylline controlled-release tablet based on artificial neural networks. *J Control Release, 68*(2), 175-186.

Trajanoski, Z., Regittnig, W., & Wach, P. (1998). Simulation studies on neural predictive control of glucose using the subcutaneous route. *Comput Methods Programs Biomed, 56*(2), 133-139.

Vapnik, V. N. (1998). *Statistical learning theory.* Wiley.

Vefghi, L., & Linkens, D. A. (1999). Dynamic monitoring and control of patient anaesthetic and dose levels: Time-delay, moving-average neural networks, and principal components analysis. *Comput Methods Programs Biomed, 59*(2), 91-106.

Vella, J. P., O'Neill, D., & Atkins, N. (1998). Sensitization to human leukocyte antigen before and after the introduction of erythropoietin. *Nephrol Dial Transplant, 13*, 2027-2032.

Wan, E. A. (1993). *Finite impulse response neural networks with applications in time series prediction.* Unpublished PhD thesis, Stanford University, Department of Electrical Engineering.

Weigend, A. S., & Gershenfeld, N. A. (1992). Time series prediction. Forecasting the future and understanding the past. *Proceedings of the NATO Advanced Research Workshop on Comparative Time Series Analysis,* Santa Fe, NM. Addison Wesley.

Zhang, X. S., Huang, J. W., & Roy, R. J. (2002). Modeling for neuromonitoring depth of anesthesia. *Critical Reviews in Biomedical Engineering, 30*(1-3), 131-173.

Zhao, S. Z., Reynolds, M. W., Lejkowith, J., Whelton, A., & Arellano, F. M. (2001). A comparison of renal-related adverse drug reactions between rofecoxib and celecoxib, based on the World Health Organization/Uppsala Monitoring Centre safety database. *Clin Ther, 23*(9), 1478-1491.

Chapter XII

Computational Fluid Dynamics and Neural Network for Modeling and Simulations of Medical Devices

Yos S. Morsi, Swinburne University, Australia

Subrat Das, Swinburne University, Australia

Abstract

This chapter describes the utilization of computational fluid dynamics (CFD) with neural network (NN) for analysis of medical devices. First, the concept of mathematical modeling and its use for solving engineering problems is presented followed by an introduction to CFD with a brief summary of the numerical techniques currently available. A brief introduction to the standard optimization strategies for NN and the various methodologies in use are also presented. A case study of the design and optimization of scaffolds for tissue engineering heart valve using the combined CFD and NN approach is presented and discussed. This chapter concludes with a discussion of the advantages and disadvantages of the combined NN and CFD techniques and their future potential prospective.

Mathematical Modeling

Introduction

Many engineering systems are of a complex nature and require techniques that relate the relevant variables in the system under consideration. Equations that express physical phenomena between quantities require absolute numerical and dimensional equality. Historically, the use of dimensional analysis of the physics observed experimentally has been very successful in adding to our understanding of the complexity of the problem in hand. Generally speaking, all physical relationships can be expressed in terms of quantities such as mass M, Length L, and time T or other related quantities such as force F, pressure P, stress τ, and so on. The application of such a system may include converting one system of units to another, developing relations or equations, reducing the number of variables required for an experimental program and, in some cases, determining the principles of model design. It should be noted that for a physical system, dimensional analysis can only indicate variables or groups of variables that are functionally related, and it does not give insight of the nature of the correlation and its complexity. One of the most common uses of dimensional analysis is in experimental planning of examining a particular phenomena or system. Moreover, the dimensional analysis does not estimate the actual behavior of the system. This requires the development of a more comprehensive mathematical model which often requires a solution to the governing equations, either ordinary differential equations or partial differential equations (ODEs/PDEs).

The Governing Equations

In recent years, the utilization of mathematical modeling to solve engineering problems has been advanced greatly by the availability of fast and user-friendly software packages. However, these models, even today, still require experimental or physical modeling results to validate and verify the numerical results. However, in general, the process of mathematical modeling may require a continuing four-stage cycle, as illustrated in Figure 1 to have a solution.

The mathematical model is constructed based on fundamental laws of physics, often by making quite a number of assumptions. Some are justified quite

Figure 1. The typical loop of mathematical modeling

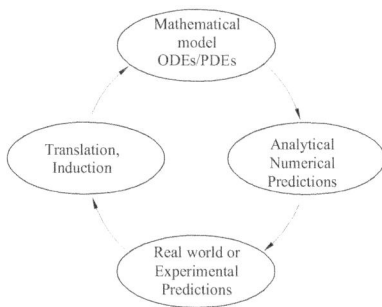

rigorously on scientific grounds, while others render the problem tractable or solvable within an economically acceptable time frame. In any case, the mathematical assumptions formulate a mathematical model, and the next two stages of the cycle are intended to test this model and modify it if need be (Figure 1). To test a model, one needs to draw certain conclusions about the real problem at hand. Such terminations are often of two types, those related to previously observed situations (*explanatory in nature*) or those related to new, not previously observed situations (*predictive in nature*). Both types are important for validating a mathematical model, though for purposes of discussion, it is reasonable to refer to both types as predictions. To obtain these outcomes, one first makes mathematical predictions, using mathematical tools, which have been previously developed or are developed for a particular mathematic model. These mathematical predictions are then translated back from the language of the model to the language of the real problem and interpreted as real-world predictions or conclusions. In the final stage, the predictions are checked against real data, either old (in the case of tests of the explanatory power of the model) or new (in the case of tests of its predictive power). On the basis of the new data, which includes the performance of the model's predictions, the model is modified, and the cycle repeats. The cyclical process is continuous and newly generated data must be validated against the explanatory power of the model or against its predictive power.

Mathematical models provide a fundamentally based quantitative relationship between process variables that provide a general insight into the overall behavior of a given system. For a new process, a mathematical model can provide guidance with respect to the general feasibility and the consistency of a new concept with both the physical and theoretical laws. If the process concept is found feasible, the model may identify critical areas that require further validation through possibly experimental investigation.

Traditionally, mathematical model development has relied on individual effort, where a scientist may have worked for a very long period of time to develop customized algorithms or a computer program, often understood by the developer alone. This imposes a major difficulty in extending the theory for further development of the program. However, in the last few decades with availability of software packages, the ready access to inexpensive computers, and the much more widespread application of modeling as a technical tool has assisted greatly in the advancement of mathematical modeling packages.

A mathematical model generally consists of algebraic or differential equations that quantitatively represent a system or process. For example, it may be a relationship that defines the time, pressure, and velocity in a pipe, defines swirling flow in an annulus, or defines the circulation patterns, fluid-structure interactions, composition of two phases in chemical equilibrium, stress distributions, and pressure drops along and across a valve or within a pump.

From the above discussion, it follows that a mathematic model may be simple differential equations or a complex set of equations, such as the coupled Navier Stokes equations with turbulence closures which may require certain expertise and advanced computer hardware to solve.

General Methodology for Model Development

A typical flowchart of a model development and implementation is shown in Figure 2. The model development involves the translation of a previously constructed physical picture into concrete mathematical terms, or more precisely, differential equations. Traditionally, problem formulation was usually performed "from scratch" by establishing a control volume and thus developing the appropriate governing equations in a differential form, by letting the dimensions of the control volume shrink to an infinitesimal size. While such a development is instructive and may indeed be appropriate for certain simple systems, at present there are rather easier and speedier ways to proceed:

- Drawing on prior experience with related systems (the rapidly growing body of modeling literature makes this possible);
- Using the "ready-made" building blocks of the key differential relationships;
- Navier-Stokes equations for fluid flow;
- Fourier's equation for heat transfer;

Figure 2. General methodology of model development

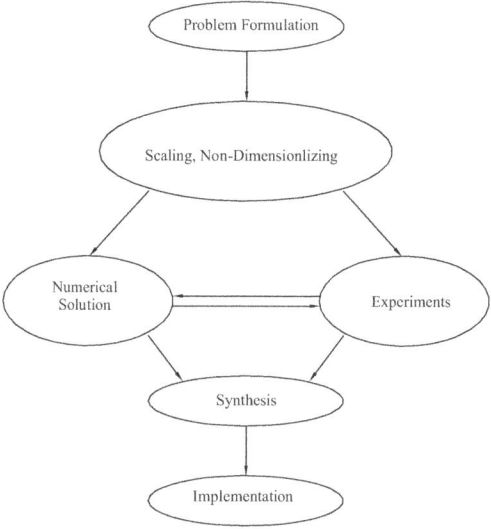

- Fick's equation for diffusion;
- Maxwell's equations for deformation processing turbulence models;
- Constitutive equations for deformation processing turbulence models.

It should be stressed that many problems involve some non-standard building blocks, such as meniscus effects, surface waves, hydrodynamic instability, surface tension, and so forth. The modeler will need to take care not to ignore these factors because the effects may have a dominant influence on the problem.

It has been shown that the critical examination of the governing equations represents the next logical step. These equations usually involve several scaled parameters as mentioned previously. Thus, the functional relationships between key process parameters, such as the solidification time proportional to the square of the characteristic dimension, the linear dependence of the melt velocities on current in induction furnaces, the relationship between the Rayleigh number and the characteristic velocity in buoyancy driven flows, Reynolds number effect on wall shear stress, and so forth, do provide a framework for interpreting data, which is unlikely to emerge from the computer output. Furthermore, the analytical solutions or functional relationships provide an excellent means for evaluating the consistency of computed solutions. The computer-generated solutions will make a much greater degree of precision possible to a whole range of process problems, such as the details of the velocity field, the thermal gradients, local values of the heat and mass transfer coefficients, and the details of mixing. Therefore, these two approaches are complementary rather than orthogonal.

At this point, it is important to stress the need to employ the correct boundary conditions because the software packages essentially solve the same types of conservation equations, and the principal factor that distinguishes individual cases is usually associated with the boundary conditions. These numerical solutions need to be checked for internal consistency, that is, by performing overall heat, mass, and momentum balances, testing sensitivity to different starting points and grid sizes, and, most importantly, checking the predictions against analytical asymptotes. The predictions will then have to be compared with experimental measurements to establish the discrepancies between these results by critical examination. If the deviation between these results is large, then it is necessary to check the appropriateness of the assumptions and to update the model.

Outline of the General Mathematical Procedures

The general principle of mathematical procedures, which can hold for any systems, can be outlined as follows:

- Define the quantity conserved, the control volume for which the equations are to be written, and select the independent and dependent variables. If only one independent variable appears, an ordinary differential equation will result.
- Apply the physical laws that yield the input and output expressions for the quantity conserved.
- Substitute these expressions into the appropriate terms in the equation.
- Develop the necessary boundary conditions.
- Solve the resulting differential equation and boundary conditions.

The above procedures can be applied to various engineering problems for design and optimization of various cardiovascular devices such as blood vessels, rotary blood pumps, ventricular assist devices, lung ventilation unit, modeling of liver stent, kidney and various other medical devices. In the following section, a case study is given to illustrate the necessary steps needed for design and optimization of model of artificial heart valves.

The success or failure of mathematical treatment of blood flow problems within cardiovascular devices depends mainly on our ability to solve the governing equations of continuity, momentum, and energy as accurately as possible. These equations contain non-linear terms and a large number of unknown variables, which makes an exact solution extremely difficult to obtain. Therefore, some assumptions of the physical phenomena must be made in order to reduce the number of unknown variables in the equations. In complex turbulent flow, a complete solution is still extremely difficult to obtain and, in attempting to solve the equations of motion, it is necessary to consider the following factors:

- The solution techniques available for the problem and their reliability;
- The methods of approximating the equations;
- The degree of accuracy requiring the validity of assumptions employed.

In general, the exact solutions for complex medical devices are difficult to obtain; moreover, the correctness of the results obtained analytically are somewhat limited due to their simplifying assumptions. With this in mind, numerical analyses have been widely used for several decades. As a result, numerical techniques have been developed to solve different combinations of ordinary/partial differential equations for various engineering and science applications. These methods are briefly summarized below:

Numerical Methods

Finite difference method (FDM), finite-volume method (FVM), and finite-element method (FEM) are widely employed to solve flow and heat transfer problems. Generally, the choice of a particular technique depends on factors such as non-linearity, geometry of boundary, and type of boundary conditions. FDM is a common and successful method used to deal with orthogonal geometries involving simple boundary conditions. In FDM methodology, discretization of the governing equations in 3D problems is simpler and the accuracy can readily be examined by the order of the truncation error in the Taylor's series expansion. However, for problems involving irregular geometry in the solution domain, FVM is more suitable. On the other hand, arbitrary and more complex geometries, involving gradient boundary conditions, FVM can be more cumbersome, and the application of FEM is preferred. Another important use of FEM is as a generalized computer algorithm, making it more advantageous than the other methods (Das & Morsi, 2003). However, development of a computer code that employs FEM is more time consuming compared to an equivalent code that uses FDM or FVM. It should be noted that the topic of "which method is good" is still the subject of debate among researchers. In reality, the choice of a particular method depends on the type of partial differential equations (PDEs) and the computational domain.

Partial Differential Equations (PDEs)

PDEs representing the physical problem may be classified as elliptic, parabolic, and hyperbolic and can be expressed in two-dimensional Cartesian form as

$$A\frac{\partial^2 \phi}{\partial x^2} + B\frac{\partial^2 \phi}{\partial x \partial y} + C\frac{\partial^2 \phi}{\partial y^2} + D\frac{\partial \phi}{\partial x} + E\frac{\partial \phi}{\partial y} + F\phi + G(x,y) = 0 \tag{1}$$

Where ϕ is the dependent variable that becomes velocity and temperature in fluid flow and heat transfer problems respectively? The mathematical character of the PDE is defined by the coefficients of A, B, and C. Other coefficients, D and E, can be functions of the spatial coordinates (x, y). The source term is represented by G. All fluid flow and heat transfer problems use a set of PDEs that are the same as the general equation shown above. However, in some situations of complex geometry, typical boundary conditions and the coefficient in the equation (1) can represent a formidable challenge in computational ability.

Computational fluid dynamics (CFD) and computer hardware during the last decade provide researchers in the field with various commercial codes of FVM and FEM such as CFX-TASCflow, FLOW3D, CFX4, CFX5, STAR-CD, Flotran, and so forth. They have helped significantly in various area of engineering to obtain reasonable approximations. However; other researchers have developed their own source codes for specific applications in fluid flow and heat transfer.

Recent improvements in the coupling library MpCCI (previously called COCOLIB) are taking place in cooperation between Computational Dynamics, Intes, GMD, and Daimler Chrysler. This capability will provide a general interface between a flow solver and a structural analysis code for estimating the fluid loads on a defined structure, particularly in multiphysics problems. Many have used this MpCCI interface to couple either their own codes or commercial codes such as fluid dynamics (CFX) with structure analysis (ANSYS, ADINA, ABACUS) and successfully simulated fluid induced large deflection problems. Several CAD development packages, such as Unigraphics, Solid-Edge, AutoCAD, Pro-

Engineer, and 3D-CAD, have become an additional advantage for developing the accurate geometries of the computational domain. The development of CPU speed has also helped to simulate more sophisticated turbulence modeling that deals with realistic geometries. Traditionally, the results generated from these codes are validated with qualitative and quantitative information gained from experimental diagnostics techniques such as partical images velocitmatry (PIV) and laser Doppler anemometry (LDA).

In general, despite all the advances in the field, the CFD approach to some typical situations remained computationally expensive in terms of time. On the other hand, it is not suitable for system simulations, particularly for optimization purposes. Moreover, when the solution demands an interactive procedure, numerical solution usually fails to provide the solutions in real time due to its iterative procedure. The major shortcomings of CFD analysis can be listed:

- The system is usually depicted in terms of the set of ordinary differential equations or partial differential equations. The mathematical representation in terms of OPDEs/PDES usually involves approximations that are not relevant to the physical model. Moreover, due to a lack of precise knowledge of the physics of the processes involved or the properties of the materials used, the mathematical model represents an ideal situation rather than a real one.

- There may be several external *disturbances,* such as a change in environmental conditions that affect the response of the system.

- The exact initial conditions to determine the state of the system may not be accurately known.

- The model may be too complicated for exact analytical solutions. Computer-generated numerical solutions may have small errors that are magnified over time.

- The solution may be inherently sensitive to small perturbations in the state of the system, in which case, any error will magnify over time.

- Numerical solutions may be too slow to be of use in real time. This is usually the case if PDEs or a large number of ODEs are involved.

Although the CFD is now increasingly used to model thermal and fluid system performance as a part of the design and engineering process, in nearly all cases, the computational time required for CFD limits its use to providing insight into the physical phenomena investigated after the basic design is chosen rather than as a design and optimization tool. This is the case where NN can be thought of as another alternative tool where a collective set of neurons can be trained with a prior knowledge database obtained from numerical CFD calculations. Thus, it was required to define an intelligent system and its collectiveness.

System Approach

A *system* may be defined as a small part of the universe that we are interested in and that has some intelligence. At this point, it is difficult to quantify the mode or the degree of intelligence that can be given to a system. However, the existing CFD/experimental data are enormous and can be one of the most important tools to create a system with some knowledge-based intelligence through various evolutionary algorithms (EAs). There are several areas where knowledge-based training approaches are applied to construct intelligent systems through evolutionary algorithms. These include instrument landing systems, automatic pilot, collision-avoidance systems, antilock brakes, smart air bags, intelligent road vehicles, medical diagnostic devices, image processing, pattern recognition, intelligent data analysis, temperature and flow control, process control, intelligent CAD, smart materials, smart manufacturing, Internet search engines, and machine translators. Neural network (NN) is one of approaches through which a knowledge-based system can be constructed.

Neurophysiologists spent many years searching for the engram, that is, the precise location in the brain for specific memories. The brain memory system has a specific structure that consists of many elements (neurons) working in parallel and in connection with one another. These sets of neurons act as a computing system for the brain. Thus, a neural network science based largely on the notion of "brain-style computation" has evolved in which a large number of very simple processing units act simultaneously on a distributed pattern of data. A trained neuron can be thought of as an expert system or a knowledge-based system in the category of information it has been given to analyze. Thus, NN that consists of several neurons has a remarkable ability to derive meaning from complicated or imprecise data that can be used to extract patterns and detect trends that are too complex to be recognized by humans or computer techniques. The application of NN to a variety of engineering applications appears to be a recent development, and a brief discussion on system development is outline below.

Simple System

A system has an input $u(t)$ and an output $y(t)$ where t is the time. A schematic representation simple open system is shown in Figure 3.

Figure 3. Schematic representation of an open system

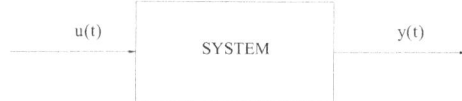

One can represent an input-output relationship by y = Ñ(u) whereÑ is an operator (addition, substraction, differential, or integral). Thus, if we know the input u(t), then the operations represented by Ñ must be carried out to obtain the output. In some situations, we may have a set of values for u(t) and y(t) and we would like to know what Ñ is. This is a *system identification* problem. If the system identifies the physics precisely, then it is called an expert/intelligent system.

For *closed-loop control*, there is a *feedback* from the output to the input of the system, as shown in Figure 4. The output of the NN model is compared with some standard value (base value). This base value can be from CFD simulation, experimental data, or analytical solution. The difference between the output and the base value can be treated as an error and minimized through a feedback closed loop approach.

Complex systems are made up of a large number of such opened/closed simple systems, each of which may be easy to understand or to solve for. Together, however, they pose a formidable modeling and computational task, and from a neurophysics point of view, each simple system behaves like a neuron.

Neural Network in CFD Application

Neural networks (NNs) have emerged as an alternative tool (Cao et al., 2004; Parlos et al., 1992) to first principle-based approaches for modeling complex

Figure 4. Closed system

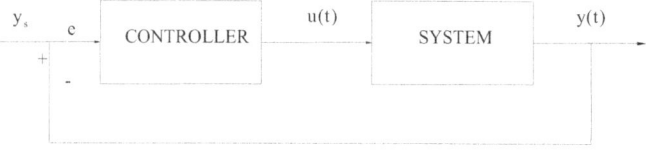

systems in a variety of engineering applications. In a particular area of CFD analysis, the volume flow rates obtained by the two-dimensional CFD analysis were used as target values for learning a neural network. By learning neural network with the target values, the values of learning results were obtained, which almost coincide with the values of CFD (Han, 2003). The authors have used backpropagation rule as a learning method with hyperbolic tangent sigmoid transfer function for connecting the input layer with the first hidden layer. Even in a particular natural convection problem, u, v, p and T, Ra, Pr can be considered as inputs and Nusselt number can be considered (heat transfer rate) as an output. Yuen and Bau (1998) used the same approach for a natural convection problem. Diaz (2000) used NN model for heat exchanger problem. Turbulence model using NN models were also reported (Gillies, 1998; Lee et al., 1997).

NN-based fluid field estimation with dimensional inputs and output has been studied by Xue and Watton (1998). The non-linear transient behavior of fluid power elements was also identified through NN modeling based upon input-output observations only. Xu et al. (1996) applied NN to model a flow through an orifice. Schreck et al. (1994) reported a non-dimensional NN configuration to characterize the unsteady, vortex-dominated flow as it develops over the wing and splitter plate of aircraft using surface pressure measurements and flow visualization. The neural network models were shown to accurately predict both temporal and spatial variations for both the unsteady separated flow fields and the aerodynamic loads. The inputs and output of the NN model were non-dimensionalized according to previous empirical and theoretical results. More recently, Cao et al. (2004) reported a non-dimensional artificial neural network (NDANN) model for accurate predictions of flow force and flow rates under the broad operating conditions of a hydraulic valve. Because of its non-dimensional characteristics, the NDANN fluid field estimator also exhibits accurate input-output scalability, which allows the NDANN model to estimate the fluid force and flow rate even when the operating condition parameter or design geometry parameters are outside the range of the training data. Sablani et. al. (2003) developed an explicit calculation of the friction factor in pipeline flow of Bingham plastic fluids. Their NN approach involved the establishment of an explicit relationship between the Reynolds number, (Re), and the friction factor, (f), under both laminar and turbulent flow conditions. In addition, EAs have also been applied to various optimization problems in thermofluid devices including airfoils, heat exchangers, fluid-structure interaction problems, and missile nozzle inlets for high-speed flow.

The overall modeling approach in NN is a black box approach, since (in principle) the development of NN models does not require prior knowledge of the process. It is sufficient to provide the network with the set of input data and the corresponding outputs. The objective is to train a model with prior knowledge input (PKI) (Chao et al., 2001; Watson et. al., 1999). However, having some idea about such relationship may provide for the fine-tuning of the NN model. In some instances, these ideas have shown exceptional improvements in NN model performance (Porru et al., 2000; Shayya & Sablani, 1998; Sablani, 2001). It is also capable of dealing with uncertainties, noisy data, and non-linear relationships. Brasquet and Le Cloirec (2000) conducted an experimental study and measured air and water pressure drops through a layer of several textile fabrics. Their study focused on the influence of specific parameters of clothes on their dynamic behavior. Using NN, they correlated fluid properties (i.e., viscosity, density, and Reynolds number) and fabric characteristics (i.e., thickness, density, number of openings, and raw material) as input neurons with pressure drop as the output neuron. The NN model they developed predicted pressure drops that closely followed the experimental values. A hybrid neural network modeling approach (Porru et. al., 2000) was proposed for the identification of the dynamic behavior of chemical reactors. They used a multilayer, feedforward neural network to correlate bulk carbon monoxide concentration and temperature with reaction rate. Their NN model was capable of describing the system kinetics over the entire range of the investigated operating conditions whereas a conventional Langmuir–Hinshelwood rate law failed to provide the correct representation. These and other studies reported in the literature underscore the importance of NN in tackling wide range of problems. However, in most of the applications of NN in modeling, a feedforward neural network is used to get a non-linear input/output mapping. A detailed methodology in the development of NN model for cardiovascular application is outlined below.

Case Study Overview: The Use of Artificial Neural Network for the Design and Optimization of Heart Valve

One of the most important applications of this area is prosthetic heart valves, which are commonly used to replace natural heart valves and are also widely used in ventricular assist devices (VAD) in total artificial hearts (TAH). The clinical success of any valve design is based on many factors including the fluid flow phenomena, particularly *in vitro* velocity profiles, shear stresses, regurgitation, and energy losses (Baldwin & Tarbell, 1991; Chandran & Cabell, 1983; Morsi et al., 2001). Thus, the optimization of the valve leaflet or wall-stress development patterns relates various parameters (Qiong et al., 2003). Moreover, if a prosthetic heart valve is to be used, the valve-related problems such as blood cell damage, thrombus formation, calcification, and infection, as well as valve durability, need consideration. In such areas, the fluid-phase is most conveniently described with respect to a Eulerian reference frame, while a Lagrangian formulation is more appropriate for the solid phase. These two formulations are not compatible, and, as a result, the numerical complexity increases manyfold.

Several numerical techniques, such as arbitrary Lagrangian Eulerian (ALE), fictitious domain/mortar element (FD//ME), and immersed boundary (IB), have been proposed recently. All these techniques solve the problem (fluid-structure) sequentially. The solution of fluid forces are obtained using conservation of law of mass and momentum equations and then the structural solution follows for each time step. In all the methods mentioned above, the deformation of the mesh poses a formidable computational task, particularly in the case of the complex geometric problems like cardiovascular application.

In the study of hemodynamics and, in particular, vascular disease, one of the most important variables is the shear stress, τ [N/m^2], at the vessel wall. Wall shear stress has considerable clinical relevance because it provides information about both the magnitude of the force that the blood exerts on the vessel wall as well as the force exerted by one fluid layer on another. Shear stress varies with flow conditions (cardiac output, heart rate, etc.) as well as with the local geometry of the vessel (curves, branches, etc.). Excessively high levels of shear stress caused, for example, by atherosclerotic lesions or artificial heart valves, may damage red blood cells (a condition called haemolysis) or the endothelium of the vessel wall. Other abnormal shear stresses, such as very low or strongly oscillatory shear stresses, may also change the biological behavior of some cells or platelets in the blood stream (leading to thrombus formation) or endothelial cells on the vessel wall. Thus, the rheology of the blood, along with the laws of conservation (basic physical laws), is important in the design and development of artificial devices.

A typical solution procedure of fully open valve is shown in Figure 5.

The mesh quality changes as the solution proceeds, as shown in Figure 6(a). Most of the time, the solution diverges due to the poor quality of mesh, and this is the case with cardiovascular problems where it needs a large deflection phenomenon. The flow dynamics are also very complex, shown in Figure 6(b), as the valve deflects from its original position.

A three dimensional mesh generation of complete tri-leaflet valve is shown in Figure 7 to give an idea of its numerical complexities (Morsi & Das, 2004). Nevertheless, few modeling approaches have been proposed using sequential weak coupling. The knowledge gained from the experimental findings also has increased our understanding in the same area.

At this point, it is impossible to carry out any numerical procedure to achieve an optimized design with the variable mentioned above. However, a neural network model can be thought of as an alternative method to deal with such optimization problems with existing numerical/experimental data. A solution can be achieved by building a model of the cardiovascular system of an individual and comparing it with the real time physiological measurements or with existing CFD simulation data. The aim is to exploit the benefits of NNs by developing an improved neural

Figure 5. Typical tri-leaflet configurations for closed and open valve

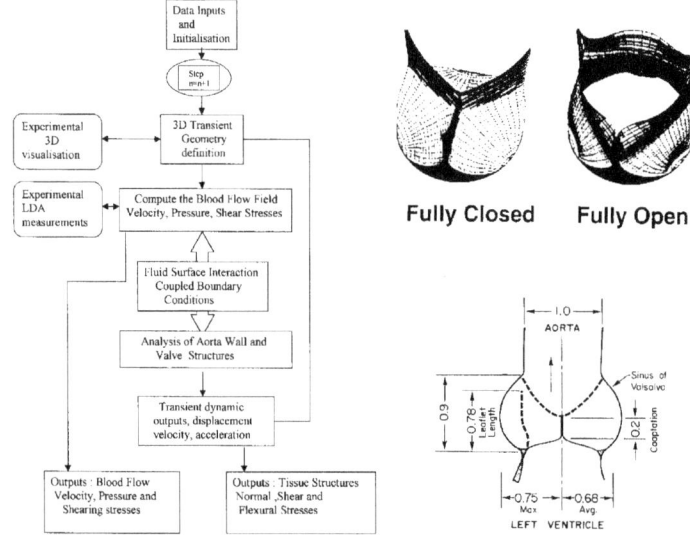

Figure 6. (a) Mesh deformation in 2D fluid-structure analysis; (b) streamline plot at peak flow condition

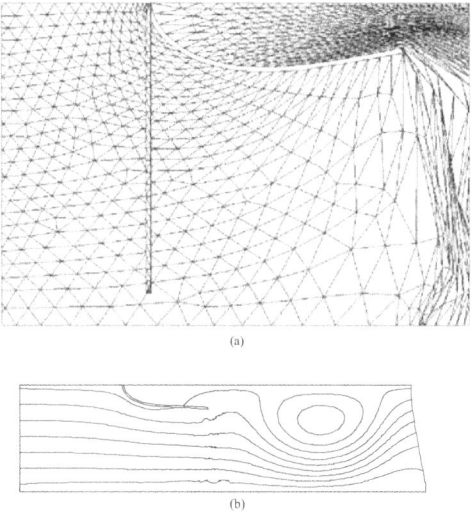

Figure 7. Computational domain for a typical fluid-structure analysis of tri-leaflet heart valve

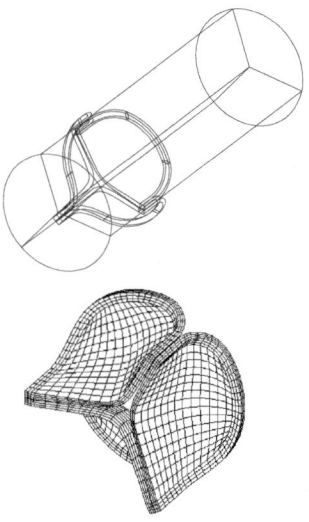

network methodology from the prior knowledge inputs for the qualitative and quantitative visualization of flow development on deformed structures.

The development of an NN model involves two basic steps. These include the generation of (or compilation of available) data required for training, the training of NN networks, and the evaluation and validation of the optimal configuration of the NN model. The procedure used for the development of the NN model is outlined below.

Step 1. Data from CFD/Experiments for Training of Artificial Neural Networks

PIV and LDA are powerful experimental techniques that enable full field velocity vectors of seeding particles suspended in a fluid to be visualized. It is effective for obtaining both qualitative and quantitative information of a flow. Particle tracking velocimetry (PTV) also uses the images of seeding particles for analysis and can give data for wide range of variables. Both these visualization data and CFD data from the numerical techniques can be used (PKI Method) to create an NN model to mimic the actual cardiovascular system for given boundary conditions.

The overall objective of the proposed NN model is to devise and evaluate an explicit procedure for estimating the heart valve leaflet deflection with time. An accurate training of a system of NN model may save computational time substantially for such a complex problem as the fluid-structure interaction of the leaflet of heart valve.

Step 2. Algorithm for Selection and Training of Neural Networks

It is necessary to design an NN model to represent the desired input-output mapping for which the following considerations should be taken into account.

- *Type of system output:* stochastic or deterministic;
- *Type of neural network connectivity:* feedforward, recurrent, or something else. This is a critical factor, especially when dealing with dynamical systems or with very large data quantities;
- *Layer transfer functions that depend on system behavior:* non-linear or linear;
- *Training routine:* gradient-based schemes or non-gradient-based schemes (Genetic Algorithms);
- *Scaling of input CFD data and output data:* both must be of constant order of magnitude.

A typical NN structure trained for modeling purposes is shown in Figure 8. A scaling unit is needed to carry the system parameters and responses into a range meaningful for NN structure considered. Once training is over, the weights and bias terms of trained NNs are saved, and NN model is used for design purposes. It has to be pointed out that even though the training phase is long, using NN model takes a very short time, as there are no complex calculations.

Neural network structure during training phase for model generating

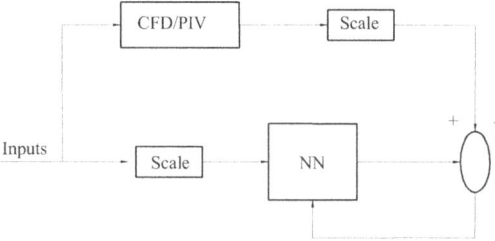

The feedforward network structure, as a possible NN model, is shown in Figure 9. There are several ways one can select the input data depending upon objective functions (Outputs). A dataset of fluid variables (u_f, v_f, P_f) and structure varibles (u_s and v_s) at all points, along with tube diameter (D), leaflet thickness (d), Reynolds number (Re), and so forth, can be used as input parameters to an NN model with deflection (δ) as an output variable. These points cover the entire domain of solution with Re varied in a large range. It is to be noted that training the NN model with a limited dataset may not capture all the information (modes non-linearities) of the physical phenomena. The input layer consisted of five neurons that corresponded to u_f, v_f, Re, D, and d, while the output layer had one neuron representing the leaflet deflection, δ. However, selecting input data in the case of a dynamic situation of fluid flow is a crucial factor because the flow changes from laminar to turbulent as time increases. Thus, enormous amounts of data are required to train an NN model with all the non-linearities that are associated with a fluid and structural member. However, the use of surface force, that is, instantaneous pressure force (as a polynomial) on the leaflet as input and the deflection as an output may reduce the number of data for a specific optimization. Neural networks are proven to be more sophisticated in analyzing non-linear functions operating on polynomial expansions.

Backpropagation algorithm is a well-known method (Haykin, 1999), as discussed above. It can be utilized for development and training. The building of a backpropagation network involved the specification of the number of hidden layers and the number of neurons in each hidden layer. Hidden layers, which can be more than one, are formed using neurons having continuously differentiable non-linear activation functions, while output neurons have linear activation functions. The number of neurons on the last layer is equal to the number of objective functions. However, in Figure 9, only one objective function is shown. All the neurons are connected to the neurons of the previous and next layers. In addition, several parameters including the learning rule, the transfer function, the learning coefficient ratio, the random number seed, the error minimization algorithm, and the number of learning cycles can be specified to improve the learning strategy. As the problem involves several non-linearities, that is, fluid flow and large material deformation, the accurate choice of these parameters is very difficult. However, a trial and error method can be used and for which several standard procedures are provided by any NNs software. Input data move ahead through the layers according to the connections, and, at the output layer, output of the NN is obtained. Thus, the major step is called training and consists in determining adequate values for these connection. The training is performed by minimizing the evaluation errors of the NN for the known points of the database entries. These outputs, y, are compared to desired values (base value), and weights are changed by means of backpropagation algorithm minimizing

Figure 9. A multilayer perceptron structure (MLP)

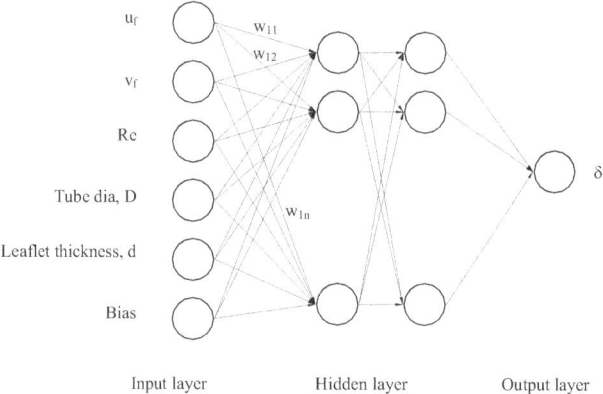

error functions depending on error, e, between desired and obtained outputs. This stage is crucial and often tedious, since this optimization exercise involves a large number of variables. It is usually performed through gradient-based methods and may suffer from local minimization, resulting in a weak training which provides a poor approximation. Moreover, the results may depend strongly on the number of layers and neurones, which is a real disadvantage for the present application, since the training should be performed automatically.

In general, as the number of hidden layers and the number of neurons within each hidden layer increased, the prediction capabilities of the network also increased. However, the number of connection weights increased significantly as the number of neurons and hidden layers increased, thereby increasing the chances of memorization of the behavior among the dataset (rather than generalization). Hence, the number of hidden layers and the neurons in the hidden layers need to be selected carefully.

The applications of NN models in fluid-structure problems may have to predominantly use the backpropagation network as it depends mostly on existing input and output data. Without the priory knowledge input (CFD data), NN model may be impossible to achieve. Thus, CFD still plays a major role in providing this information for NN models. However, developing the model through these data may save the computational or optimization time significantly.

Conclusion

In this chapter, development of an NN model with the existing CFD/experimental results is discussed particularly in the area where a multiphysics phenomena (fluid-structure) along with a complex geometry. Emphasis is given to the backpropagation technique with multilayer perceptron (MLP) because backpropagation techniques are the most suitable for training non-linear data structures. At this stage, the NN models are not widely used in CFD analyses because of the longer time involved in the training procedure with such a large non-linear data range. However, soon we will achieve a convenient mode of training procedure with evolutionary algorithms.

References

Baldwin, J. T., & Tarbell, J. M. (1991). Mean velocities and Reynolds stresses within regurgitant jets produced by tilting disc valves. *ASAIO Transactions, 37*, 348-349.

Brasquet, C., & Le Cloirec, P. (2000). Pressure drop through textile fabrics-experimental data modeling using classical models and neural networks. *Chemical Engineering Sciences, 55*, 2767-2778.

Cao, M., Wang, K. W., & DeVries, L. (2004). Steady state hydraulic valve fluid field estimator based on non-dimensional artificial neural network. *Journal of Computing and Information Science in Engineering, 4*, 257-270.

Cao, M., Wang, K. W., Fujii, Y., & Tobler, W.E. (2004). A hybrid neural network approach for the development of friction component dynamic model. A*SME Journal of Dynamic Systems, Management and Control, 126*(1), 144-153.

Chandran K. B., & Cabell, G. N. (1983). Laser anemometry measurements of pulsatile flow past aortic valve prostheses. *Journal of Biomechanics, 16*, 865-873.

Chao, L., Jun, X., & Liangjin, X. (2001). Knowledge-based artificial neural network models for Fin line. *International Journal of Infrared and Millimeter Waves, 22*, 2.

Das, S., & Morsi, Y. (2003). Natural convection in domed porous enclosures: Non-Darcian flow. *Journal of Porous Media, 6*(3), 159-175.

Diaz, G. (2000). *Simulation and control of heat exchangers using artificial neural networks.* PhD thesis, University of Notre Dame, Department of Aerospace and Mechanical Engineering.

Gillies, E. A. (1998). Low-dimensional control of the circular cylinder wake. *Journal of Fluid Mechanics, 371*, 157-178.

Han, S. Y., & Maeng, J. S. (2003). Shape optimization of cut-off in a multi-blade fan/scroll system using neural network. *International Journal of Heat and Mass Transfer, 46*, 2833-2839.

Haykin, S. (1999). *Neural networks: A comprehensive foundation.* New York: Macmillan.

Lee, C., Kim, J., Babcock, D., & Goodman, R. (1997). Application of neural networks to turbulence control for drag reduction. *Physics of Fluids, 9*(6), 1740-1747.

Lin, Q., Morsi, Y. S., Smith, B., & Yang, W. (2004). Numerical simulation and structure verifications of Jellyfish heart valve. *International Journal of Computer Applications in Technology, 21*(1-2), 2-7.

Morsi, Y. S., Zhou, Z., & Hassan, A. (2001). A three dimensional computational investigation of turbulent flow through aortic valve. *Frontiers of Medical and Biomedical Engineering, 11*(1), 1-11.

Parlos, A. G., Atiya, A. F., Chong, K. T., & Tsai, W. K. (1992). Nonlinear identification of process dynamics using neural networks. *Nuclear Technology, 97*(1), 79-96.

Porru, G., Aragonese, C., Baratti, R., & Servida, A. (2000). Monitoring of a CO oxidation reactor through a grey model-based EKF observer. *Chemical Engineering Sciences, 55*, 331-338.

Qiong, L., Morsi, Y.S., Benjamin, S., & William, Y. (2003). Numerical simulation and structure verification of jellyfish heart valve. *International Journal of Computer Applications in Technology, 20*, 1-6.

Sablani, S. S. (2001). A neural network approach for non-iterative calculation of heat transfer coeMcient in fluid-particle systems. *Chemical Engineering and Processing, 40*, 363-369.

Sablani, S. S., Shayya, W. H., & Kacimov, A. (2003). Explicit calculation of the friction factor in pipeline flow of Bingham plastic fluids: A neural network approach. *Chemical Engineering Science, 58*, 99-106.

Schreck, S. J., & Helin, H. E. (1994). Unsteady vortex dynamics and surface pressure topologies on a finite pitching wing. *Journal of Aircraft, 31*(4), 899-907.

Shayya, W. H., & Sablani, S. S. (1998). An artificial neural network for non-iterative calculation of the friction factor in pipeline flow. *Computers and Electronics in Agriculture, 21*(3), 219-228.

Watson, P. M., Gupta, K. C., & Mahajan, R. L. (1999). Applications of knowledge-based artificial neural network modeling to microwave components. *International Journal of RF and Microwave CAE, 9,* 254-260.

Xu, P., Burton, R. T., & Sargent, C. M. (1996). Experimental identification of a flow orifice using a neural network and the conjugate gradient method. *ASME Journal of Dynamic Systems, Measurements and Control, 118*(2), 272-277.

Xue, Y., & Watton, J. (1998). Dynamics modeling of fluid power systems applying a global error descent algorithm to a self-organizing radial basis function network. *Mechatronics, 8*(7), 727-745.

Yuen, P. K., & Bau, H. H. (1998). Controlling chaotic convection using neural nets-theory and experiments. *Neural Networks, 11*(3), 557-569.

Chapter XIII

Analysis of Temporal Patterns of Physiological Parameters

Balázs Benyó, Széchenyi István University, Hungary and
Budapest University of Technology and Economics, Hungary

Abstract

This chapter deals with the analysis of spontaneous changes occurring in two physiological parameters: the cerebral blood flow and respiration. Oscillation of the cerebral blood flow is a common feature in several physiological or pathophysiological states and may significantly influence the metabolic state of the brain. Our goal was to characterize the temporal blood flow pattern before, during, and after the development of CBF oscillations. Investigation of this phenomenon may not only clarify the underlying regulatory mechanisms and their alterations under certain conditions but also lead to the development of novel clinical diagnostic tools for early identification of developing cerebrovascular dysfunction in pathophysiological states such as brain trauma or stroke. A disturbance in normal breathing may occur in several nervous and physical diseases. In the present study, we introduce a reliable online method which is able to recognize abnormal sections of respiration, that is, the most common breathing disorder, the sleep apnea syndrome, based on a single time signal, the nasal air flow. There are several common features of the above problems and signals under investigation that imply similar solutions. The chapter introduces the systematic way of selecting proper feature extraction method and optimal classification procedure. The introduced approach can be generalized for the analysis of similar time series featuring physiological parameters.

Introduction

This chapter deals with the analysis of spontaneous changes occurring in two physiological parameters: the *cerebral blood flow* and *respiration*. Oscillation of the cerebral blood flow (CBF) is a common feature in several physiological or pathophysiological states and may significantly influence the metabolic state of the brain. These low-frequency oscillations may be influenced by pharmacological interventions (inhibition of the nitric oxide synthesis) and by pathologic conditions (ischemia, large, and small artery disease). Our goal was to characterize the temporal blood flow pattern before, during, and after the development of CBF oscillations. The physiological parameter in this case was measured by laser-Doppler flowmetry recording the movement of red blood cells in the brain tissue. Investigation of this phenomenon may not only clarify the underlying regulatory mechanisms but also lead to the development of novel clinical diagnostic tools for early identification of developing cerebrovascular dysfunction in pathophysiological states such as brain trauma or stroke.

A disturbance in normal breathing may occur in several nervous and physical diseases. The most common breathing disorder is the sleep apnea syndrome (SAS). By definition, an episode of apnea occurs if someone's breathing ceases for a certain period of time. A commonly used and reliable diagnostic method for the detection of apnea is the polysomnographic (PSG) assay which is a multichannel signal record measured during the whole sleeping process. The standard diagnostic nocturnal PSG consists of 9 to 12 physiological parameters. Even the limited-channel version of PSG records—recorded by portable devices—contain 5 different physiological signals. The evaluation method for PSG records is frequently off-line. An online evaluation opportunity is more frequent in the case of portable devices. The typical specificity and sensitivity of apnea detection is 80%-90% and somewhat lower for hypnea (Clark et al., 1998). Most of the methods work on a multisignal basis and process several signals simultaneously.

In the present study, we address the development of a reliable online method that is able to recognize abnormal sections of respiration (i.e., apnea and hypnea events) based on a single time signal, the nasal air flow. This method could make the diagnosis of sleeping disorders easier and cheaper.

The common features of the CBF and respiratory signals are as follows:

- Flow signals are measured,
- The frequency of the phenomena under investigation is low (below 1 Hz),
- The methods found to be efficient in analyzing these signals are similar.

Beyond the similarities, the introduced cases present two typical classes of biomedical signal analysis problems:

- In the case of the respiration analysis, we are looking for local or temporary features of the signals existing for dozens of seconds and processing the signals online.
- In the case of CBF signal characterization, we are aiming at the detection of long-term features of the flow signal, characterizing the signals for a few minutes and carrying out the analysis off-line.

In the solution of the two problems above we could not use the methods found in literature. The most frequently analyzed signals in similar studies are the electrocardiogram (ECG), an electrical recording of the heart activity used in the investigation of heart disease, and the electroencephalogram (EEG), used to detect abnormalities in the electrical activity of the brain (Li et al., 1995; Senhadji et al., 1995). The typical frequency of these signals is significantly higher (above 1 Hz) than the signals in our study (typically less than 1 Hz); therefore, the methods used for the analysis of EEG and ECG signals cannot be applied directly in our case.

In the initial part of this chapter, we will introduce both of the physiological phenomena under investigation. The subsequent section deals with the questions of selecting a proper feature extraction method and an optimal classification procedure. Afterwards, the results will be presented. The discussion of the results and the summary conclude the chapter.

Physiological Phenomenon under Investigation

Analysis of two physiological phenomena are addressed in this chapter:

- Characterization of cerebral blood flow signals and
- Detection of sleeping abnormalities (apnea) based on the respiration signals.

From the engineering point of view, we were faced with the following difficulties in both cases:

- No analytical model verified by physiologists describing the physiological phenomenon.
- A limited number of experiments, and/or the experiments were disturbed by other symptoms similar to the phenomenon under investigation.

Cerebral Blood Flow Characterization

Low-frequency oscillations of the cerebral hemodynamics and metabolism have been documented in several physiological or pathophysiological states (Intaglietta, 1990; Mayhew et al., 1996; Obrig et al., 2000). Although their origin is controversial, they share some common features. First, they are characterized by their spontaneity (i.e., they occur without any overt stimulus). Second, they can be differentiated from other oscillatory phenomena such as high-frequency oscillations (e.g., the heartbeat or respiratory cycles) because of their slowness. Third, they are influenced by pharmacologic conditions (inhibition of nitric oxide synthesis) and pathologic conditions (ischemia, large and small artery disease), as well as by hypercapnia, and by functional stimulation (for reviews see Obrig et al., 2000). Particularly, spontaneous low-frequency oscillations (LFOs) occurring at approximately 0.1 Hz might be distinguished from spontaneous very-low-frequency oscillations (VLFOs) centered at approximately 0.04 Hz. These spontaneous oscillations were observed with functional near-infrared spectroscopy, laser-Doppler-flowmetry, transcranial Doppler-sonography, and functional magnetic resonance imaging. Hudetz et al. (1998) suggested that spontaneous oscillations in cerebral hemodynamics may represent autoregulatory processes of cerebral blood flow (CBF) and that they might be of myogenic origin. This concept is supported by observations in cerebral arteries showing spontaneous tension changes (vasomotion) in vitro.

In many experimental contexts, vasomotion is problematic since it is frequently unpredictable and difficult to reproduce. Inhibition of nitric oxide (NO) synthesis reportedly evokes CBF oscillations, although the mechanism of this action has not been clarified yet. In isolated rat middle-cerebral arteries, it has been recently demonstrated that the induction of vasomotion after a blockade of the NO synthesis is mediated mainly by the thromboxane-pathway (Lacza et al., 2001). In a subsequent in-vivo study, the vulnerability of the cerebral circulation to thromboxane-induced CBF-oscillations has been reported in the absence of NO (Lenzsér et al., 2003). Therefore, simultaneous NO synthase blockade and stimulation of thromboxane receptors is an effective method for the induction of cerebral vasomotion both in-vitro and in-vivo.

The aim of the present study was to characterize the temporal pattern of this vasomotion. Investigation of this phenomenon may not only clarify the underlying cellular mechanism but also lead to the development of novel clinical diagnostic tools for early identification of developing cerebrovascular dysfunction in pathophysiological states such as brain trauma or stroke.

Experimental Method

The experiments in this study were carried out on anesthetized (urethan, 1.3 g/kg ip.), spontaneously breathing adult male Wistar rats. The heads of the animals were fixed in a stereotaxic head holder, and the skull was thinned over the parietal cortex on both sides where two laser Doppler (LD) probes were placed in predefined positions as described previously by Lacza et al. (2000). A 5-min segment of the LD flux (LDF) recording was evaluated before the administration of the NO synthase (NOS) inhibitor N^G-nitro-L-arginine methyl ester (L-NAME, 100 mg/kg iv.). After 75 minutes, the thromboxane receptor-agonist U-46619 was applied intravenously in a dose of 1 µg/kg. The pattern of the LDF recording was evaluated before and 25 minutes after the administration of U-46619. The time signal generated by the LD probes was sampled at 200 Hz (see Figure 1).

Medical experts have defined three classes of CBF signals based on their qualitative features (Benyó et al., 2004a; Lenzsér et al., 2003):

- *Class A*: Normal blood flow signals before applying any drugs, without any oscillation.
- *Class B*: Blood flow signals after the administration of L-NAME, before the administration of U-46619. Oscillation can be seen in these signals.

Figure 1. Typical CBF signal

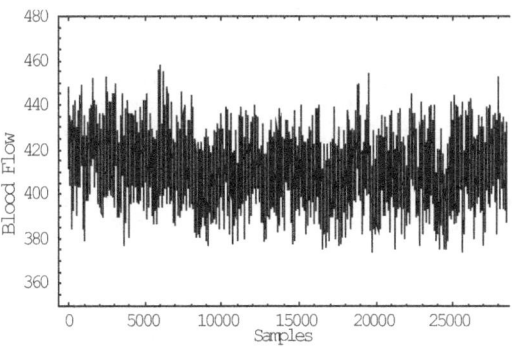

Figure 2. Different sections of the CBF signal; Class A: *no drugs;* Class B: *after the administration of L-NAME;* Class C: *after the administration of U-46619*

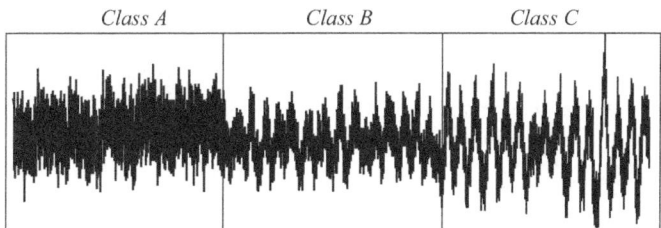

- *Class C*: Blood flow signals after the administration of U-46619. Strong oscillation can be seen in these signals.

Typical sections of the signal belonging to the above three classes are shown in Figure 2. In this study, we addressed the development of a method to distinguish these three classes of CBF signals.

Detection of Apnea

The apnea syndrome occurs if the patient breathing stops for a certain period of time, if the magnitude of the respiration movements decrease for at least ten seconds to less than 5% of the physiological values (Köves, 1996; Saunders & Sullivan, 1994). In medical literature, the mild version of apnea is called *hypnea*, where the movements decrease below half of the normal values. The occurrence of sleep apnea episodes might be physiological. They would usually be regarded as pathological only if more than five episodes of apnea occur per sleeping hour (Köves, 1996; Kryger et al., 2000). The origin of apnea can be *central*, caused by the lack of central moto-neural respiration drive, or can be *obstructive*, caused by the occlusion of the upper airways (Guilleminault & Partinen, 1990).

A commonly used and reliable diagnostic method for the detection of apnea is the polysomnographic (PSG) assay which is a multichannel signal record measured during the whole sleeping process. The standard diagnostic nocturnal PSG consists of the following vital parameters (Standards of Practice Committee, 1997): electroencephalogram (EEG), electrooculogram (EOG), electromyogram (EMG), nasal airflow (NAF), abdominal and/or thoracic movements, body position, snore microphone, electrocardiogram (ECG), and blood oxygen saturation (SO_2). A limited-channel version of PSG is also frequently used for apnea screening, especially in portable devices, including only the following signal channels: NAF, abdominal and/or thoracic movements, SO_2, heart rate (HR), and systolic blood pressure (SBP) (Ferber et al., 1994). An example for the signals used for apnea detection can be seen in Figure 3.

Figure 3. Breathing signals used for apnea detection: nasal airflow (NAF), abdominal and/or thoracic movements (REP), blood oxygen saturation (SO_2), heart rate (HR), systole blood pressure (SBP) (Várady, 2002)

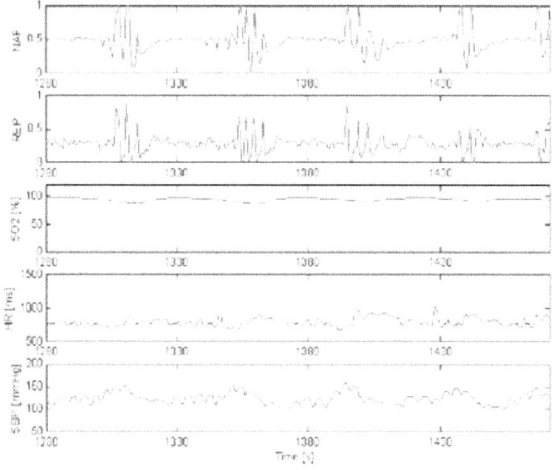

The diagnosis procedure for apnea includes several methods: the detection of apnea and hypnea events, the determination of their origin (central/obstructive), and the calculation of the respiration disorder index (RDI), that is, the number of apnea and hypnea events per sleeping hour (Köves, 1996).

The evaluation method for PSG records is frequently off-line and done in the time domain. Generally, the vendor of the recording device provides an evaluation package. An online evaluation opportunity is more frequent in the case of portable devices. The typical specificity and sensitivity of apnea detection is 80%-90% and somewhat lower for hypnea (Clark et al., 1998). Most of the methods work on a multisignal basis and process several signals simultaneously.

In the present study, we address the development of a reliable online method able to recognize apnea and hypnea events based on a single time signal, the nasal air flow. We were not aiming at the determination of the origin of the apnea, that is, whether it is central or obstructive.

Respiration Records

In our apnea detection experiments, we used the breathing records of the MIT-BIH PSG database (Goldberger et al., 2000; Moody, n.d.). The actually used dataset contains 18 PSG records having lengths from 1 hour up to 7 hours (4 hours on average). We selected 16 records out of the 18 from 16 different patients. The selected records contain other physiological signals besides the NAF signal; however, these signals were used only for testing the efficiency of our method and calculating the selectivity and sensitivity of the method.

Feature Extraction

The most important problem in the case of the analysis of time sequences is the reduction in the number of dimensions of the signals. The time signals under investigation generally contain some thousand samples in the time domain; however, the most sophisticated classification methods can efficiently process only dozens of inputs. This makes it necessary to extract the important features from the signals and process this derived information by classification methods. This information compression is generally possible since the time series signals are redundant in the sense that the consecutive values of the time series are not independent but highly correlated (Rangayyan, 2002).

The method of this information compression or dimension reduction is called, in general, feature extraction (FE). Accordingly, the data vector, the result of the FE, is called a feature vector (FV).

There are many application domain-specific FE methods (Baura, 2002); however, the most popular scheme in the FE methods consists of two steps: (1) transform the time signal to the frequency domain and (2) discard the non-important coefficients.

Signal Transforms

It is well known that a periodic signal may be written as a series expansion of sinusoids (or equivalently complex exponentials). More generally, a signal $f(t)$ may be expressed as the superposition:

$$f(t) = \sum_k a_k \Psi_k(t)$$

where k is an integer index of the finite or infinite summation, a_k are the real or complex valued expansion coefficients, and $\Psi_k(t)$ are members of a set of real or complex functions called expansion functions. If the expansion is unique, the set is called a basis for the class of signals under investigation. The set members $\Psi_k(t)$ are known as the basis functions of the series of expansion. It is desirable to have an orthogonal basis, which means that

$$\int \Psi_k(t)\Psi_l^*(t)dt = \begin{cases} 0, k \neq l \\ 1, k = l \end{cases}.$$

Discrete Fourier Transform

The discrete-time Fourier transform (DTFT) of a discrete time signal is a representation of the signal in terms of complex exponential signal $e^{-j\omega n}$, where ω is a real frequency variable. The one dimensional DTFT is defined by the following equations:

$$X(\omega) = \sum_{n=-\infty}^{\infty} x[n]e^{-j\omega n}$$

Figure 4. The DTFT (the curve) and the corresponding DFT (dots)

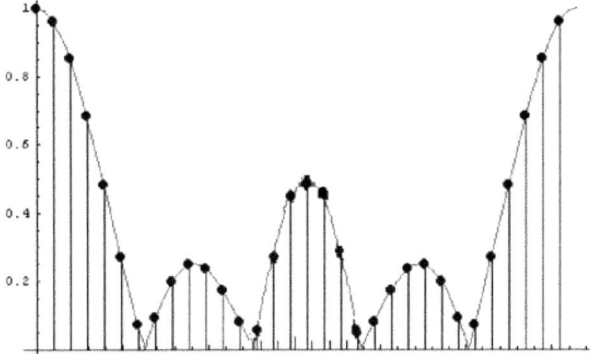

$$x(n) = \frac{1}{2\pi} \int_{-\pi}^{\pi} X(\omega)e^{-j\omega n} d\omega$$

where n is an integer time variable and ω is the real radial frequency.

The discrete Fourier transform (DFT) is a frequency domain representation of finite-extent sequences. The DFT is a decomposition of finite-extent sequence by a family of complex exponential sequences. The DFT of a discrete-time sequence of length N is itself a sequence of length N. The values of DFT are evenly spaced samples of the DTFT. Given a finite-length sequence x[n] (i.e., x[n]=0 for n≠0, 1, ..., N-1) we get

$$X[k] = X(\omega), \varpi = \frac{2\pi}{N} k$$

where X[k] is the N-point DFT and X(ω) is the DTFT of x[n], see Figure 4.

Wavelet Transform

The wavelet-based analysis is similar to the Fourier analysis where sinusoids are chosen as the basis function. The wavelet analysis is also based on a decomposition of a signal using an orthogonal family of basis functions. Because of the used basis function, the wavelets are well suited for the analysis of transient, time-varying signals. The wavelet expansion is defined by a two-parameter family of functions:

$$f(t) = \sum_k \sum a_{j,k} \Psi_{j,k}(t)$$

where j and k are integers, the $\Psi_{j,k}(t)$ are the wavelet expansion functions. The wavelet expansion (or basis) functions based on the mother wavelet of the formula

$$\Psi_{j,k}(t) = 2^{j/2} \Psi(2^j t - k)$$

where j is the translation parameter and k is the dilation parameter.

The expansion coefficients $a_{j,k}$ are called the discrete wavelet transform (DWT) coefficients of $f(t)$. The coefficients are given by the following equation

$$a_{j,k} = \int f(t) \Psi_{j,k}(t) dt .$$

The DFT and the DWT are the two most commonly used techniques for the signal transformation to the frequency domain. More details of the transforms can be found in Li et al. (1995) and Senhadji et al. (1995).

Feature Vector Definition

The selection of the coefficients representing the signals in the FV is highly problem specific. Alternative techniques (Mörchen, 2003) are:

- Selection of the first few coefficients. Generally, these are the most relevant coefficients.
- Selection of the largest coefficients representing the highest energy components of the signal.

In the second case, the selected coefficients are generally supplemented in the FV with the corresponding frequency value.

If the application does not allow any of the coefficients to be neglected, an alternative option is to compact the coefficients by dividing the frequency domain into sections and calculating the average of the subsequent coefficients in these segments (Goswami & Chan, 1999).

The FE is a very sensitive step in the time series analysis. No general rules can be formed for the selection of the optimal FE technique (Berthold & Hand, 2003). All of them have advantages and disadvantages, and so each have their own optimal field of application.

FE for Cerebral Blood Flow Characterization

Fourier Transform

The CBF signal classes are shown in Figure 2. The Fourier Spectra of the signals from these classes are shown in Figure 5. The oscillation of the *Class B* and *Class C* signals can be easily recognized. The Fourier Spectra of these signals,

Figure 5. Discrete Fourier Spectra of CBF signals; Class A*: no drugs;* Class B*: after the administration of L-NAME;* Class C*: after the administration of U-46619*

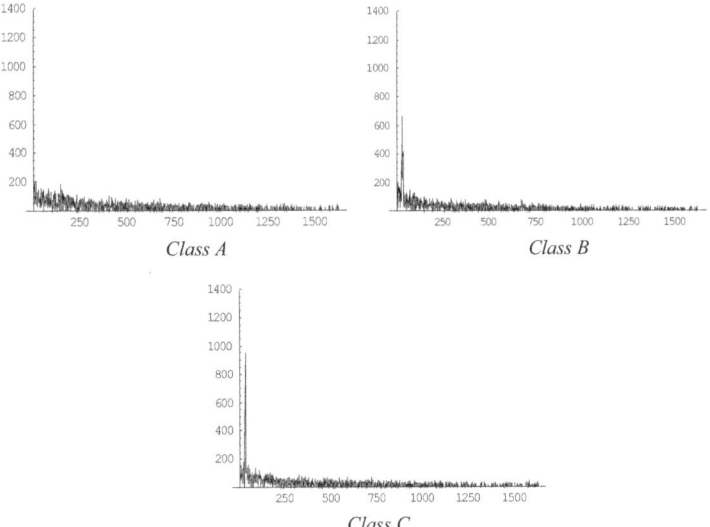

Class A   Class B

Class C

Figure 6. Normalized feature space of CBF signals in the case of DFT based FE: Class A *(triangle): normal blood flow;* Class B *(box): before administration of U-46619;* Class C *(star): after administration of U-46619*

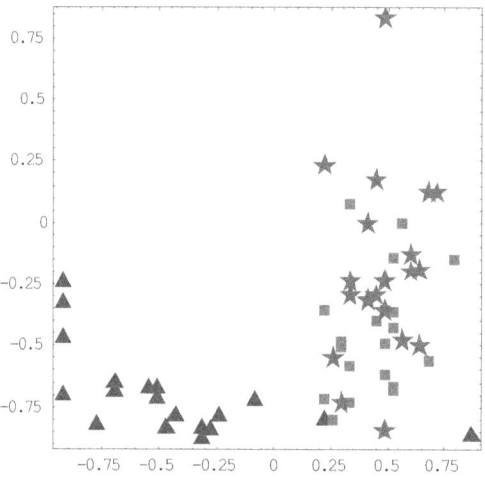

in most cases, contain a "tiny" spike, probably responsible for the observable oscillation of the time signal (Figure 2). The difficulty in recognition is caused by the fact that the frequency and the amplitude (or the signal/noise proportion) of the spike varies from case to case. Otherwise, it would be easy to identify the signal via traditional signal processing methods, that is, with a low-pass filter.

Based on these obtrusive features in the signals, a very simple feature vector can be constructed: the largest coefficient of the Discrete Fourier Spectrum and the corresponding frequency, as suggested by Lenzsér et al. (2003).

The FVs can be visualized on the so-called feature space (FS). In this case, the FS is a two-dimensional vector with elements of the spike position in frequency and the amplitude of the spike. The points on the two-dimensional plane represent the FVs belonging to the experiments. The elements of the vector are normalized to the interval {-1;1}. The FS is shown in Figure 6. Triangles represent the normal blood flow signals (*Class A*), boxes represent the signals after the administration of L-NAME (*Class B*), and stars represent the signals after the administration of U-46619 (*Class C*).

In the preliminary works (Benyó et al., 2004a; Lenzsér et al., 2003) several, much more sophisticated FE methods and FVs are tested, as suggested by authors of similar studies:

- Different numbers of the largest DFT coefficients and their frequencies and
- The average of the subsequent coefficients in different frequency ranges.

These experiments showed that the most adequate DFT-based FE method is the most simple one, defined in Lenzsér et al. (2003). The misclassification rate was much higher in all other cases.

Wavelet Transform

In order to confirm the result of the classification using the DFT-based FE, we were looking for a more general FE method. According to the literature (Goswami & Chan, 1999; Szilagyi et al., 1997), the Discrete Wavelet Spectra reflect the signal features better if the features are "local" in the frequency domain; that is, the differences between two signals are limited to a certain range of the frequency. In the second phase of our studies, we used the DWT-based FE method.

Employing Daubechies filter of second order for the 2^n samples of the time signal, DWT decomposes the signal into n resolution levels, into one approximation subband and $n-1$ wavelet subbands. In our case $n = 16$, see the phase space plot (PSP) of DWT of the time signal on Figure 7.

Figure 7. Phase space plot of the DWT of the CBF signal (n = 16)

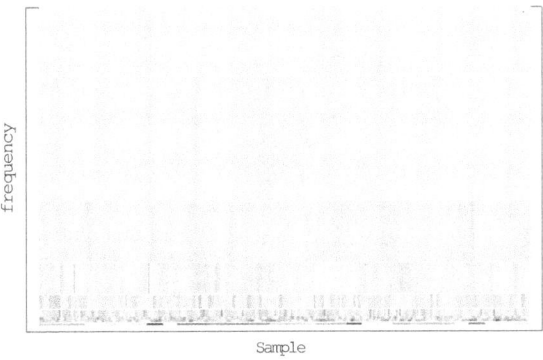

Figure 8. The phase space plot of the DWT of the time signal (n = 8)

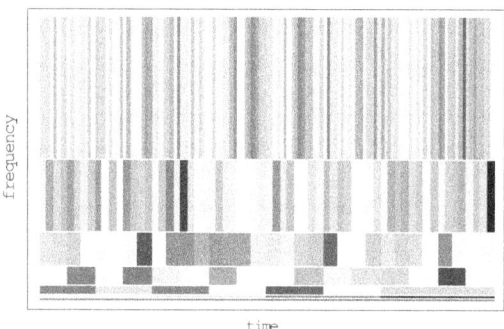

In the PSP, each rectangle represents a wavelet coefficient (vertical direction) and the darker a rectangle, the larger the absolute value of the corresponding wavelet coefficient. The residual trend is plotted in the bottom row, and the finest detail in the top row.

The PSP in the case of $n = 8$ is also shown in the Figure 8 in order to better show the structure of the PSP.

It can be seen in the PSP (Figure 7, n = 16) that the upper part of the figure is lighter than the bottom part, which means that the higher order coefficients are significantly smaller than the first few ones. It follows from this that the average energy content of the coefficients at higher resolution is very low; therefore, these coefficients can be neglected.

In this case, the average coefficients of the two lowest subbands were considered as the feature vector. The DWT-based feature vector can be visualized on a two-dimensional plane, on an FS as seen in Figure 9. In Figure 9, the class A signals (triangles) can be easily separated from the other signals. This suggests that the DWT-based feature vector will have strong discriminatory ability between the Class A signals and the other signals. However, the points representing the Classes B and C (stars and boxes) are overlapping so much that the discriminatory ability of this FV between these two classes is very low. We also note that the points representing the feature vectors are placed very close to the diagonal line which means that the ratio of the two components of the FV— that is, the two largest coefficients of the DWT—is very similar in each experiment. The physiological interpretation of this phenomena has not yet been clarified.

Figure 9. Normalized feature space of CBF signals in the case of DWT-based FE: Class A *(triangle): normal blood flow;* Class B *(box): before administration of U-46619;* Class C *(star): after administration of U-46619*

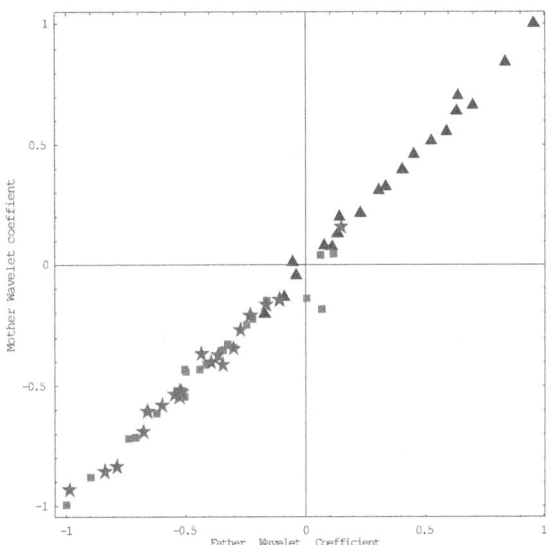

FE for Apnea Detection

FE in Time Domain

An obvious idea when recognizing apnea events is to transform the signals to the frequency domain. The episode of apnea lasts for 10-40 seconds which poses the question: which portion of the time signal should be transformed? If we use too short portions (e.g., less than 10 sec), we will increase the computational complexity (computation time) and decrease the specificity of the spectra. If we transform longer portions of the time signal (e.g., more than 10 sec), then the method will ignore any short apnea events. This is the main reason why the apnea detection algorithms in the frequency domain have moderate success (Várady, 2002).

The other option for the FE is to use the segments of the time signal directly. The main problem is that the normal breathing of patients varies greatly over time. It highly depends on the physiological and mental state of the patient. This results in high instability of recognition using the time signals directly.

The solution is preprocessing the time signals and using the segments of these derived signal as FV. The FE suggested by Várady (2002) copies the human recognition strategy. Two signals are extracted from the normalized respiration (nasal air flow) signal: an instantaneous respiration amplitude (IRA) and an instantaneous respiration interval (IRI).

The IRA signal will be correlated with the amplitude of the corresponding respiration signal. It will change if the amplitude of the respiration changes rapidly. The IRI signal will be correlated with the time distance between two breaths and will change if the rhythm of the breathing changes. Both the IRA and IRI signals were normalized and spanned over the continuous time (see Figure 10).

The exact algorithm of the generation of IRI and IRA signals has been described (Várady & Bongár, 2001). Both derived signals have a limited "memory", which helps to emphasize the apnea events.

Classification Methods
via ANN and the Results

There are two important factors influencing the efficiency of the classification: characterization of the elements to classify (i.e., feature extraction) and the classification model to apply.

Figure 10. Nasal air flow (at the top) and the derived IRI and IRA signals in the case of episodes of apnea (at the left side) and in the case of normal sleeping (at the right side)

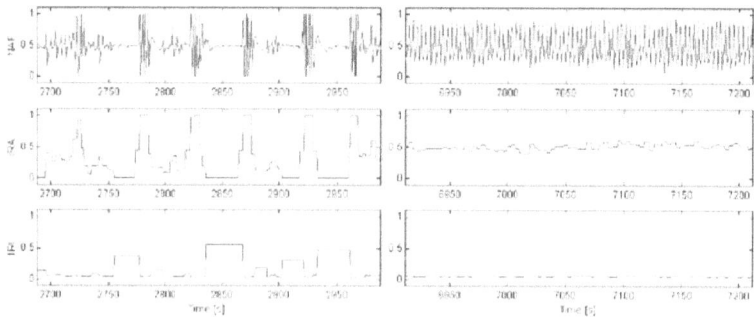

The application field of the most simple linear classification models is very much limited; they can be applied only if the elements to classify are linearly separable. In any other case, we have to use a non-linear classification model.

The selection of the proper classification model is particularly difficult if we do not know the theoretical description (i.e., the theoretical model) of the physical phenomenon under investigation. The physiological processes frequently belonging to this category of problems, the biological systems, are very complex systems, and their complexity significantly exceeds the complexity of technical ones. In these cases, we necessarily use a general classification model with an adaptive learning phase that provides the opportunity of selecting the optimal classification model which is appropriate to our problem. The ANNs are one of these general classification models whose universal approximation feature has been theoretically proven. This was the main reason of applying ANNs in the case of our physiological signal classification problems.

There is a number of general classification methods (Duda et al., 2001) offering the opportunity to divide datasets into distinguished classes. Typical situations, worth considering the use of artificial neural networks (ANN), are if the system under investigation is non-linear or stochastic and the signals to be analyzed are noisy.

The above conditions are fulfilled in the cases of both problems introduced in this chapter, which was a further reason for the application of the ANNs.

The analysis process of the CBF signals is divided into three phases:

- In the first phase, a Kohonen neural network with unsupervised learning is used.
- In the second phase, a backpropagation neural network with supervised learning is used.
- In the third phase, a radial basis function (RBF) neural network with supervised learning is used.

The goal of the analysis in the different phases is shown in Table 1.

The Kohonen network was selected because it can be used with the unsupervised learning phase. This allows us to verify whether the selected FE is an appropriate characterization of the elements to classify. The backpropagation network and the RBF network had been successfully applied in the solution of many physiological signal analysis problems (Baura, 2002; Szilágyi & Benyó, 2003). This focused our attention to these networks during the selection of the proper general classification model.

Table 1. The three phases of CBF signal analysis

	Kohonen Network Unsupervised Learning	Backpropagation Network	RBF Network
FE method applied	1. DFT-based FE 2. DWT-based FE	1. DFT-based FE 2. DWT-based FE	DFT-based FE
Goal of the analysis	Basic classification and verification of the FE method.	Signal characterization and generation of an analytical form for classification.	More sophisticated signal characterization for easier interpretation of results.

In the case of the apnea detection problem, the FE verification phase was unnecessary since the clinical results showed that the abnormal and normal respiration signal segments (i.e., segments with the episode of apnea and without) can be separated. Thus, we were able to skip the first verification step. The requirement of the online detection of apnea made it necessary to use as simple a classification model as possible. The backpropagation network is one of the most simple ANN-based classifiers. Since the result of the classification was satisfactory using the backpropagation network, the results obtained by the RBF network are also omitted.

The experiments introduced in the chapter are summarized in Table 2.

Characterization of Cerebral Blood Flow Signals

Unsupervised Network

DFT-Based FE

The result of the classification using the Kohonen neural network is shown in Figure 11. The classes are separated by straight lines reflecting the linear nature of the Kohonen network. The circles in the middle of the ranges are the codebook vectors belonging to the given class.

Table 2. Experiments introduced in the chapter

	Kohonen Network Unsupervised Learning	Backpropagation Network	RBF Network
CBF Characterization	1. DFT-based FE 2. DWT-based FE	1. DFT-based FE 2. DWT-based FE	DFT-based FE
Apnea Detection	–	IRI and IRA based FE	–

Figure 11. Classes generated by Kohonen neural network using unsupervised learning. The circles are the codebook vectors belonging to the given class.

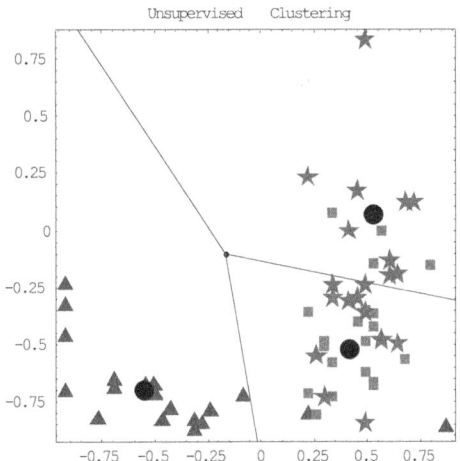

Table 3. Misclassification rate of Kohonen NN

	Class A (triangle)	Class B (square)	Class C (star)
Kohonen ANN	2/20 = 10%	4/20 = 20%	11/20 = 55%

This classification method could efficiently separate the signals of *Class A* from the signals of other two classes. Since the learning phase of the classification was unsupervised, this result validates the use of the selected feature extraction method.

This classification method could not differentiate between the *Class B* and *Class C* signals. Based on the number of misclassified signals (Table 3), these two classes seem to be overlapping in this classification scheme.

DFT-Wavelet-Based FE

In order to verify that the chosen feature vector is an acceptable representation of the time signal, unsupervised classification via neural network was carried out

Figure 12. Unsupervised classification of signals of right brain side

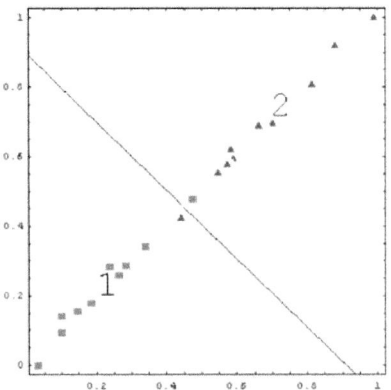

Figure 13. Unsupervised classification of signals of left brain side

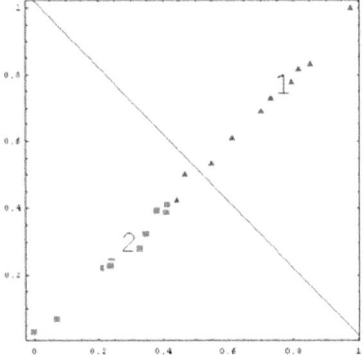

for the 20 signals resulting from the measurements of the right side of the brain, belonging to the two different classes (normal state and state affected by drug injection). Only two signals that were very close to the separation surface (see Figure 12) were misclassified. The same classification was carried out for the signals of the left side of the brain; see Figure 13.

Figure 14. Unsupervised classification of signals of right and left brain side

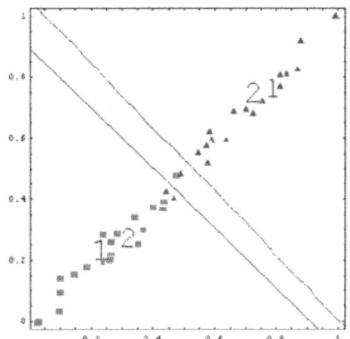

Here again, two signals—clearly seen in neighborhood of the separation surface—were misclassified. In addition, it turned out that signals from the right and left side of the brain do not differ from each other considerably; only a narrow band contains misclassified signals; see Figure 14.

These results show that the applied feature representation can be accepted, especially considering that these signals resulted from direct measurements of different experiments.

Backpropagation Network

DFT-Based FE

In the case of using backpropagation network, at first, we have to define the structure of the network: the number of output nodes, the number of hidden layers, and the number of nodes in the hidden layer. The number of input nodes generally equals the number of components of the FV. There are many theoretical and practical considerations that help us in this heuristic process of network structure definition:

- The number of teaching samples limits the number of nodes to use. If the number of nodes is not significantly less than the number of teaching samples, then it generally leads to uncertain classification.
- In order to increase the classification power of the network by hidden layers, the number of nodes in the hidden layer should include at least as

many nodes as the output layer does. Generally, it is nonsense to use more than two hidden layers.

- If we do not allow hierarchical (i.e., iterative) classification, then the number of classes to distinguish equals the number of output nodes.

In our case, we wanted to differentiate three classes of signals; therefore, we used three output nodes. Since the number of teaching samples was limited to 60, we decided to use only one hidden layer with different number of nodes. Networks with 6 and 12 nodes in the hidden layer and 3 nodes in the output layer for the three classes—{1,0,0}, {0,1,0}, and {0,0,1}, respectively—have been applied; see Figures 15 and 16.

Figure 15. The result of the classification with six nodes in the hidden layer

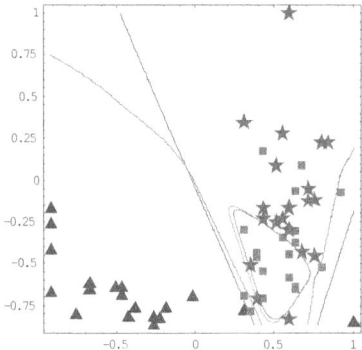

Figure 16. The result of the classification with 12 nodes in the hidden layer

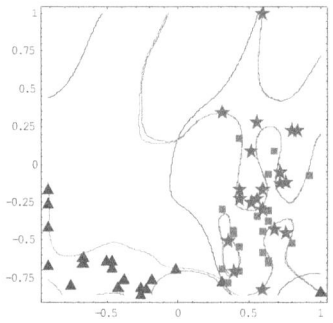

These figures indicate clearly that the backpropagation network was not able to separate the strongly overlapping *Class B* and *Class C* when there were only six nodes in the hidden layer. Increasing the number of nodes in the hidden layer makes the misclassification rate significantly lower. However, in this case, the borders of the classification fields (indicated by curves in Figures 15 and 16) will be very close to the points representing the signals on the FS. This means that the classification is not robust. Any kind of noise that moves the points on the FS just slightly will result in misclassification. Thus, the backpropagation network-based classification with more than six nodes in the hidden layer is unusable in the practice.

DWT-Based FE

In order to develop a model for classifying the CBF signals using DWT-based FE, we employed a supervised backpropagation neural network with sigmoid activation functions. As indicated above, this FE was insufficient to distinguish between Class B and Class C signals. Therefore, we used this classification model to separate Class A and Class B signals. Because of this, considering the rules listed in the above section, the network has two input and two output nodes. We wanted to define the structure of the network as simply as possible; thus, we used only one hidden layer with two additional nodes. The teaching set consists of 75% of the total number of signals (30 signals), and the rest served for testing (10 signals).

The network learned the teaching set; however, one inconsistent signal was recovered; see Figure 17.

Figure 17. Supervised classification with a backpropagation network with two hidden nodes

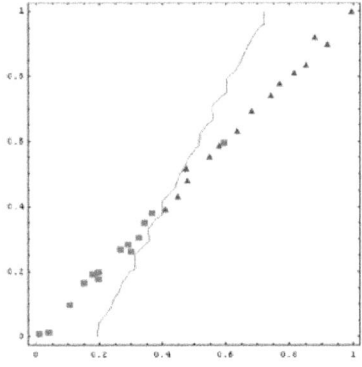

Figure 18. Supervised classification with a backpropagation network with three hidden nodes

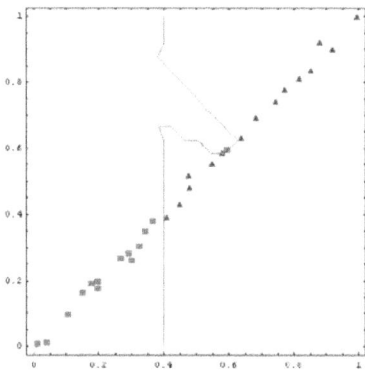

More than two hidden nodes resulted in overlearning; see Figure 18. This figure shows that the neural network also tried to learn the outlier signal.

Our ANN model for signal classification can be expressed in analytical form, thanks to the symbolic algebra built in the *Mathematica* kernel:

$$\left\{ -272.322 + \frac{272.422}{1 + e^{-33.9811 - 176.416\,w1 - 97.6414\,w2}} + \right.$$
$$\frac{273.155}{1 + e^{34.0373 - 176.736\,w1 + 97.8106\,w2}},$$
$$273.322 - \frac{272.422}{1 + e^{-33.9811 + 176.416\,w1 - 97.6414\,w2}} -$$
$$\left. \frac{273.155}{1 + e^{34.0373 - 176.736\,w1 - 97.8106\,w2}} \right\}$$

where *w1* and *w2* are the wavelet coefficients of the approximation subband of the DWT of the time signal. This function, after rounding, gives {1, 0} and {0, 1} as output for the two classes, respectively.

Employing this model, only 2 signals were misclassified from the 10 elements of the testing set that were not involved in the teaching process.

Figure 19. Result of radial basis function neural network classification. The learning phase was supervised.

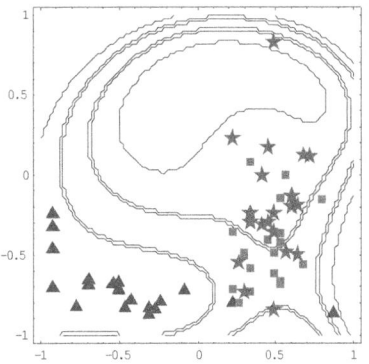

RBF Network

DFT-Based FE

The result of Radial Basis Function neural network-based classification is shown in Figure 19. This method gave significantly better results in classification of the signals after the administration of L-NAME; that is, the separation of signals in *Class B* and *Class C* were significantly better. This is the benefit of the non-linear nature of the RBF neural networks.

The number of misclassified signals is significantly less than in the case of using the backpropagation ANN; however, the classification is not perfect.

Apnea Detection

Backpropagation Network

The FV used for apnea detection contains 50 values: 25 from the corresponding IRA signal and 25 from the corresponding IRI signal. Therefore, the ANN used for classification had 50 input nodes. There were two hidden layers with 10 and 4 nodes, and 2 output nodes. In the hidden and the output nodes, we used sigmoid-like activation functions. The network is implemented by *Mathematica 5*.

For the training, we selected 380 vectors from nine different patients. There were 120 apnea, 120 hypnea, and 140 normal patterns. We used binary output

Figure 20. Histogram of the classification error

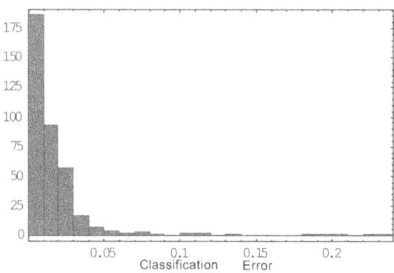

on the network. The first output node distinguished the apnea and normal signal parts; the second output distinguished the hypnea and apnea patterns.

The teaching was extremely fast. We considered the output of the network as a two-dimensional vector and calculated the error as a distance of the vectors. The histogram in Figure 20 shows that the error (distance between the actual output and the required value) was very small (< 0.05) in most cases.

The result of the classification can be seen in Figure 21. The apnea and hypnea segments are clearly recognized.

The statistical evaluation of the apnea detection method using IRI-like and IRA-like FE and similar ANN has been described by Várady (2002). The specificity of the recognition of apnea, hypnea, and normal sleeping is 88%-94%. The sensitivity of the recognition of normal and apnea events was 97%-98%, and it was 78% in the case of hypnea.

Discussion and Conclusion

Characterization of CBF Signals

In this study, three CBF signal classification methods are introduced. All three methods gave an opportunity for the systematic classification of the given time signals. The misclassification rate steadily decreased when using more advanced and more sophisticated classification algorithms.

The DFT-based FV allowed us to separate the defined classes of signals. The number of misclassified cases is shown in Table 4. It can be clearly seen that the

Figure 21. The result of event recognition. The record contains episodes of apnea (network output = 2), hypnea (network output = 1), and normal sleeping phases (network output = 0).

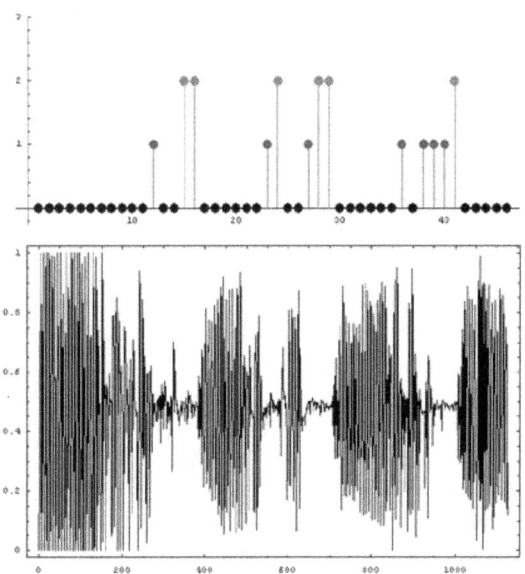

Table 4. Misclassification rate using DFT-based FV

	Class A (triangle)	Class B (square)	Class C (star)
Kohonen ANN	2/20 = 10%	4/20 = 20%	11/20 = 55%
Backpropagation ANN	1/20 = 5%	3/20 = 15%	9/20 = 45%
RBF ANN	1/20 = 5%	6/20 = 30%	4/20 = 20%

Class A signals could be efficiently separated from the signals of the other two classes with all three classification methods. This means that the separation of *Class A* signals from the other signals is much easier based on the selected FE method. On the other hand, the separation of the heavily overlapping classes (*Class B* and *Class C* signals) was much worse.

The efficiency of the Kohonen ANN-based classification was relatively low, especially regarding the *Class B* and *C* signals. However, the robustness of the method could be advantageous in the case of noisy signals. The Kohonen ANN classification shows a relatively high tolerance toward signal uncertainty.

The successful classification by Kohonen network with unsupervised learning phase validated the use of our FE method. This validation is always important if we do not have detailed model of the physical phenomenon under investigation and we develop a sophisticated FE whose physical interpretation is difficult or impossible.

The results of the RBF network-based classification seem easy to interpret, since the class domains are continuous. Based on these experiments, the RBF ANN-based classification proved to be the best candidate to apply in practice. However, more measurements are required to get an absolutely precise general classification model. It is likely that the separation of *Class B* and *Class C* signals requires an improvement in the FE method. These two classes seem to be overlapping in the feature space.

A fundamental benefit of the use of the DWT-based feature extraction was to give an independent and alternative method for the classification of CBF signals. We experienced that the effect of the CBF oscillations was limited to a certain range of the frequency. The DWT-based FV was able to reflect this phenomenon better than the DFT-based FV; therefore, the DWT-based FV resulted in a lower misclassification rate with the same type of ANN.

The medical interpretation of the results of the CBF signal classification is a challenging task. Although the physiological mechanism of the spontaneous oscillation of the vascular tone (called vasomotion) is studied intensively (Nilsson & Aalkjær, 2003), the biophysical model of vasomotion is not yet known. The generation of the analytical form of the classification function may help us to understand the nature of the underlying physiological phenomenon, to develop an adequate biophysical model for vasomotion and to define the model parameters.

Apnea Detection

The developed apnea detection method was found to be robust and patient-independent, which is the most important feature in clinical practice. The efficiency of event recognition measured by the selectivity and sensitivity is found to be high. The application of the method is relatively easy; it uses only one respiration signal, the nasal air flow. The developed method is not computation-intensive; thus, it is a promising candidate to apply in mobile, online apnea detection devices.

Summary

According to these results, the ANN proved to be an effective tool for the temporal analysis of physiological signals like cerebral blood flow and respiration.

The relatively simple backpropagation ANN proved to be a very efficient classification engine in the case of apnea detection problem, although for the CBF signal analysis, the RBF ANN was found to be a better classifier.

Proper selection of the FE significantly affects the success of the entire signal analysis. The utilization of the unsupervised Kohonen ANN is a valuable and important tool for the validation of the selected FE method.

On the one hand, the more dimensions the feature space has, the better the classification result should be. On the other hand, the number of FV dimensions is constrained by the number of measurements. In order to teach and test the ANN properly, the number of independent experiments should considerably exceed the number of FS dimensions. For instance, in the case of CBF signal analysis, the number of experiments was 60 and a two-dimensional FV was applied, while for apnea detection, the FV dimension was 50 and the number of measurements was more than 500.

The number of experiments in medical practice is always limited. Until the above-mentioned requirement is satisfied, the ANN will be a promising candidate for medical signal analysis. If the requirement is not fulfilled, then a different classification method should be considered, for example, Support Vector Machine classifiers (Benyó et al., 2004b, Burgers, 1998; Hearst, 1998).

Acknowledgments

The research was supported by the Hungarian National Research Fund, Grant No. OTKA F046726, T042990, T037386.

References

Baura, G. D. (2002). *Systems theory and practical applications of biomedical signals.* New York: John Wiley & Sons.

Benyó, B., Lenzsér, G., & Paláncz, B. (2004a, July 25-29). Characterization of the temporal pattern of cerebral blood flow oscillations. *Proceedings of the 2004 International Joint Conference on Neural Networks* (pp. 468-471).

Benyó, B., Benyó, Z., Somogyi, P., & Paláncz, B. (2004b). Classification of cerebral blood flow oscillation using SVM classifiers with different kernels. In W. Elmenreich, J. A. Tenreiro Machadó, & Imre Rudas (Eds.), *Intelligent systems at the service of mankind.* Ubooks.

Berthold, M., & Hand, D. J. (Eds.). (2003). *Intelligent data analysis: An introduction.* Berlin: Springer.

Burgers, C. J. C. (1998). A tutorial on support vector machines for pattern recognition. *Data Mining and Knowledge Discovery, 2,* 121-167.

Clark, S. A., Wilson, C. R., Satoh, M., Pegelow, D., & Dempsey, J. A. (1998). Assessment of inspiratory flow limitation invasively and noninvasively during sleep. *American Journal of Respiratory and Critical Care Medicine, 158*(3), 713-22.

Duda, R. O., Hart, P. E., & Stork, D. G. (2001). *Pattern classification.* New York: John Wiley & Sons.

Ferber, R., Millman, R., & Coppola, M. (1994). Portable recording in the assessment of obstructive sleep apnea. *Sleep, 17,* 378-392.

Goldberger, G., et al. (2000). Physiobank, physiotoolkit, and physionet: Components of a new research resource for complex physiologic signals. *Circulation, 101*(23), 215-220.

Goswami, J. C., & Chan, A. K. (1999). Fundamentals of wavelets. *Theory, algorithms, and application.* New York: John Wiley & Sons.

Guilleminault, C., & Partinen, M. (1990). *Obstructive sleep apnea syndrome: Clinical diagnosis & treatment.* New York: Raven Press.

Hearst, M. A. (1998). Support vector machines. *IEEE Intelligent Systems, 35,* 18-28.

Hudetz, A. G., Biswal, B. B., Shen, H., Lauer, K. K., & Kampine, J. P. (1998). Spontaneous fluctuations in cerebral oxygen supply. In A. G. Hudetz & D. F. Bruley (Eds.), *Oxygen transport to tissue XX* (pp. 551-559). New York: Plenum Press.

Intaglietta, M. (1990). Vasomotion and flowmotion: Physiological mechanisms and clinical evidence. *Vasc Med Rev, 1,* 101-112.

Köves, P. (Ed.). (1996). *Obstructive sleep apnea syndrome.* Budapest, Hungary: Springer Verlag.

Kryger, M. H., Roth, T., & Dement, W. C. (Eds.). (2000). *Principles and practice of sleep medicine* (3rd ed.). Philadelphia: W.B. Saunders.

Lacza, Z., Erdös, B., Görlach, C., Wahl, M., Sándor, P., & Benyó, Z. (2000). The cerebrocortical microcirculatory effect of nitric oxide synthase blockade is dependent upon baseline red blood cell flow in the rat. *Neuroscience Letters, 291*, 65-68.

Lacza, Z., Hermán, P., Görlach, C., Hortobágyi, T., Sándor, P., Wahl, M., & Benyó, Z. (2001). NO synthase blockade induces chaotic cerebral vasomotion via activation of thromboxane receptors. *Stroke, 32*, 2609-2614.

Lenzsér, G., Hermán, P., Komjáti, K., Sándor P., & Benyó, Z. (2003). Nitric oxide synthase blockade sensitizes the cerebrocortical circulation to thromboxane-induced CBF oscillations. *Journal of Cerebral Blood Flow and Metabolism, 23*, 88.

Li, C., Zeng, C., & Tai, C. (1995). Detection of ECG characteristic points using wavelet transforms. *IEEE Transactions on Biomedical Engineering, 42*, 21-28.

Mayhew, J.E., Askew, S., Zheng, Y., Porrill, J., Westby, W.M., Redgrave, P., Rector, D.M., & Harper, R.M. (1996). Cerebral vasomotion: A 0.1-Hz oscillation in reflected light imaging of neural activity. *Neuroimage, 4*, 183-193.

Moody, G. B. (n.d.) *The MIT-BIH polysomnograph database: Description of signals and annotations*. Retrieved October 10, 2005, from http://www.physionet.org

Mörchen, F. (2003). *Time series feature extraction for data mining using DWT and DFT.* Data Bionics Group, Philipps-University Marburg, Marburg, Germany.

Nilsson, H., & Aalkjær, C. (2003). Vasomotion: Mechanisms and physiological importance. *Molecular Interventions, 3*, 79-89.

Obrig, H., Neufang, M., Wenzel., R., Kohl, M., Steinbrink, J., Einhäupl, K., & Villringer, A. (2000). Spontaneous low frequency oscillations of cerebral hemodynamics and metabolism in human adults. *Neuroimage, 12*, 623-639.

Rangayyan, R. M. (2002). *Biomedical signal analysis.* New York: John Wiley & Sons.

Saunders, N. A., & Sullivan, C. E. (1994). *Sleep & breathing* (2nd ed.). Lung Biology in Health & Disease, vol. 71. New York: Marcell Dekker.

Senhadji, L., et al. (1995). Comparing wavelet transforms for recognizing cardiac patterns. *IEEE EMBS Magazine, 14*, 167-173.

Standards of Practice Committee of the American Sleep Disorders Association. (1997). Practice parameters for the indications for polysomnography and related procedures. *Sleep, 20*, 406-422.

Szilágyi, L., & Benyó, Z. (2003, August). Epileptic waveform recognition using wavelet decomposition and artificial neural networks. *Proceedings of the 5th IFAC Symposium on Modeling and Control in Biomedical Systems* (pp. 301-303), Melbourne, Australia.

Szilágyi, S. M., Szilágyi, L., & Dávid, L. (1997, October). Comparison between neural-network-based adaptive filtering and wavelet transform for ECG characteristic points detection. *Proceedings of 19th Annual International Conference of IEEE Engineering in Medicine and Biology Society* (pp. 272-274), Chicago, Illinois.

Várady, P. (2002). *New methods for the analysis of vital parameters and for the integration of the methods to the diagnostic system* (in Hungarian). PhD thesis. Budapest University of Technology and Economics, Budapest, Hungary.

Várady, P., & Bongár, S. Z. (2001). Detection of airway obstruction and sleep apnea by analyzing the phase relation of respiration movement signals. *Proceedings of the IEEE IMTC International Conference, 1*, 185-190.

About the Authors

Rezaul Begg received BSc and MSc engineering degrees in electrical and electronic engineering from Bangladesh University of Engineering and Technology (BUET), Dhaka, Bangladesh, and a PhD in biomedical engineering from the University of Aberdeen, UK. Currently, he is a faculty member at Victoria University, Melbourne, Australia. Previously, he worked with Deakin University and BUET. He researches in biomedical engineering, biomechanics, and machine learning areas, and has published more than 100 research papers in these areas. He is a regular reviewer for several international journals and was on the TPC for a number of major international conferences. He received several awards, including the BUET Gold Medal and the Chancellor Prize for Academic Excellence.

Joarder Kamruzzaman received a BSc and an MSc in electrical engineering from Bangladesh University of Engineering & Technology, Dhaka, Bangladesh (1986 and 1989, respectively), and a PhD in information system engineering from Muroran Institute of Technology, Japan (1993). Currently, he is a faculty member in the Faculty of Information Technology, Monash University, Australia. His research interest includes computational intelligence, computer networks, and bioinformatics. He has published more than 90 refereed papers in international journals and conference proceedings. He is currently serving as a program committee member of a number of international conferences.

Ruhul Sarker obtained a PhD from DalTech (former TUNS), Dalhousie University, Halifax, Canada. He is currently a senior academic at the School of Information Technology and Electrical Engineering, University of New South Wales (UNSW), Canberra, Australia. Before joining UNSW, Dr. Sarker worked with Monash University and Bangladesh University of Engineering and Technology. He has published more than 100 refereed technical papers in the international journals, edited reference books, and conference proceedings. He has written two books, edited six reference books, and several proceedings, and served as guest editors and technical reviewers for a number of international journals. Dr. Sarker was a technical co-chair of IEEE-CEC2003 and served many international conferences in the capacity of chair, co-chair, or PC member.

*   *   *

Harjeet Bajaj (Bachelor of Engineering, McMaster) is currently a master's candidate in electrical and computer engineering at McMaster University, Canada. His background is in electrical and computer engineering with a special interest in analysis of physiological signals through advanced signal processing and artificial neural networks. In the past, he has worked on high profile projects such as a nationally collaborated initiative to find causes of tinnitus. He was instrumental in developing a computer model of biological neural networks to find a potential cause of tinnitus. In addition, he has helped develop smart designs for hearing aids that have been taken to market. Outside of modeling of biomedical systems, he has experience in clinical aspects of biomedical engineering, including: gastrointestinal stimulation, hemodynamic signal processing, and myoelectric sympathetic nerve activity mapping.

Norman D. Black is acting pro-vice-chancellor (teaching and learning) at the University of Ulster at Jordanstown, Northern Ireland. He is past president of the European Society for Engineering and Medicine, sits on the Council of the RSM's Forum for Telemedicine & Telecare and has contributed to a variety of national and international committees, including Technology Foresight Healthcare Panel on Information Technology. Professor Black has worked in the area of bioengineering for the past 17 years and has research interests in knowledge-based systems and telemedicine. Professor Black is a fellow of the Royal Society of Medicine and member of the IEEE.

Balázs Benyó is an associate professor of information technology and vice dean for research and foreign affairs at Széchenyi István University, Hungary. He is also affiliated as a research fellow to the Budapest University of Technology and

Economics, Hungary. He holds CSc and PhD degrees in computer science. He is a member of the IEEE Computer Society. He conducts research on biological signal processing and design and verification methods of safety-critical diagnostic systems. He has participated in more than 20 research projects. Currently, he is leading four projects sponsored by Hungarian and European funds. He has published more than 70 scientific papers.

Nan Bu received his BE and ME degrees in mechanical engineering from Dalian University of Technology, China, in 1998 and 2001, respectively, and the doctor of engineering degree in systems engineering from Hiroshima University, Japan, in 2005. He is currently a postdoctoral research fellow in the Department of Artificial Complex Systems Engineering at Hiroshima University, Japan. His research interests include neural networks, pattern classification, and bioelectric signal analysis. Dr. Bu is a member of the IEEE.

G. Camps-Valls was born in València, Spain in 1972, and received a BSc degree in physics (1996), a BSc degree in electronics engineering (1998), and a PhD degree in physics (2002) from the Universitat de València, Spain. He is currently an assistant professor in the Department of Electronics Engineering at the Universitat de València, where teaches electronics, advanced time series processing, and digital signal processing. His research interests are neural networks and kernel methods for hyperspectral data analysis, health sciences, and safety-related areas. He is the author (or co-author) of 20 journal papers, several book chapters, and more than 50 international conference papers. He is a referee of several international journals and has served on the scientific committees of several international conferences. Visit http://www.uv.es/~gcamps for more information.

Kap Luk Chan received the PhD degree in robot vision from Imperial College of Science, Technology and Medicine, University of London, UK., in 1991. He is now an associate professor with the School of Electrical and Electronic Engineering, Nanyang Technological University, Singapore. He also holds a joint appointment in the Division of Bioengineering, School of Chemical and Biomedical Engineering. His research interests are in image analysis and computer vision, and biomedical signal and image analysis. He is a consultant to local and multinational companies in Singapore. He is a member of the IEEE and IEE.

Robert T. Davey gained an MSc with distinction in computing at the University of Ulster in 2001. His dissertation involved designing and implementing an MS Windows-based display program for the auditory brainstem response (ABR).

After spending 6 months as a research assistant exploring the use of fourth generation graphical programming languages for data acquisition, he began 3 years' PhD research using digital signal processing techniques and software modeling as a means of automating the analysis of the ABR waveform. Currently, he is working in City University, London, UK, in the Department of Language and Communication Science.

Subrat Das is presently working as research engineer in the School of Engineering and Industrial Science at Swinburne University of Technology, Australia. He received his BE and ME from South Gujarat University, India, and submitted his PhD thesis in 2001. His research interests are finite element methods, porous media flow, fluid-structure interaction, ultrasonic and laser Doppler techniques for flow measurements. Currently, he is working on "three dimensional numerical simulation of trileaflet valve using weak coupling."

Mark P. Donnelly received a computer science degree from the University of Ulster at Jordanstown, Northern Ireland, in 2004 and is currently undertaking a PhD within the Recognised Medical Informatics Research Group at the same institution. His research aims to investigate the use of computerized techniques for the diagnosis of cardiovascular disease. Specifically, this includes an investigation into the use of body surface potential mapping for data acquisition and employing state-of-the-art intelligent data analysis techniques, such as neural networks, to identify those characteristics exhibited by specific cardiac abnormalities. Other areas of interest include electromyography analysis for the control of artificial hands.

Dewar Finlay holds a Bachelor of Engineering degree in electronic engineering. He is currently employed as a research assistant in the School of Computing and Mathematics at the University of Ulster at Jordanstown, Northern Ireland. His main research interest is in the application of artificial intelligence to the interpretation of electrocardiogram data. He has published several papers and is currently perusing a PhD in this area. Dewar's other research interests include the application of mobile and wireless technology to remote healthcare delivery.

Sheng Fu received the PhD degree in Nanyang Technological University, Sinagpore, in 2004. He worked as an anaesthetist in the Anaesthesia Department of Baogang Hospital from 1991 to 1998. His research interests include early colorectal cancer diagnosis and analysis of cancer tissue structure, confocal laser scanning image of cell and tissue analysis, and clinical anaesthesia. He is now a research fellow in the Biomedical Engineering Research Centre, Nanyang Technological University, Sinagpore.

Osamu Fukuda received his BE degree in mechanical engineering from Kyushu Institute of Technology, Japan, in 1993, and the ME and PhD degree in information engineering from Hiroshima University, Japan in 1997 and 2000. From 1997 to 1999, he was a research fellow of the Japan Society for the Promotion of Science. He joined the Mechanical Engineering Laboratory, Agency of Industrial Science and Technology, Ministry of International Trade and Industry, Japan, in 2000. Since 2001, he has been the member of the Assistive Device Technology Group, Institute for Human Science and Biomedical Engineering, National Institute of Advanced Industrial Science and Technology, Japan. His main research interests are the human interface and the neural network. Dr. Fukuda is a member of Japan Society of Mechanical Engineers, Robotics Society of Japan.

J. F. Guerrero-Martínez has been working for the University of Valencia, Spain, since 1985. He achieved his PhD in 1988. He is a member of the IEEE Engineering in Medicine and Biology Society, the International Federation for Medical & Biological Engineering, the International Society for Holter & Non-Invasive Electrocardiology and the Spanish Society of Biomedical Engineering. He has collaborated in several research projects: four on telematics applications (secure data transmision, database development for telematic services, etc.), and 10 of them related with biomedical engineering (medical instrumentation, acquisition systems, digital processing of biomedical signals), in collaboration with staff from different hospitals of Valencia (Hospital Clínico, La Fe, Hospital Dr. Peset). He is the author (or co-author) of many journal papers, several book chapters, and more than 100 international conference papers.

H. Glen Houston is a principal audiological scientist at the Royal Victoria Hospital, Belfast, Northern Ireland. He graduated from Queen's University Belfast with a BSc in physiology (1976) and MSc in audiology, University of Salford (1980). He has worked for over 25 years in audiology and has significant experience in the recording and interpretation of auditory evoked potentials. His interests include personalized digital hearing aids and teaching audiology to UU students, BSc clinical physiology. He is a registered clinical scientist and member of the British Academy of Audiology.

Jörg M. Jäger is a research staff member in the Department of Training and Movement Science at the Westfälische Wilhelms-University of Münster, Germany. His interests include pattern recognition, artificial neural networks, and statistical shape analysis. Jäger studied mathematics and sports at the Philipps-University of Marburg and the Justus-Liebig-University of Gießen. He received his state certificate in 2000 and worked until 2002 in Davos, Switzerland, in the field of sport rehabilitation and healthcare. Since 2002, he has worked in research projects in the Institute of Sport Science in Münster.

Markad V. Kamath, PhD (IIT, Madras), PhD (McMaster), PEng, is an associate professor in the Department of Medicine at McMaster University, Hamilton, Ontario, Canada. Dr. Kamath has graduated more than 12 master's-level students and is supervising two PhD students. His research interests focus on applications of signal processing and pattern recognition methods toward understanding physiological processes, especially those related to disease states. He has worked with EEG analysis and cortical evoked potentials recorded in response to esophageal stimulation. He is a professional engineer in the province of Ontario, Canada.

Shankar M. Krishnan received his PhD degree from the University of Rhode Island and has worked in academia, healthcare industry, and hospitals in the United States. He has been the director of Biomedical Engineering Research Center and the head of Division of Biomedical Engineering at the Nanyang Technological University, Singapore. His research interests are medical instrumentation, image processing, telemedicine, bio-optics, and medical robotics. Dr. Krishnan served as a member of the National Medical Research Council of Singapore and is also actively involved in IEEE EMBS and the Biomedical Engineering Society of Singapore. He was also a consultant on several medical projects.

Peng Li received the Bachelor of Engineering and Master of Engineering degrees from North China Electric Power University, China, in 1993 and 1998, respectively. He was a lecturer in Power Engineering Department, North China Electric Power University from July 1998 to April 2002. He is now a PhD candidate at the School of Electrical and Electronic Engineering of Nanyang Technological University, Singapore. His research interests include pattern recognition, computer vision, machine learning, and signal processing, particularly in ensemble learning, kernel-based methods, and novelty detection. He is a student member of IEEE.

J. D. Martín-Guerrero was born in Valencia, Spain in 1974. He received a BS degree in physics (1997), a BS degree in electronics engineering (1999), a MS degree in electronics engineering (2001), and a PhD degree in electronics engineering (2004) from the University of Valencia, Spain. He is currently an assistant professor at the University of Valencia. His research interests are related to the application of soft-computing to a number of different fields, such as medicine, image processing, marketing, or Web mining. He is a member of the European Neural Network Society.

H. Gerry McAllister holds a BSc and MSc in electrical and electronic engineering and a PhD in computing science. He is currently head of School of Computing and Mathematics at the University of Ulster, Northern Ireland, where he has been employed, formerly as lecturer, since 1987. Prior to that, he was senior research officer in the Faculty of Medicine, Queens University Belfast. His research interests throughout have been in recording and analysis methods of EEG and evoked potentials and new methods of detection and correction for hearing acuity. He is also director of the National Higher Education Academy Information and Computer Science Subject Centre, a chartered engineer, member of the Institution of Electrical Engineers and the British Computer Society.

Paul J. McCullagh received a BSc (1979) and PhD (1983) in electrical and electronic engineering at Queen's University Belfast. He is currently a senior lecturer in computing and mathematics at the University of Ulster, Northern Ireland. He coordinates the Ulster Institute of eHealth, which is a collaboration between the University of Ulster and the Ulster Commuity and Hospitals Trust. Prior to that, he was a research officer at the Department of Mental Health, Queens University Belfast. His research interests include signal and image processing and data mining in medicine. He is also interested in medical informatics education. He is a council member of European Society for Engineering & Medicine, a chartered engineer, member of the Institution of Electrical Engineers and the British Computer Society.

Yos S. Morsi has wide-ranging internationally recognized expertise in the area of modeling and simulations, and design of special devices. His recent work concentrates on the use of rapid prototyping FDM for the production of Scaffolds. This work has led to techniques that, for the very first time, permit construction of the manufacturing of the first Australian Tri-leaflet (aortic) heart valve scaffold made from biodegradable biocompatible materials. In 2003, he established the tissue engineering laboratories at IRIS which consist of the Biofluids section for modeling and producing scaffolds and cell dynamic conditioning. He has published more than 80 refereed articles in international journals and conferences.

Chris Nugent has a degree in electronic systems and DPhil in biomedical engineering both attained from the University of Ulster at Jordanstown, Northern Ireland. He is currently employed as a Senior Lecturer in the School of Computing of Mathematics at the University of Ulster. His research areas focus on the application of artificial intelligence to medical decision support systems, computerized electrocardiology, and the evolving usage of the Internet as a means of innovative healthcare delivery.

Skip Poehlman, PhD (McMaster), PEng, is an associate professor in the computing and software (CAS) Department of McMaster University in Hamilton, Ontario, Canada. As head of the Applied Computersystems Research Group (ACsG), he has graduated six PhD students and more than 30 Master's level students. Research focus areas include intelligent performance support systems, knowledge-based user modeling & graphical user interface (GUI) development, and intelligent network management systems. Main collaboration research efforts with McMaster's Department of Medicine are ongoing. A number of peer-reviewed papers have been published in AI journals, distributed systems journals, IEEE transactions and computer-human interaction journals as well as related conferences. Skip is a professional engineer and a member of the ACM, American Association of Artificial Intelligence (AAAI), and Canadian Information Processing Society (CIPS), as well as a senior member of the IEEE.

Wolfgang I. Schöllhorn, chair of the Department of Training and Movement Science at the University of Münster, Germany, since 2000. His major interests are in motor learning, stochastic resonance, pattern recognition, and system dynamics. He studied physics and sports at the University of Mainz, Frankfurt and Cologne. He received his diploma in sports in 1985, the state certificate in physics 1991, his PhD in biomechanics in 1990, and his venia legendi for movement and training science 1995. From 1997 to 2000, he was an assistant professor at the University of Leipzig, Germany, and had several guest professorships in Canada, Austria, and Taiwan. In 1999, he received the Myashita performance award from the International Society of Biomechanics for the introduction of a new learning approach, the differential learning.

Robert Spaziani (M.D. FRCP(C)) is a clinical scholar with the Department of Medicine, McMaster University, Canada, and is a practicing gastroenterologist at St. Joseph's Hospital (Hamilton, Ontario, Canada). Dr. Spaziani, a Canada scholar, has a background in pharmacology. Dr. Spaziani has been an active member of a multidisciplinary research group at McMaster University for 10 years, investigating the role of autonomic nervous system in diseases of the cardiovascular, gastroenterological, neurological, and respiratory systems. Dr. Spaziani has been invited to present at several international conferences and has received both local and international scientific awards.

Yoshiyuki Tanaka received his BE degree in computer science and systems engineering from Yamaguchi University in 1995, and his ME and Doctor of Engineering degrees in information engineering from Hiroshima University in 1997 and 2001, respectively. From 2001 to 2002, he was a research associate with the Faculty of Information Sciences, Hiroshima City University. He is currently a research associate in the Department of Artificial Complex Systems Engineering at Hiroshima University, Japan. His research interests include biological motor control and human-machine interaction. Dr. Tanaka is a member of the Robotics Society of Japan, Institute of Electrical Engineering of Japan, the Society of Instrumentation and Control Engineers in Japan, and the Institute of Electrical and Electronics Engineers.

Toshio Tsuji received his BE degree in industrial engineering in 1982, his ME and Doctor of Engineering degrees in systems engineering in 1985 and 1989, all from Hiroshima University. He was a research associate from 1985 to 1994, and an associate professor, from 1994 to 2002, in Faculty of Engineering at Hiroshima University. He was a visiting professor of University of Genova, Italy for one year from 1992 to 1993. He is currently a professor in the Department of Artificial Complex Systems Engineering at Hiroshima University, Japan. Dr. Tsuji won the Best Paper Award from the Society of Instrumentation and Control Engineers in 2002, and the K. S. Fu Memorial Best Transactions Paper Award of the IEEE Robotics and Automation Society in 2003. His current research interests have focused on human-machine interface, and computational neural sciences, in particular, biological motor control. Dr. Tsuji is a member of the IEEE, the Japan Society of Mechanical Engineers, the Robotics Society of Japan, and the Society of Instrumentation and Control Engineers in Japan.

Koji Tsujimura received his BE and ME degrees in electrical, computer and systems engineering from Hiroshima University in 2002 and 2004. He currently works at Sensing Technology Laboratory of OMRON Corporation, Japan. His main research interest is to develop a new sensor based on radio frequency and optical sensing technologies.

Adrian R. Upton (MA, MB, B.Chir., LRCP, MRCS, FRCP(C), FRCP(E), FRCP(G)) is a professor of medicine and biomedical sciences and is the director of clinical neurology at McMaster University, Canada. During his 40 years experience as a neurologist, Dr. Upton has trained dozens of physicians, residents, and scientists in neurology. As an investigator, Dr. Upton has published over 400 peer-reviewed papers and several book chapters in the field. His research includes diagnosis of herpes encephalitis, motor unit counting, the double crush syndrome, control of tremor with primidone, evoked potentials, and neurostimulation. Over 30 years, he has pioneered the use of new forms of neurostimulation (cerebellar, thalamic, vagal), culminating in the receipt of a number of patents on new pacemakers for the brain, involving responsive stimulation that corrects abnormal electrical activity in epilepsy, Parkinson's disease, movement disorders, migraine, and pain. These new pacemakers are in controlled trials in the USA.

Jie Wu, BEng., MS (Singapore), MS (Leuven), is currently a PhD candidate in computer science at McMaster University, Hamilton, Canada. She received her B.Eng. degree in 1998 in computer engineering from the East China Shipbuilding Institute. In 2002, she received an MS degree in computer science from the National University of Singapore. A year later, she obtained an Advanced Studies Master's degree of Industrial Management from Katholieke Universiteit Leuven, in Belgium. She has applied artificial neural networks to differentiate between real world photographs and computer rendered images. Jie is now working on pattern recognition, medical imaging, and medical information systems at McMaster.

Index

I

image analysis 27
immersed boundary 275
input layer 5
instantaneous respiration amplitude (IRA) 300
instantaneous respiration interval (IRI) 300
IRA (see instantaneous respiration amplitude)
isointegral maps 66
isopotential maps 66

J

jack-knifing 96
joint angle 221

K

k-nearest neighbor 22
Karush-Kuhn-Tucker (KKT) 115
kinematic 219
kinetic 219
knowledge-based neural nets 24

L

laser doppler (LD) 288
laser doppler anemometry (LDA) 270
LD (see laser doppler)
LD flux (LDF) 288
LDA (see laser doppler anemometry)
learning algorithms 2
learning vector quantization 47, 180
learning-based approach 109
likelihood ratio method 181
linear Bayes normal classifier 123
linear discriminant analysis 36, 70, 222
local linear maps 29
log-linearized Gaussian mixture network 133, 155
logistic discriminant analysis 70
logistic regression 24
low back pain 34
low-frequency oscillations 287

M

magnetic resonance imaging (MRI) 31
maximum likelihood 133
mean absolute error 254
mean error 254
medical decision support systems 2
MFNN (see multilayer feedforward neural network)
minimum toe clearance 222
MLP (see multi-layered perceptron)
model development 94
model selection 116
motion-discrimination 170
motor neuron disease 14
MRI (see magnetic resonance imaging)
multi-layered perceptron (MLP) 22, 69, 132, 246
multilayer feedforward neural network (MFNN) 224
myocardial infarction 22, 87
myocardial ischemia 88

N

nasal airflow 290
nearest mean classifier 123
nerve-based visual prosthesis 42
network architecture 136
network self-organizing map 88
neural cell detection system 29
neural computation 3
neural filter 133
neural network (NN) 4, 13, 31, 132, 240, 262, 271
neurological 179
neuromuscular 34
neurons 3
nitric oxide (NO) 288
NN (see neural network)
non-dimensional artificial neural network (NDANN) 273
non-invasive electrocardiography 82
non-linear model predictive control 242
non-stationarity 245
non-uniform Sampling 245

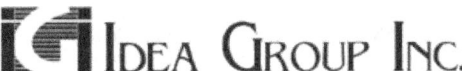

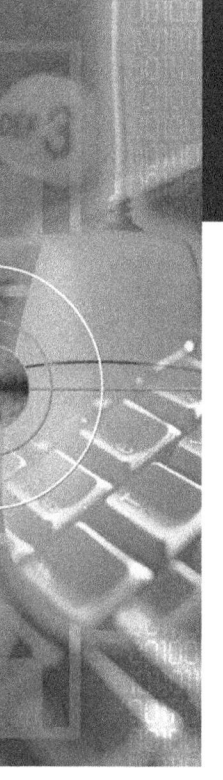
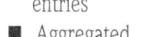
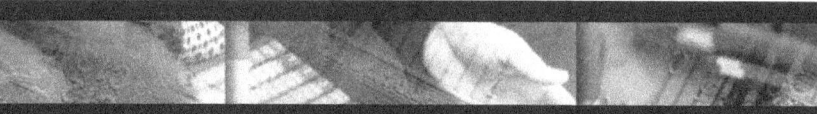